Mastering the Techniques of
Laparoscopic Suturing & Knotting

Mastering the Techniques of
Laparoscopic Suturing & Knotting

SECOND EDITION

RK Mishra
Director and Chief Surgeon, World Laparoscopy Hospital, Gurugram, Haryana, India
Director and Chief Surgeon, World Laparoscopy Training Institute, DHCC, Dubai, UAE
Director and Chief Surgeon, World Laparoscopy Training Institute, Orlando, Florida, USA
Professor and Head of Minimal Access Surgery, TGO University
Member, Indian Medical Association (IMA)
Member, Association of Surgeons of India (ASI)
Member, Indian Association of Gastrointestinal Endosurgeons (IAGES)
Member, International College of Surgeons (ICS)
Member, Endoscopic and Laparoscopic Surgeons of Asia (ELSA)
Fellow of International Medical Sciences Academy (IMSA)
General Secretary, World Association of Laparoscopic Surgeons (WALS)
General Secretary, International College of Robotic Surgeons (ICRS)
Member, European Association for Endoscopic Surgery (EAES)
Member, European Association for Transluminal Surgery (EATS)
Member, Society of American Gastrointestinal and Endoscopic Surgeons (SAGES)
Member, American Society for Metabolic and Bariatric Surgery (ASMBS)
Member, American Association of Gynecologic Laparoscopists (AAGL)
Member, International Society for Gynecologic Endoscopy (ISGE)
Member, Society of Laparoendoscopic Surgeons (SLS)
Member, Society of Robotic Surgery (SRS)
Member, Clinical Robotic Surgery Association (CRSA)
Editor-in-Chief, World Journal of Laparoscopic Surgery (WJOLS)
First University Qualified Master Minimal Access Surgeon of India (M.MAS)

Foreword
Ray L Green

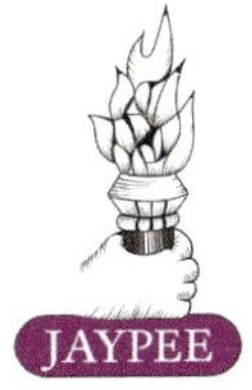

JAYPEE BROTHERS MEDICAL PUBLISHERS
The Health Sciences Publisher
New Delhi | London

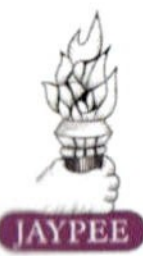 **Jaypee Brothers Medical Publishers (P) Ltd**

Headquarters
EMCA House
23/23-B, Ansari Road, Daryaganj
New Delhi 110 002, India
Landline: +91-11-23272143, +91-11-23272703
+91-11-23282021, +91-11-23245672
E-mail: jaypee@jaypeebrothers.com

Overseas Office
JP Medical Ltd.
83, Victoria Street, London
SW1H 0HW (UK)
Phone: +44-20 3170 8910
E-mail: info@jpmedpub.com

Corporate Office
Jaypee Brothers Medical Publishers (P) Ltd.
4838/24, Ansari Road, Daryaganj
New Delhi 110 002, India
Phone: +91-11-43574357
Fax: +91-11-43574314
E-mail: jaypee@jaypeebrothers.com

EU GPSR Authorised Representative
Logos Europe, 9 rue Nicolas Poussin
17000, La Rochelle, France
Phone: +33 (0) 6 67 93 73 78
E-mail: Contact@logoseurope.eu

Website: www.jaypeebrothers.com
Website: www.jaypeedigital.com

© 2025, Jaypee Brothers Medical Publishers

Inquiries for bulk sales may be solicited at: jaypee@jaypeebrothers.com

Mastering the Techniques of Laparoscopic Suturing & Knotting

First Edition: 2009
Second Edition **2025**
Reprint **2026**
ISBN: 978-93-5696-716-8

Printed in India

Dedicated to

Great Surgeon
&
My Loving Father

Foreword

Suturing is one of the oldest and most basic techniques in surgery. It serves as the foundation for wound closure, tissue approximation, and hemostasis. Proficiency in suturing is essential for performing even the simplest surgical procedures and is critical for more complex operations. Without a solid grasp of suturing, surgeons cannot effectively manage wounds, repair tissues, or perform many types of laparoscopic surgeries.

Mastering suturing skills is a cornerstone of minimal access surgical practice. Despite the advent of advanced technologies and devices, the ability to suture effectively remains a fundamental and indispensable competency for surgeons. The significance of developing suturing skills in surgery extends across multiple dimensions.

It is with immense pride and satisfaction that I introduce this second edition of Professor Mishra's exemplary work. This updated version of *Mastering the Techniques of Laparoscopic Suturing and Knotting* continues to serve as a definitive guide on crucial laparoscopic skills.

This book offers an in-depth exploration of all major and emerging laparoscopic knot-tying techniques used in both gynecological and general surgical procedures. It provides comprehensive details on indications, patient preparation, positioning, and step-by-step suturing techniques for a range of minimally invasive surgeries.

Manual suturing provides laparoscopic surgeons with a level of precision and control that is unmatched by automated devices. The ability to carefully place sutures in minimally invasive surgery allows for meticulous tissue approximation, minimizing tension and promoting optimal healing. This precision is particularly important in delicate procedures, such as vascular surgery, microsurgery, and reconstructive surgery, where fine control over tissue manipulation is essential.

The author of the updated version of *Mastering the Techniques of Laparoscopic Suturing and Knotting* in this second edition has skillfully addressed the common challenges and intricacies associated with laparoscopic suturing and knotting. By incorporating clinical scenarios and practical tips, this book bridges the gap between theory and practice, making it an invaluable reference for daily surgical practice. Additionally, the inclusion of patient preparation, positioning, and postoperative care provides a holistic view of the surgical process.

The purpose of any medical text is to deliver a cohesive report that enhances understanding of key issues. This book of suturing and knotting succeeds in that aim, assisting us in refining our techniques, making judicious use of knotting skills, and providing optimal care to our patients in a cost-effective manner.

The illustrations in this second edition, both photographs and line drawings, are of exceptional quality. The chapters are concise, effectively using subheadings, and are well referenced. Each section begins with a balanced discussion of the clinical application of knots in relation to laparoscopic procedures.

I hope that readers of this excellent book will approach this vital art with the respect, humility, and enthusiasm that minimally invasive surgery warrants. This remarkable resource is a pleasure to read, and its design, style, and content will surely provide satisfaction to anyone involved in surgical intervention. Professor Mishra has created an outstanding and state-of-the-art review of suturing techniques in laparoscopy, and this book is highly recommended for all practicing minimally invasive surgeons.

Ray L Green
Diplomate of the American Board of Obstetrics and Gynecology
Fellow of the American College of Obstetricians and Gynecologists
President, World Association of Laparoscopic Surgeons (USA)

Preface to the Second Edition

I am thrilled to introduce my latest work, *"Mastering the Techniques of Laparoscopic Suturing and Knotting"*, to surgeons and gynecologists worldwide. While my initial book, "Textbook of Practical Laparoscopic Surgery," touched upon these vital skills, the encouragement and requests from students globally inspired me to dedicate an entire volume to the art and science of suturing and knotting.

The field of minimal access surgery has witnessed remarkable evolution in less than two decades. The shift from traditional open surgeries, which have been the cornerstone of internal organ access and disease treatment for over a century, to laparoscopic techniques highlights the significant benefits of minimizing bodily trauma.

Innovation is at the heart of every surgical specialty, continually introducing new methods that enhance the application of sutures and knots scientifically. Proficiency in laparoscopic suturing and knotting is indispensable for any surgeon, enabling precise tissue approximation and embodying the ethos that the future of surgery is inherently tied to suturing. The importance of mastering these techniques extends beyond patient benefits, such as secured hemostasis, to heralding advancements in healthcare that are both cost-effective and outcome-oriented, reducing the reliance on expensive staplers and adhesives.

This book opens new doors for surgeons and gynecologists by equipping them with the knowledge and skills for advanced minimally invasive suturing and knotting techniques. It is designed to guide readers through the nuances of these techniques, setting the stage for new frontiers in surgical and gynecological practice.

Accompanied by full-color photographs, detailed procedural descriptions, and video footage, this book offers a comprehensive learning experience. This blend of visual and textual elements, along with surgical commentary, provides an immersive approach to mastering complex skills outside the operating room. This work is poised to be a valuable addition to any medical library, offering insights into both common and advanced procedures now being performed in leading centers worldwide.

Focused exclusively on procedural techniques, this book provides clear, concise descriptions alongside introductory insights, deliberately steering away from an exhaustive literature review to maintain a sharp focus on practical skills.

As we present this detailed, high-quality resource, we aim for it to be recognized for its uniqueness and excellence in the field. While every effort has been made to ensure accuracy and clarity, I welcome any constructive feedback and acknowledge that, despite our best efforts, oversights may occur. Your insights and critiques are not only appreciated but also essential for the continuous improvement of this scientific endeavor.

RK Mishra

Preface to the First Edition

I am very happy to present my second book *Mastering the Techniques of Laparoscopic Suturing and Knotting* to surgeons and gynecologists of the whole world. Although I have discussed laparoscopic suturing and knotting in my first book *Textbook of Practical Laparoscopic Surgery* but this book is a result of pressure and demand of my students from all over the world to write a book exclusively on suturing and knotting.

In less than fifteen years, so much has happened in the very young field of minimal access surgery. The gradual change from the large incision surgery, used successfully for over 100 years in providing access to internal organs and in treating disease, has paved the way for the use of laparoscopic surgeries and all the inherent advantages of minimal trauma to the body.

Every surgical specialty is seeing new and innovative methods using different types of surgical skills including scientific way of using suture and knots. Laparoscopic suturing and knotting is one of the most important skills for every laparoscopic surgeon and with this skill he can do proper tissue approximation. This is very true that there is no future without suture. Suturing and knotting is so important not only because of the benefit to patients in the form of better secured hemostasis but also because of the promise it holds in providing improved health care in a cost effective, outcome oriented way without the use of costly staplers and glue.

Many procedures that previously required a laparotomy are now performed using laparoscopy if the surgeon or gynecologist has confidence in suturing and knotting. Readers of this book will gain an understanding of advanced minimally invasive suturing and knotting techniques and learn about the development and delivery of relevant skill. I hope that the mastering suturing and knotting techniques in this book will be helpful in directing new frontier for surgeons and gynecologists.

Over actual surgical footage is included an accompanying DVD with spoken commentary about all types of suturing and knotting techniques commonly used anywhere in the world. The reader will also be able to review a procedure with full color photographs and then view selected procedures on video. The combination of photographs, written text, surgical footage and spoken commentary is one of the most realistic approaches to understanding a complex surgical skill without actually scrubbing into the case. This book represents an important work and is an excellent addition to any reference library.

In addition to the commonly performed major procedures using suture, I have also illustrated many advanced procedures currently performed only at specialized centres throughout the world. The text in this book is limited to procedural descriptions of suturing and knotting and succinct introductory paragraphs explaining general indications without a comprehensive review of the literature. This text is strictly focused on procedures, as will become apparent to the reader. We have attempted to design a high-quality, comprehensive book and hope that the reader appreciates its distinctiveness and merit.

Although I have taken every care to make this book error free, nonetheless grammatical mistakes may have been overlooked in this scientific book. I will be grateful for any constructive criticism.

RK Mishra

Acknowledgments

I extend my heartfelt gratitude to all those who made the creation of *"Mastering the Techniques of Laparoscopic Suturing and Knotting"* possible. My journey began with the invaluable encouragement from the Department of Minimal Access Surgery at the University of Dundee, United Kingdom, whose support was instrumental in embarking on this academic endeavor.

My appreciation extends to the dedicated staff of World Laparoscopy Hospital, Gurugram, Haryana, for their assistance in conducting the necessary research and allowing the use of departmental data. I am equally grateful to my students, whose relentless enthusiasm and support have been a constant source of motivation.

Special thanks are owed to Professor Sir Alfred Cuschieri, whose guidance, insightful suggestions, and encouragement were pivotal throughout my research and the writing process. My colleagues from the Department of Surgery at Ninewells Hospital and Medical School, University of Dundee, Scotland, United Kingdom, deserve recognition for their support and contribution to my research efforts.

I am deeply thankful to my best friend, Professor Steven D Wexner, President of SAGES in 2007 and Professor of Surgery at Ohio State University, Ohio, USA, for his moral support and encouragement in completing this book. My gratitude also goes to my fellow surgeons and gynecologists for their invaluable assistance, interest, and insightful advice.

I owe a debt of gratitude to Mr Sumit Kumar Sinha for his meticulous proofreading and support during the challenging phases of my clinical and teaching responsibilities. My assistant, Mr Raghubir Singh, along with Bubble and Naina, has been instrumental in refining the final manuscript, enhancing its readability and grammatical precision. I extend my sincere thanks to the entire staff at Laparoscopy Hospital, New Delhi, for their contributions to this project.

I express my appreciation to the team at Jaypee Brothers Medical Publishers (P) Ltd., especially for their unique work culture and commitment to excellence. I especially appreciate the constant support and encouragement of Mr Jitendar P Vij (Group Chairman) and Mr Ankit Vij (Managing Director) of M/s Jaypee Brothers Medical Publishers (P) Ltd, New Delhi, India, in publishing the book and also their associates, particularly Ms Chetna Malhotra (Senior Director—Professional Publishing, Marketing, and Business Development) , and Ms Pragati Singh (Development Editor) who have been prompt, efficient, and most helpful.

Lastly, but most importantly, I dedicate my profound thanks to my wife, Sadhana, whose endless love and support were the backbone of my perseverance and completion of this work.

Contents

Video Contents

Chapter 12: Role of Correct Port Position in Laparoscopic Suturing and Knotting

Video 20: Video Lecture of Abdominal Access Technique

Chapter 13: Comparison of Laparoscopic Knots

Video 21: Comparison of Laparoscopic Knots

Chapter 14: Prevention of Postoperative Adhesion Formation

Video 22: Adhesion Prevention in Laparoscopic Surgery

Chapter 15: Glues and Adhesive in Laparoscopic Tissue Approximation

Video 23: Glue in Laparoscopic Surgery

Chapter 16: Impact of Training on Laparoscopic Suturing and Knotting

Video 24: How to Avoid Mistakes and Errors in Minimal Access Surgery

Video 25: Contraindication of Laparoscopic Surgery

Chapter 17: Robotic Suturing and Knotting

Video 26: Robotic Suturing and Knotting

1

Introduction

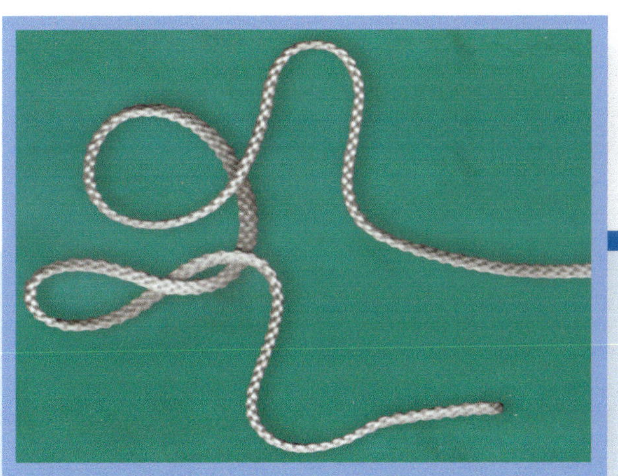

■ INTRODUCTION

Laparoscopic surgery, also known as minimally invasive surgery, has revolutionized the field of medicine by offering patients shorter recovery times, reduced pain, and smaller scars compared to traditional open surgery. However, the success of laparoscopic procedures heavily relies on the surgeon's ability to suture and knot effectively within the confined space of the body. In this chapter, we will explore the critical importance of suturing and knotting techniques in laparoscopic surgery.

■ CHALLENGE OF LAPAROSCOPIC SUTURING AND KNOTTING

Laparoscopic surgery involves making small incisions through which a camera and specialized instruments are inserted to perform intricate procedures inside the body. Unlike open surgery, where surgeons have a direct line of sight and a greater range of motion, laparoscopic surgeons must work within a limited visual field and with instruments that have restricted movement. This makes suturing and knotting in laparoscopy a highly demanding skill.

■ WHY SUTURING AND KNOTTING MATTER

- *Tissue closure and hemostasis:* Suturing is essential for closing incisions or punctures in organs or vessels. Proper suturing ensures that tissues are securely sealed, preventing postoperative complications such as bleeding and infection.
- *Organ reconstruction:* In some laparoscopic surgeries, organs may need to be reconstructed or repaired. Suturing allows surgeons to meticulously restore the structure and function of organs, ensuring the patient's well-being.
- *Securing instruments:* Laparoscopic instruments, such as clips, graspers, or staplers, may not always be suitable for certain tasks. Suturing provides a versatile method for securing tissues, vessels, or structures when other instruments are not ideal.
- *Minimizing scarring:* Laparoscopic surgery is renowned for its minimal scarring. Precise suturing techniques help achieve this by minimizing tissue trauma and ensuring a cosmetically pleasing outcome for the patient.
- *Preventing herniation:* Properly sutured incisions reduce the risk of herniation, where tissues or organs protrude through the surgical site after the procedure.

This complication can be painful and may require further surgery to correct.

■ TECHNIQUES FOR EFFECTIVE SUTURING AND KNOTTING IN LAPAROSCOPY

- *Precision:* Laparoscopic suturing demands precision and accuracy. Surgeons must place sutures exactly where needed to achieve the desired tissue closure or reconstruction.
- *Knot security:* Knots in laparoscopic surgery must be exceptionally secure to prevent them from slipping or loosening inside the body. Surgeons often employ knot-tying techniques specific to laparoscopy, such as the "Roeder" or "Smyth" knots.
- *Instrument familiarity:* Proficiency with laparoscopic instruments is crucial. Surgeons should be well-versed in the various types of needle holders, graspers, and needle drivers to effectively manipulate sutures.
- *Depth perception:* Laparoscopic surgeons must develop a keen sense of depth perception, as they are working in a two-dimensional visual field. Training and experience play a vital role in honing this skill.
- *Continuous learning:* Laparoscopic surgery is a constantly evolving field. Surgeons must stay up-to-date with the latest techniques and technologies through continuous education and training.

In laparoscopic surgery, suturing and knotting are not merely technical skills; they are the cornerstone of successful procedures. The ability to suture precisely and tie secure knots within the confined space of the body ensures patient safety, optimal outcomes, and minimal postoperative complications. As laparoscopic surgery continues to advance, the mastery of suturing and knotting techniques remains a fundamental skill that every laparoscopic surgeon must cultivate and refine to provide the best possible care to their patients.

Sutures are the thread or stitch used by surgeons. Once the suture is satisfactorily placed, it must be secured with a knot. Knotting is a method for fastening or securing suture by tying or interweaving. Knotting and suturing as a method for closing wounds is one of the oldest skill acquired by primitive human and the technique of suturing is thousands of years old. Today's laparoscopic knots are basically a modification of knots used by seamen, fishermen, weavers or hangmen. Knotting skills to the surgeon were transmitted by sailors, scouts, climbers, cavers, arborists, rescue professionals, and fishermen.

Many surgeons of modern medicine have given their name for different knots and they claim that they have developed a new knot, which is a rarity. Almost all the knots in the world (3,854 of them) are described and illustrated in a reference book by Clifford W Ashley, first published in 1944. Knots, splices, hitches, hooks, beckets, toggles, and sinnets are included in the Ashley Book of Knots.

Although suture materials and aspects of the technique have changed, the goals remain the same, closing dead space, supporting and strengthening wounds until healing increases their tensile strength, approximating skin edges for an aesthetically pleasing and functional result, and minimizing the risks of bleeding and infection.

As more knots are learned, patterns begin to become evident in their structure and methods of tying **(Fig. 1)**. The learning of knots rewards practice and patience. They must be strong (so they do not break), nontoxic and hypoallergenic (to avoid adverse reactions in the body), and flexible (so they can be tied and knotted easily). In addition, they must lack the so called "wick effect" which means that sutures must not allow fluids to penetrate the body through them from outside, which could easily cause infections.

Knots are essential in all industrial, occupational, recreational, and domestic settings. Even simple activities such as running a load from the hardware store to home can result in disaster if a clumsy twist in a cord passes for a knot. Knots can save the spelunker from foolishly becoming buried under millions of tons of rock. Whatever the activity, such as sailing on the water or climbing on a cliffside rock, learning well-tested knots prior to some hazardous activity introduces a critical measure of safety. For surgeons, wrongly applied knot is disastrous and can lead to increased risk of morbidity and mortality. In addition to safety, appropriate knots can prevent the necessity of cutting lines. Even if the suture does not break, a knot may still fail to hold. A knot which holds firm under a variety of adverse conditions is said to be more secure than one that does not.

■ FAILURES OF KNOTS

Understanding why knots fail in laparoscopic surgery: Laparoscopic surgery has revolutionized the medical field by offering patients less invasive procedures, shorter recovery times, and smaller scars compared to traditional open surgery. However, within this realm of minimally invasive surgery, the challenge of knot failure is a critical concern. In this chapter, we will delve into the various factors that contribute to knot failure in laparoscopic surgery and explore the strategies employed to mitigate these risks.

The significance of knots in laparoscopic surgery: Knots play a pivotal role in laparoscopic surgery, just as they do in open surgery. They are used to secure sutures, ligate vessels, close tissue incisions, and maintain the integrity of the surgical site. A well-tied knot is essential for ensuring hemostasis, preventing leaks, and ultimately achieving a successful surgical outcome.

Common reasons for knot failure:
- *Inadequate tension:* One of the primary reasons for knot failure is inadequate tension on the suture. If the suture is not pulled tight enough, the knot may not hold, leading to potential complications such as bleeding or leakage.
- *Slippage:* Knots can slip if they are not properly secured. This is more likely to occur in laparoscopic surgery due to the confined workspace and limited visibility, making it challenging to ensure that knots are firmly tightened.
- *Suture material:* The choice of suture material matters. Some materials may be more prone to knot slippage or failure than others. Surgeons must select the appropriate suture material for the specific surgical task.

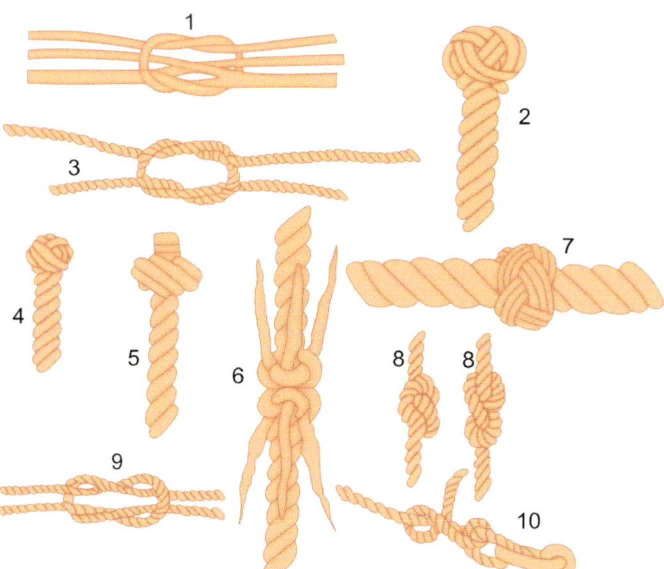

Fig. 1: Different types of nonsurgical knots: (1) Splice; (2) manrope knot; (3) granny knot; (4) rosebud stopper knot; (5) Matthew Walker knot; (6) shroud knot; (7) Turks head knot; (8) overhand knot, figure-of-eight knot; (9) reef knot or square knot; and (10) two half-hitches (see round turn and two half hitches).

- *Knot type:* Different knot types are used in laparoscopic surgery, such as square knots or sliding knots. The choice of knot type should match the surgical situation. An improperly selected knot may not provide the necessary security.
- *Tissue tension:* The tension on the tissues being sutured can affect knot security. Tissues that are under excessive tension or are too friable may compromise the integrity of the knot.
- *Instrument handling:* Laparoscopic instruments require precision in handling. Errors in instrument manipulation, such as twisting or kinking the suture, can weaken the knot.

Strategies to prevent knot failure:
- *Proper training:* Surgeons and surgical teams must receive thorough training in laparoscopic suturing and knot-tying techniques. Proficiency in these skills is vital for success.
- *Instrument mastery:* Familiarity with laparoscopic instruments is essential. Surgeons should practice using needle drivers and graspers to ensure precise suture manipulation.
- *Tension management:* Maintaining appropriate tension on the suture during knot tying is crucial. Surgeons should develop a keen sense of the right amount of tension required for each knot.
- *Knot selection:* Selecting the correct knot for the task at hand is imperative. Surgeons should have a repertoire of knots and choose the one best suited for the specific surgical situation.
- *Continuous learning:* Laparoscopic surgery is continually evolving. Surgeons should stay updated on the latest techniques and technologies to improve their skills and reduce the risk of knot failure.

Knot failure in laparoscopic surgery is a critical concern that can lead to complications and compromised patient outcomes. Surgeons must be acutely aware of the factors that contribute to knot failure and employ strategies to minimize these risks. Through proper training, instrument mastery, tension management, and knot selection, laparoscopic surgeons can enhance their ability to tie secure knots, ensuring the success of minimally invasive procedures and the safety of their patients.

Slipping

The tension from the tissue causes the suture to work back through the knot in the direction of the tissue plane. If this continues far enough, the working end will pass into the knot and the knot unravels and fails. This behavior can be worsened when the knot is repeatedly strained and let slack, dragged over rough terrain.

Capsizing

Capsizing (or spilling) a knot is changing its form, rearranging its parts, usually by pulling on specific ends in specific ways. Some knots when used in an inappropriate way tend to capsize easily or even spontaneously. Often, the capsized form of the knot offers little resistance to slipping or unravelling. For an excellent example of a knot that capsizes dangerously is when instead of surgeon's knot, the surgeon applies reef knot if he or she does not cross the hand.

Sliding

In knots that are meant to secure vessels, failure can be defined as the knot moving relative to the vessel being gripped. While the knot itself does not fail, it ceases to perform the desired function. For example, a simple rolling hitch tied around an artery and pulled parallel to the artery might hold to a certain tension and then start sliding. Sometimes, this can be corrected by working up the knot tighter before subjecting it to load, but usually, a knot with more wraps or a different size or type of suture needs to be used.

In much of the literature on laparoscopic surgery, the learning curve for performing the technique is described as steep. In fact, laparoscopy is more than a new technique; it is a completely different way of operating as far as tissue approximation is concerned. The visualization is different, the instruments are different, and the tactile aspects are very different. Laparoscopic suturing and knotting is a skill that requires a great deal of practice: "As a young surgeon in training, you sit up all night, night after night, tying knots over and over and over again until it becomes perfect."

■ COMPONENTS OF KNOT

Bight

Bight is the center part of a length of suture as opposed to the ends. A "bight" is any curved section, slack part, or loop between the ends of a suture. The phrase "in the bight" implies a U-shaped section of suture is itself being used in making a knot. Many knots can be tied either with the end or in the bight (**Fig. 2**).

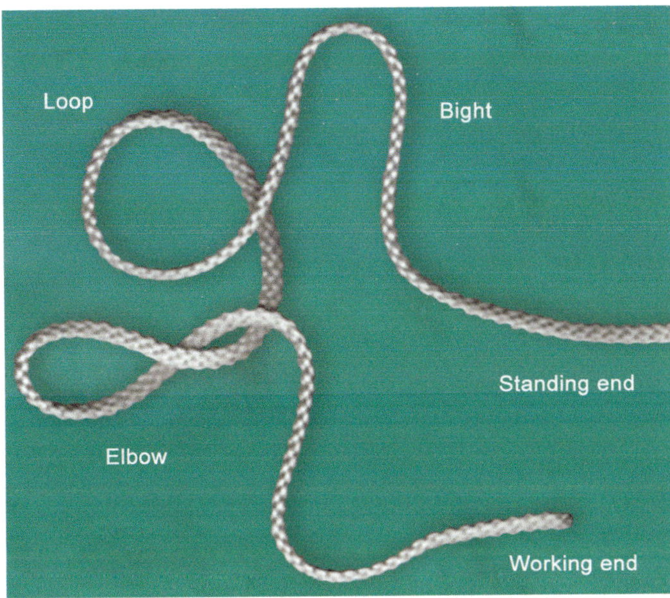

Fig. 2: Main components of knot.

Loop

A full circle formed by passing the working end over itself. The term "loop" is also used to refer to a category of knots.

Elbow

Elbow is two crossing points created by an extra twist in a loop.

Standing End

Standing end is the end of the suture not involved in making the knot, often shown as unfinished or long end.

Standing Part

Standing part of knot is the section of line between knot and the standing end.

Turn

A turn or single turn is a single pass behind or through an object. A round turn is the complete encirclement of an object, which requires two passes. Two round turns circle the object twice, which require three passes.

Working End

Working end is the active end of a line used in making the knot. It may also be called the "running end" or "live end" or tail end.

Working Part

Working part of knot is the section of line between knot and the working end.

■ TYPES OF SUTURE

Monofilament versus Multifilament Strands

Sutures are classified according to the number or strands of which they are comprised.

Monofilament sutures are made of a single strand of material. Because of their simplified structure, they encounter less resistance as they pass through tissue than multifilament suture material. They also resist harboring organisms which may cause suture line infection. These characteristics make monofilament sutures well-suited to vascular surgery, for example, polyamide (nylon) and polypropylene.

Multifilament sutures consist of several filaments, or strands, twisted or braided together. This affords greater tensile strength, pliability, and flexibility. Multifilament sutures may also be coated to help them pass relatively smoothly through tissue and enhance handling characteristics, for example, polyglycolic acid (PGA), silk, and polyester.

Note: Catgut is multifilament in construction; however, due to polishing, it gives a finish of monofilament.

Sutures traditionally have been classified into natural (i.e., naturally occurring) and synthetic (man-made). The use of natural sutures is declining for a number of reasons. Examples of natural sutures include catgut and silk. Suture material is also classified into absorbable and nonabsorbable.

■ SUTURE MATERIALS

Choosing the right suture material for laparoscopic surgery—preferences and considerations: Laparoscopic surgery, with its numerous advantages, has become a standard approach for many surgical procedures. The success of these minimally invasive surgeries depends on various factors and one crucial aspect is the choice of suture material. Surgeons must carefully consider several factors when selecting the appropriate suture material for each specific case. In this chapter, we explore the preferences and considerations that guide the selection of suture material in laparoscopic surgery.

Understanding suture material types: Suture materials come in a variety of types, each with its unique characteristics. The two primary categories of suture materials are:

- *Absorbable sutures*: These sutures break down and are absorbed by the body over time. They are often used for internal tissues that do not require long-term support.
- *Nonabsorbable sutures*: These sutures do not break down in the body and may need to be removed after a certain period. They are often used for tissues that require long-term support or for closing external incisions.

Preferences in laparoscopic surgery:
The choice of suture material in laparoscopic surgery depends on several key factors:

- *Tissue type:* Different tissues have varying characteristics. Delicate tissues may require finer, less traumatic sutures, while tougher tissues may demand stronger sutures for secure closure.
- *Location:* The location of the surgical site is crucial. For internal structures, absorbable sutures are commonly used as they do not require removal. Nonabsorbable sutures are preferred for closing external incisions.
- *Suture size (gauge):* The size of the suture, often referred to as the gauge, is chosen based on the tissue's thickness and the surgeon's preference for handling. Thinner sutures are used for delicate tissues, while thicker sutures provide greater strength.
- *Material strength:* Different materials have varying tensile strengths. Surgeons may choose materials such as polypropylene or nylon for stronger tissues, while tissues with less tensile strength may require materials such as PGA or chromic gut.
- *Allergies and reactions:* Some patients may have allergies or sensitivities to specific suture materials. Surgeons should consider the patient's medical history and any known allergies when making their choice.
- *Duration of support:* If long-term tissue support is required, nonabsorbable sutures are favored. In contrast, absorbable sutures are chosen for tissues that will heal and regain strength relatively quickly.
- *Knot security:* Certain suture materials hold knots better than others. Surgeons often prefer materials such as silk or polypropylene for their knot-tying reliability.
- *Handling characteristics:* Surgeons have personal preferences for the feel and handling of different suture materials. Some materials are more pliable and easier to work with, while others may be stiffer.

Considerations in laparoscopic suture material selection: In addition to the preferences mentioned earlier, several considerations influence the choice of suture material in laparoscopic surgery:

- *Infection risk:* Suture materials should not promote infection. Nonabsorbable sutures may be associated with a slightly higher risk of infection due to their persistence, so this factor must be carefully evaluated.
- *Biocompatibility:* Suture materials should not provoke an adverse tissue response. Biocompatible materials reduce the risk of complications.
- *Cost:* The cost of suture materials can vary significantly. Surgeons often need to balance the benefits of a particular material with the cost to healthcare institutions and patients.
- *Surgical technique:* The surgeon's skill and preferred technique can influence suture material choice. Some techniques may work better with specific materials.

The selection of suture material in laparoscopic surgery is a nuanced decision that involves numerous factors, including tissue type, location, patient history, and surgical technique. Surgeons must carefully consider the individual needs of each case to ensure optimal outcomes and patient safety. By understanding the preferences and considerations surrounding suture materials, surgeons can make informed choices that contribute to the success of laparoscopic procedures and the well-being of their patients.

Absorbable and Nonabsorbable Sutures

Absorbable versus nonabsorbable suture material in laparoscopic surgery—making the right choice:
Suturing is a fundamental skill in surgery and choosing the appropriate suture material is critical to achieving successful outcomes in laparoscopic procedures. In laparoscopic surgery, two broad categories of suture materials are commonly used—absorbable and nonabsorbable. This chapter delves into the characteristics, advantages, and considerations of both types to help surgeons make informed decisions in laparoscopic settings.

Absorbable suture material: Absorbable sutures are designed to gradually degrade and be absorbed by the body over time. These sutures offer several advantages in laparoscopic surgery:

- *Tissue healing:* Absorbable sutures are often used for internal structures, such as the abdominal cavity, where the sutures will eventually be absorbed by the body as the tissues heal. This eliminates the need for suture removal, reducing patient discomfort and risk of infection.

- *Long-term support:* Some absorbable sutures, such as PGA or polylactic acid (PLA), provide sufficient strength for tissue approximation during the critical healing period. They gradually lose tensile strength as the tissues regain their strength.
- *Reduced tissue reaction:* Absorbable sutures tend to provoke fewer tissue reactions compared to nonabsorbable materials. This makes them suitable for tissues where minimal inflammation is desired.
- *Precise closure*: Absorbable sutures are often finer in diameter, allowing for precise tissue apposition without excessive trauma to the tissues.

Nonabsorbable suture material: Nonabsorbable sutures, as the name suggests, do not degrade and must be removed from the body after a specified period. These sutures have their own set of advantages in laparoscopic surgery:

- *Strength and durability:* Nonabsorbable sutures, such as nylon or polypropylene, are known for their high tensile strength and durability. They are preferred for tissues that require long-term support or where greater strength is needed.
- *Tissue approximation:* Nonabsorbable sutures can hold tissues together for extended periods, making them suitable for situations where the tissues may take longer to heal.
- *Precise knot tying:* These sutures often have better knot-holding capabilities, ensuring secure tissue closure, especially in laparoscopic procedures where knot security is crucial.
- *Easy removal:* Surgeons can easily remove nonabsorbable sutures once the tissues have healed, which can be less painful and less prone to complications than absorbable sutures breaking down over time.

Considerations for choosing between absorbable and nonabsorbable sutures in laparoscopic surgery: The choice between absorbable and nonabsorbable sutures in laparoscopic surgery depends on several factors:

- *Tissue type:* Consider the type of tissue being sutured. Delicate or friable tissues may benefit from absorbable sutures, while nonabsorbable sutures may be necessary for tougher tissues.
- *Location:* Internal tissues often benefit from absorbable sutures, while nonabsorbable sutures are typically used for external closures and areas that require long-term support.
- *Healing time:* Assess the expected healing time of the tissues. Absorbable sutures are suitable for tissues that will regain strength relatively quickly, while nonabsorbable sutures may be needed for tissues with a more extended healing process.
- *Knot security:* Evaluate the importance of knot security. Nonabsorbable sutures often provide better knot-tying security, making them ideal for situations where the sutures must withstand significant tension.
- *Patient factors:* Consider the patient's medical history, allergies, and potential sensitivities to suture materials when making the choice.

In laparoscopic surgery, the choice between absorbable and nonabsorbable suture materials is a crucial decision that can significantly impact patient outcomes. Surgeons must carefully assess the characteristics of each material, the specific surgical context, and the patient's needs when selecting the appropriate suture material. By making informed choices, surgeons can contribute to the success of laparoscopic procedures, patient comfort, and overall surgical excellence.

Sutures are divided into two kinds—those which are absorbable and will break down harmlessly in the body over time without intervention and those which are nonabsorbable and must be manually removed if they are not left indefinitely. The type of suture used varies on the operation, with the major criteria being the demands of the location and environment **(Table 1)**.

Sutures to be placed in a stressful environment, for example, the heart (constant pressure and movement) or the bladder (adverse chemical presence), may require specialized or stronger materials to perform their role; usually such sutures are either specially treated or made of special materials and are often nonabsorbable to reduce the risk of degradation.

Absorbable Sutures

Absorbable sutures are made of materials which are broken down in tissue after a given period of time, which depending on the material can be from 10 days to 8 weeks. They are used therefore in many of the internal tissues of the body. In most cases, 3 weeks is sufficient for the wound to close firmly. The suture is not needed any more and the fact that it disappears is an advantage, as there is no foreign material left inside the body and no need for the patient to have the sutures removed.

TABLE 1: Characteristic of different suture material.

Properties	Plain catgut	Chromic catgut	Polyglycolic acid (PGA)	Polydioxanone (PDS)
Description	• Absorbable biological suture material—plain is an absorbable suture made by twisting together strands of purified collagen taken from bovine intestines • The natural plain thread is precision ground in order to achieve a monofilament character and treated with a glycerol-containing solution • Plain is absorbed by enzymatic degradation	• Absorbable biological suture material—chromic is an absorbable suture made by twisting together strands of purified collagen taken from bovine intestines • Due to undergoing a ribbon stage chromicization (treatment with chromic acid salts), the chromic offers roughly twice the stitch-holding time of plain catgut • The natural chromic thread is precision ground in order to achieve a monofilament character and treated with a glycerol-containing solution • Chromic is absorbed by enzymatic degradation	• It is a synthetic absorbable suture material • Braided synthetic absorbable multifilament made of PGA and coated with N-laurin and L-lysine, which render the thread extremely smooth, soft, and knot safe	• It is a synthetic absorbable suture material • Monofilament synthetic absorbable suture, prepared from the polyester, poly (p-dioxanone)
Composition	?	Natural purified collagen	PGA	Polyester and poly (p-dioxanone)
Tensile strength	Strength retention for at least 7 days	?	?	?
Structure	Monofilament	Monofilament	Braided	Monofilament
Origin	Bovine serosa surface finish	Bovine serosa	Synthetic	Synthetic through the critical wound
Treatment	?	Treatment with a glycerol-containing solution and chromic acid salts	Coated with magnesium stearate	Uncoated
Type of absorption	Proteolytic enzymatic digestion complete by 90 days	Proteolytic enzymatic digestion complete in 70 days. Absorption by enzymatic digestion and starts losing tensile strength on implantation from 18 to 21 days of catgut chromic	Absorption by hydrolysis complete between 60 and 90 days. Always predictable and reliable	Wound support can remain up to 6 weeks; however, tensile strength decreases to about 70% at 14 days and 25% at 42 days
Tissue reaction	Moderate—plain catgut enjoys lower tissue reaction as compared to chromicized	Moderate	?	?
Thread color	Straw	Brown	Violet	Violet
Size available	USP 6–0 (1 metric) to USP 3 (7 metric)	USP 6–0 (1 metric) to USP 3 (7 metric)	USP 6–0 (1 metric) to USP 2 (5 metric)	USP 6–0 (1 metric) to USP 2 (5 metric)
Sterilization	Ethylene oxide (E.O.) gas	E.O. gas	E.O. gas	E.O. gas

Contd…

Contd...

Properties	Plain catgut	Chromic catgut	Polyglycolic acid (PGA)	Polydioxanone (PDS)
Advantages	Very high knot pull tensile strength, good knot security due to special excellent handling features	Very high knot pull tensile strength, good knot security due to special surface finish, improved smoothness due to the dry presentation of the thread, excellent handling features	• High initial tensile strength, good holding power through the critical wound-healing period • Smooth passage through tissue, easy handling, excellent knotting ability, secure knot tying	Tensile strength retention, guaranteed holding power
Indications	For all surgical procedures, especially when tissues that regenerate faster are involved. General closure, gynecology, and gastrointestinal tract surgery	For all surgical procedures, especially for tissues that regenerate faster	Subcutaneous, intracutaneous closures, abdominal and thoracic surgeries	The PDS is particularly useful where the combination of an absorbable suture and extended wound support is desirable
Contraindications	Not recommended for incisions that require the sustaining of the tissues for a prolonged period of time	Not recommended for an incision that requires sustaining of the tissues for a prolonged period of time	This suture being absorbable should not be used where extended approximation of tissue is required	This type of suture being absorbable is not to be used where prolonged approximation of tissues under stress is required and/or in conjunction with prosthetic devices
Precautions	• Special precautions should be taken in patients with cancer, anemia, and malnutrition conditions • They tend to absorb the sutures at a higher rate • Cardiovascular surgery due to the continued heart contractions • It is absorbed much faster when used over mucous membrane or in the vagina, due to the presence of microorganisms • Avoid using where long-term tissue approximation is needed. Absorption is faster in infected tissues	• It is absorbed much faster when used in the mouth and in the vagina, due to the presence of microorganism • Cardiovascular surgery, due to the continued heart contractions • Special precautions should be taken in patients with cancer, anemia, and malnutrition conditions • They tend to absorb this suture at a higher rate	• Special precautions should be taken in elderly patients and patients with history of anemia and malnutrition conditions • As with any suture material, adequate knot security requires the accepted surgical technique of flat and square ties	• The PDS suture knots must be properly placed to be secure • Mucosal sutures remaining in place for extended periods may be associated with localized irritation • Subcuticular sutures should be placed as deeply as possible in order to minimize the erythema and induration normally associated with absorption

Absorbable sutures were originally made of the intestine of sheep, the so called catgut. The manufacturing process was similar to that of natural musical strings for violins and guitar and also of natural strings for tennis racquets. The inventor, a 10th century surgeon named al-Zahrawi reportedly discovered the dissolving nature of catgut when his lute's strings were eaten by a monkey. Today, gut sutures are made of specially prepared beef and sheep intestine and may be untreated (plain gut), tanned with chromium salts to increase their persistence in the body (chromic gut), or heat treated to give more rapid absorption (fast gut). However, the major part of the absorbable sutures used are now made of synthetic polymer fibers, which may be braided or monofilament; these offer numerous advantages over gut sutures, notably ease of handling, low cost, low tissue reaction, consistent performance, and guaranteed nontoxicity. In Europe and Japan, gut sutures have been banned due to concerns over bovine spongiform encephalopathy (BSE) (mad cow disease), although the herds from which gut is harvested are certified BSE-free. Each major suture manufacturer has its own proprietary formulations for its brands of synthetic absorbable sutures; various blends of PGA (vicryl, for example), lactic acid, or caprolactone are common. Occasionally, absorbable sutures can cause inflammation and be rejected by the body rather than absorbed.

The natural absorbable sutures (catgut) tend to have unpredictable rates of absorption and tissue reaction. For the most part, these sutures have short half-lives, so they are not good for wound closure where strength is desirable. Their use is being discontinued.

The synthetic absorbable sutures are broken down by hydrolyzation. They generally have a longer half-life, less tissue reaction, and a more consistent breakdown rate. The synthetic absorbable, PGA (Dexon®) or polyglactin 910 (Vicryl®), have decreased tissue reaction compared to the natural absorbable. Knot security is fair and can be used for extracorporeal knotting.

Polyglactin 910 (vicryl) keeps 75% of its tensile strength for about 2 weeks and 50% by 3 weeks. The coated sutures decrease the drag through tissue, so it is easier to use, but there are variable rates of absorption. Polyglactine is good suture material for intracorporeal suturing.

Poliglecaprone 25 (Monocryl®) is a monofilament product that has easy passage through tissue, good handling, and is inert. It keeps tensile strength for only a week but stays in the wound for almost 4 months. It is good for anastomosis, gynecologic work, and small vessel ligation and epithelial approximation. This material can be used for both extra- and intracorporeal suturing.

The delayed absorbable monofilament sutures such as polydioxanone (PDS®) and polyglyconate (Maxon®), used for abdominal wound closure have good tensile strength and low tissue reaction, but the knots are not as strong. PDS is considered as ideal material for extracorporeal knotting by many surgeons and gynecologists.

Polydioxanone is also good for contaminated fields because it has a low affinity for bacteria. It is good for general use, tissue approximation, biliary work, anastomosis, fascial closures, heart surgery, and orthopedics.

Panacryl® is a braided synthetic absorbable suture. It has good tensile strength, low tissue reaction, and fairly good knot security. It maintains 60% of its tensile strength at 6 months. It may be a good substitute for a nonabsorbable suture because it has complete absorption in 2.5 years. It is good for fascial closures, closing tissues under tension, and it might have a role in the compromised patient where you presume there is going to be inadequate or delayed wound healing.

Nonabsorbable Sutures

The natural nonabsorbable materials, cotton and silk, should be relegated to the past. Even though they have good knot security and are easy to tie, they provoke a lot of tissue reaction.

Synthetic nonabsorbable sutures in common use include nylon, polyester, and stainless steel. The role of this material in laparoscopic surgery is very limited and can be used if the other materials are not available.

Nonabsorbable sutures are made of materials which are not metabolized by the body and are used therefore either on skin wound closure, where the sutures can be removed after a few weeks, or in some inner tissues in which absorbable sutures are not adequate. This is the case, for example, in the heart and in blood vessels, whose rhythmic movement requires a suture which stays longer than 3 weeks, to give the wound enough time to close. Other organs, such as the bladder, contain fluids which make absorbable sutures disappear in only a few days, too early for the wound to heal. Inflammation caused by the foreign protein in some absorbable sutures can amplify scarring, so if other types of suture are less antigenic (i.e., do not provoke as much of an immune response), it would represent a way to reduce scarring.

There are several materials used for nonabsorbable sutures. The most common is a natural fiber, silk, which undergoes a special manufacturing process to make it adequate for its use in surgery. Other nonabsorbable sutures are made of artificial fibers, such as polypropylene, polyester, or nylon; these may or may not have coatings to enhance their performance characteristics. Finally, stainless steel wires are commonly used in orthopedic surgery and for sternal closure in cardiac surgery.

Nonabsorbable sutures are those which are not digested by body enzymes or hydrolyzed in body tissue. They may be used in a variety of applications:

- Exterior skin closure—to be removed after sufficient healing has occurred
- Within the body cavity, where they will remain permanently encapsulated in tissue
- Patient history of reaction to absorbable sutures, keloidal tendency, or possible tissue hypertrophy

- Prosthesis attachment (i.e., defibrillators, pacemakers, and drug delivery mechanisms)
- Where lifelong support is required like in cardiovascular surgeries

These sutures may be uncoated or coated, uncolored or naturally colored or dyed, with Food and Drug Administration- (FDA)-approved dyes to enhance visibility.

■ SIZE AND TENSILE STRENGTH

Size denotes the diameter of the suture material:

- The accepted surgical practice is to use the smallest diameter suture that will adequately hold the mending wounded tissue. This practice minimizes trauma as the suture is passed through the tissue to effect closure. It also ensures that the minimum mass of the foreign material is left in the body.
- Suture size is stated numerically; as the number of 0s in the suture size increases, the diameter of the strand decreases. For example, size 5–0, or 00000 is smaller in diameter than size 4–0, or 0000. The smaller the size, the less tensile strength the suture will have. **Table 2** shows different diameters of sutures.

- Knot tensile strength is measured by the force, in kilograms force (kgf), which the suture strand can withstand before it breaks when knotted.
- The tensile strength of the tissue to be mended (its ability to withstand stress) determines the size and tensile strength of the suturing material the surgeon selects. The accepted rule is that the tensile strength of the suture need never exceed the tensile strength of the tissue. However, sutures should be at least as strong as normal tissue through which they are being placed.

If the tissue reduces suture strength over time, the relative rates at which the suture loses strength and the wound gains strength are important. If the suture biologically alters the healing process, these changes must also be understood.

■ SUTURE CHARACTERISTICS

If an ideal suture material could be created, it would be:
- Sterile
- Highly uniform tensile strength, permitting use of finer sizes

TABLE 2: Different diameter of suture.

USP designation	Collagen metric diameter (mm)	Synthetic absorbable metric diameter (mm)	Nonabsorbable metric diameter (mm)	American wire gauge
11–0			0.01	
10–0	0.02	0.02	0.02	
9–0	0.03	0.03	0.03	
8–0	0.05	0.04	0.04	
7–0	0.07	0.05	0.05	
6–0	0.1	0.07	0.07	38–40
5–0	0.15	0.1	0.1	35–38
4–0	0.2	0.15	0.15	32–34
3–0	0.3	0.2	0.2	29–32
2–0	0.35	0.3	0.3	28
0	0.4	0.35	0.35	26–27
1	0.5	0.4	0.4	25–26
2	0.6	0.5	0.5	23–24
3	0.7	0.6	0.6	22
4	0.8	0.6	0.6	21–22
5		0.7	0.7	20–21
6			0.8	19–20
7				18

- High tensile strength retention in vivo, holding the wound securely throughout the critical healing period, followed by rapid absorption
- Consistent uniform diameter
- Predictable performance
- Noncapillary, nonallergenic, and noncarcinogenic
- Easy to handle, ties down well, provides optimum knot security
- Minimally reactive in tissue and not predisposed to bacterial growth
- Capable of holding tissue layers throughout the critical wound healing period securely when knotted without fraying or cutting
- Resistant to shrinking in tissues
- Absorbed completely with minimal tissue reaction after serving its purpose

However, because the ideal all-purpose suture does not yet exist, the surgeon must select a suture that is at least as close to the ideal as possible.

PERSONAL SUTURE PREFERENCE

Most surgeons have a basic "suture routine," a preference for using the same material(s) unless circumstances dictate otherwise. The laparoscopic surgeon acquires skill, proficiency, and speed in handling by using one suture material repeatedly and may choose the same material throughout his or her entire career.

A number of factors may influence the choice of materials:
- His or her area of specialization
- Wound closure experience during clinical training
- Professional experience in the operating room
- Knowledge of the healing characteristics of tissues and organs
- Knowledge of the physical and biological characteristics of various suture materials
- Patient factors (age, weight, overall health status, and the presence of infection)

PRINCIPLES OF SUTURE SELECTION

Among the many decisions that face the surgeon in the operating room, suture selection for the procedure at hand may be one of the most critical. Personal preference will of course play a role. But the final choice will depend upon various patient factors that influence the healing process, the characteristics of the tissues involved, and potential postoperative complications.

The wide variety of suturing materials available can make it difficult to choose the most appropriate suture for a given task.

Following are the principles (guide) for selecting a suture material:
- When a wound reaches maximal strength, sutures are no longer needed. Therefore, slow-healing tissues (skin, fascia, and tendons) should be secured with nonabsorbable sutures or long-lasting absorbable sutures and fast healing tissues (stomach, colon, and bladder) should be healed with absorbable sutures.
- Foreign bodies in potentially contaminated tissues may convert contamination into infection. Therefore, multifilament sutures which may convert contaminated wound into an infected one should be avoided. Monofilament sutures or absorbable sutures should be used in infected wound which resist harboring infection.
- Where cosmetic results are important, close and prolonged apposition of tissues and avoidance of irritants will produce the best results. Therefore, smallest inert monofilament suture materials (nylon and polypropylene) should be used and using skin sutures alone should be avoided and surgeon should use subcuticular closure whenever possible.
- Foreign bodies in the presence of fluids containing high crystalloid concentrations may cause precipitation and stone formation. Hence, absorbable sutures in the urinary and biliary tracts should be used to avoid stone formation.
- Regarding suture size, the finest sized sutures should be used which commensurate with the natural strength of the tissue to be sutured. Retention sutures should be used to reinforce appropriately sized primary sutures if the patient is at risk of producing sudden strains on the suture line postoperatively. The retention sutures should be removed as soon as that risk is reduced.

SURGICAL NEEDLES

There are different types of needle used in laparoscopic surgery.

Traumatic needles are needles with holes or eyes which are supplied to the hospital separate from their suture thread. The suture must be threaded on site, as is done when sewing at home.

Atraumatic needles with sutures comprise an eyeless needle attached to a specific length of suture thread. The suture manufacturer swages the suture thread to the eyeless atraumatic needle at the factory. There are several advantages to having the needle premounted on the suture. The doctor or the nurse does not have to spend time threading the suture on the needle. More important, the suture end of a swaged needle is smaller than the needle body. In traumatic needles with eyes, the thread comes out of the needle's hole on both sides. When passing through the tissues, this type of suture rips the tissue to a certain extent, thus the name traumatic. Nearly all modern sutures feature swaged atraumatic needles.

There are several shapes of surgical needles including:

Cutting Needles

Cutting needles have at least two opposing cutting edges **(Fig. 3)**. They are sharpened to cut through tough, difficult-to-penetrate tissue. Cutting needles are ideal for skin sutures that must pass through dense, irregular, and relatively thick connective dermal tissue. Due to the sharpness of the cutting edge, care must be taken in some tissue (tendon sheath or oral mucous membrane) to avoid cutting through more tissue than desired.

Conventional Cutting Needles

In addition to the two cutting edges, conventional cutting needles have a third cutting edge on the inside concave curvature of the needle. The shape changes from a triangular cutting blade to that of a flattened body on both straight and curved needles **(Fig. 4)**. This needle type may

be prone to cutout of tissue because the inside cutting edge cuts toward the edges of the incision or wound.

The inside and outside curvatures of the body are flattened in the needle-grasping area for greater stability in the needle holder.

Reverse Cutting Needles

These needles were created specifically for tough, difficult-to-penetrate tissue such as skin, tendon sheath, or oral mucosa. Reverse cutting needles are used in ophthalmic and cosmetic surgery where minimal trauma, early regeneration of tissue, and little scar formation are primary concerns. The reverse cutting needle is as sharp as the conventional cutting needle, but its design is distinctively different. The third cutting edge is located on the outer convex curvature of the needle.

This offers several advantages as follows:
- Reverse cutting needles have more strength than similar-sized conventional cutting needles.
- The danger of tissue cutout is greatly reduced.
- The hole left by the needle leaves a wide wall of tissue against which the suture is to be tied.

Round Body Needles

Round body needles pierce and spread tissue without cutting it. The needle point tapers to a sharp tip. The needle body then flattens to an oval or rectangular shape. This increases the width of the body to help prevent twisting or turning in the needle holder. Round body needles are usually used in easily penetrated tissue such as the peritoneum, abdominal viscera, myocardium,

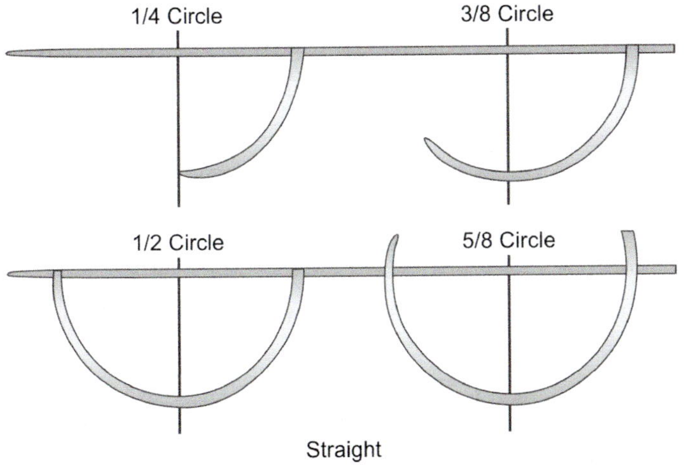

Fig. 3: Cutting needles.

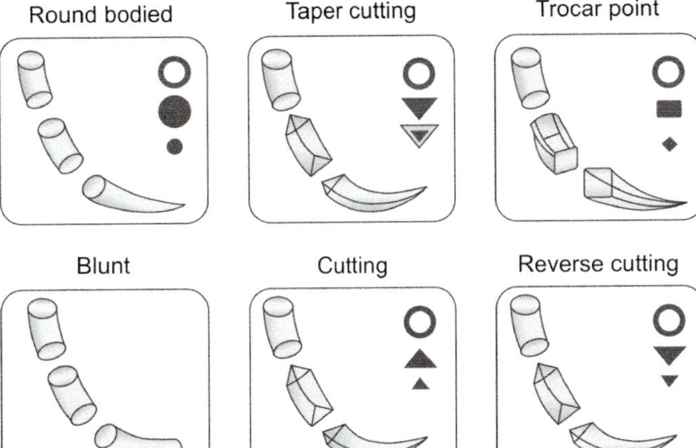

Fig. 4: Conventional cutting needles.

and subcutaneous layers. They are preferred when the smallest possible hole in the tissue and minimum tissue cutting are desired. They are also used in the internal anastomoses to prevent leakage which can subsequently lead to contamination of the abdominal cavity. In the fascia, round body needles minimize the potential for tearing the thin connective tissue lying between parallel and interlacing bands of denser, connecting tissue.

Mayo Needle

The Mayo needle has a round body but heavier and more flattened body than conventional taper needles. This needle was designed for use in dense tissue, particularly for gynecological procedures, general closure, and hernia repair.

Taper Cutting Needles

Taper cutting needles combine the features of the reverse cutting edge tip and round body needles. Three cutting edges extend approximately 1/32" back from the point. These blend into a round taper body. All three edges are sharpened to provide uniform cutting action. The point readily penetrates dense, tough tissue. The objective should be for the point itself not to exceed the diameter of the suture material. The taper body portion provides smooth passage through tissue and eliminates the danger of cutting into the surrounding tissue. Although initially designed for use in cardiovascular surgery on sclerotic or calcified tissue, the taper cutting needle is widely used for suturing dense, fibrous connective tissue—especially in fascia, periosteum, and tendon where separation of parallel connective tissue fibers could occur with a conventional cutting needle.

Blunt Point Needles

Blunt point (BP) needles can literally dissect friable tissue rather than cutting it. They have a taper body with a rounded BP that will not cut through tissue. They may be used for suturing the liver and the kidney. In addition, BP needles for general closure are especially helpful when performing procedures on at-risk patients.

Endoski Needle

The distal end is tapered half circle and proximal shaft of the needle is straight. The shaft of the needle is 1.5 times the length of curved portion of Endoski needle. In our day-to-day practice, we can convert half-circled needle into

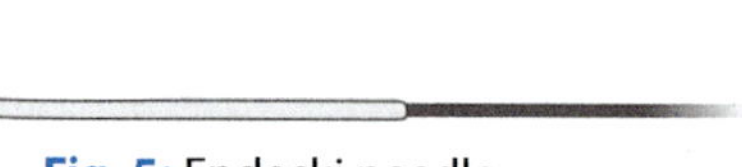

Fig. 5: Endoski needle.

BOX 1: Different sliding knots.

- Two half-hitches
- Reversed half-hitches
- Practical knot (simple version)
- Practical knot (advanced version)
- Nicky's knot or taut-line hitch
- Giant knot
- Modified tautline hitch
- Tennessee slider
- Clinch knot, Wendel Knoten, and Vale knot
- Locking knot
- Secure knot
- Tonsillectomy knot
- Noose loop
- Duncan loop, blood slip knot, Hangman's knot, easy loop, ordura knot
- Triad knot
- Three-twist knot
- Figure-of-eight noose
- Hangman's knot
- Hangman's tie
- Mid-ship knot

Endoski shaped by making proximal half of the needle straight.

With increasing proficiency, curved needle can also be used, but in laparoscopic surgery, most intuitive needle is Endoski needle. Endoski has advantage of both straight and curved needle (**Fig. 5**).

■ TYPES OF KNOT

The type of extracorporeal knot chosen to complete the loop depends on the clinical situation and the material used.

Types of Extracorporeal Knot

More than 22 different sliding knots were used by the surgeons worldwide (**Box 1**).

Commonly used extracorporeal knots in laparoscopic surgery are:

- Square knot
- Roeder's knot
- Meltzer's knot
- Mishra's knot

- Weston's knot
- Tayside knot

Commonly used intracorporeal knot:
- Square knot
- Surgeon's knot
- Tumble square knot
- Continuous suturing with Dundee jamming knot and Aberdeen termination

■ GENERAL PRINCIPLES OF KNOT TYING

The type of knot tied will depend upon the material used, the depth and location of the incision, and the amount of stress that will be placed upon the wound postoperatively.

Multifilament sutures are generally easier to handle and tie than monofilament sutures. The surgeon must work slowly and meticulously.

Speed in knot tying frequently results in less-than-perfect placement of the strands.

When tying a knot, the surgeon must consider the amount of tension he or she is placing upon the incision and must allow for postoperative edema.

The general principles of knot tying which apply to all suture materials are:
- The completed knot must be firm to virtually eliminate slippage.
- The simplest knot for the material used is the most desirable.
- Tie the knot as small as possible and cut the ends as short as possible. This helps to prevent excessive tissue reaction toward absorbable sutures and to minimize foreign body reaction to nonabsorbable sutures.
- Friction ("sawing") between strands may weaken suture integrity and it should be avoided.
- Damage to the suture material during handling should be avoided, especially when using surgical instruments in instrument ties.
- Excessive tension which may break sutures and cut tissue should be avoided. This practice will lead to successful use of finer gauge materials.
- Sutures used for tissue approximation should not be tied too tightly, as this may contribute to tissue strangulation. Approximate; do not strangulate.
- Traction should be maintained at one end of the strand after the first loop is tied to avoid loosening of the throw.
- The final throw should be made as nearly horizontal as possible.

- Surgeon should not hesitate to change stance or position in relation to the patient in order to place a knot securely and flat.
- Extra throws do not add to the strength of a properly tied knot but only adds to its bulk. Some procedures involve tying knots with the fingers, using one or two hands; others involve tying with the help of instruments. Perhaps, the most complex method of knot tying is done during endoscopic procedures, when the surgeon must manipulate instruments from well outside the body cavity.

Steps of Knotting

There are three steps of knot tying:
1. Configuration (tying)
2. Shaping (drawing)
3. Securing (locking or snuggling)

"It is important to remember that knot is either exactly right or is hopelessly wrong; it is never nearly right."

■ HOW TO LEARN LAPAROSCOPIC AND SUTURING AND KNOTTING?

Learning laparoscopic surgery, suturing, and knotting requires dedication, practice, and proper guidance. Following is a step-by-step guide to help you get started on your journey to mastering these skills:

1. *Educational foundation:*
   a. *Basic medical knowledge:* Start by building a strong foundation in anatomy, physiology, and surgical principles. Understanding the human body's structures and functions is essential.
   b. *Medical school or medical assistant training:* Enrolling in medical school or a medical assistant program can provide you with the foundational knowledge necessary for surgical training.
2. *Online resources:*
   a. *Online courses:* Numerous online platforms offer laparoscopic surgery courses. Websites such as Coursera, edX, and Khan Academy provide valuable resources and lectures on medical topics.
3. *Formal laparoscopic training:*
   a. *Medical residency:* If you are a medical student, consider pursuing a surgical residency program. This offers hands-on experience and structured training in various surgical techniques, including laparoscopy.

b. *Fellowship programs:* Some institutions offer laparoscopic surgery fellowships specifically designed to provide advanced training in minimally invasive techniques.
4. *Hands-on experience:*
   a. *Simulation training:* Laparoscopic simulators are valuable tools for practicing skills in a controlled environment. Look for institutions or courses that offer access to these simulators.
   b. *Cadaver laboratories:* Some medical schools or surgical programs provide opportunities to practice on cadavers, which can enhance your understanding of human anatomy.
5. *Suturing and knot-tying workshops:*
   a. *Surgical skills workshops:* Attend workshops that focus on suturing and knot-tying techniques. These often provide guidance from experienced surgeons and ample hands-on practice.
   b. *Suture practice kits:* Invest in suture practice kits available online. These kits typically include sutures, needles, and synthetic tissues to simulate real surgical scenarios. Practice regularly to improve your skills.
6. *Mentorship and preceptorship:*
   a. *Find a mentor:* Seek out experienced laparoscopic surgeons who can serve as mentors. Their guidance and expertise will be invaluable as you learn these skills.
   b. *Preceptorship:* Consider participating in a preceptorship program, where you can shadow an experienced surgeon to gain practical insights into laparoscopic surgery.
7. *Attend conferences and workshops:*
   a. *Medical conferences:* Attend medical conferences, particularly those focused on minimally invasive surgery. These events offer opportunities to learn from experts, observe live surgeries, and network with professionals.
8. *Certification and continuing education:*
   a. *Board certification:* If you are pursuing a career as a surgeon, work toward board certification in your chosen specialty. Certification typically requires demonstrating proficiency in laparoscopic techniques.
   b. *Continuing education:* Stay current in your field by attending workshops, courses, and conferences throughout your career. Laparoscopic surgery continues to evolve and ongoing education is essential.
9. *Practice, practice, and practice:*
   a. Regular and deliberate practice is crucial for skill development. Focus on perfecting your suturing and knot-tying techniques through repetition.
10. *Safety and ethical considerations:*
   a. Always prioritize patient safety and ethical standards in your practice. Adhere to the highest ethical and professional standards in healthcare.

Remember that learning laparoscopic surgery and mastering suturing and knot-tying skills is a continuous process. It requires dedication, patience, and a commitment to ongoing education and improvement. Seek opportunities for mentorship, hands-on experience, and formal training to become proficient in these essential surgical techniques.

■ CONCLUSION

In conclusion, laparoscopic surgery represents a significant advancement in modern medicine, offering numerous benefits such as reduced recovery times, minimized pain, and smaller scars. However, the success of these minimally invasive procedures heavily relies on the surgeon's expertise in suturing and knotting within the confined space of the body. Mastery of these skills is essential for ensuring effective tissue closure, maintaining hemostasis, and preventing complications like bleeding, infection, and herniation. Understanding the different types of knots, their potential failures, and the appropriate suture materials is crucial. Surgeons must continuously refine their techniques and stay updated with the latest advancements to achieve optimal patient outcomes. As the field of laparoscopic surgery continues to evolve, the ability to perform precise suturing and secure knotting remains a fundamental and indispensable skill for every laparoscopic surgeon.

■ BIBLIOGRAPHY

1. Al Fallouji M. Making loops in laparoscopic surgery: State of the art. Surg Laparosc Endosc. 1993;3:477-81.
2. Balg F, Boileau P. The mid-ship knot: A new simple and secure sliding knot. Knee Surg Sports Traumatol Arthrosc. 2007;15:217-8.
3. Bardana DD, Burks RT, West JR. The effect of suture anchor design and orientation on suture abrasions: An in-vitro study. Arthroscopy. 2003;19:274-81.
4. Brouwers JE, Oosting H, DeHaas D, Klopper PJ. Dynamic loading of surgical knots. Surg Gynecol Obstet. 1991;173:443-8.

5. Budworth G. The Book of Practical Fishing Knots. Mechanicsburg, PA: Stackpole Books; 2003. ·

6. Burkhart SS, Wirth MA, Simonich M, Salem D, Lanctot D, Athanasiou K. Knot security in simple sliding knots and its relationship to rotator cuff repair: How secure must the knot be? Arthroscopy. 2000;16:202-7.

7. Burkhart SS, Wirth MA, Simonich M, Salem D, Lanctot D, Athanasiou K. Loop security as a determinant of tissue fixation security. Arthroscopy. 1998;14:773-6.

8. Campbell DF, Nassar AHM, Tamijmarane A. The vale knot—an intracorporeal slipknot. Surg Endosc. 2000;14: 90-1.

9. Carpenter EM, Hendrickson DA, James S, Franke C, Frisbie D, Trostle S, et al. A mechanical study of ligature security of commercially available pre-tied ligatures versus hand tied ligatures for use in equine laparoscopy. Vet Surg. 2006;35(1):55-9.

10. Chan KC, Burkhart SS, Thiagarajan P, Goh JCH. Optimization of stacked half-hitch knots for arthroscopic surgery. Arthroscopy. 2001;17:752-9.

11. Chan KC, Burkhart SS. How to switch posts without rethreading when tying half-hitches. Arthroscopy. 1999;15:444-50.

12. Croce E, Olmi S. Intracorporeal knot-tying and suturing Techniques in laparoscopic surgery: technical details. JSLS. 2000;4:17-22.

13. De Beer JF, van Rooyen K, Boezaart AP. Nicky's knot: A new slip knot for arthroscopic surgery. Arthroscopy. 1998;14:109-10.

14. Delimar D, Korzinek K, Hancevic J. Initial throw locking internal knotting technique. Surg Endosc. 1998;12:1184-5.

15. Delimar D. A secure arthroscopic knot. Arthroscopy. 1996;12:345-7.

16. Elkousy HA, Sekiya JK, Stabile KJ, McMahon PJ. A biomechanical comparison of arthroscopic sliding and sliding-locking knots. Arthroscopy. 2005;21:204-10.

17. Fischer SP. How to make sense out of arthroscopic knot-tying. Available from http://www.aana.org/pdf/FallCourse/2006%20knot%20tying%20handout.pdf [Last accessed May, 2024].

18. Fleega BA, Sokkar SH. The giant knot: A new one-way self-locking secured arthroscopic slip knot. Arthroscopy. 1999;15:451-2.

19. Gunderson PK. The half-hitch knot: A rational alternative to the square knot. Am J Surg. 1987;154:538-40.

20. Hage JJ. How Capsizing, Flipping, and flyping of traditional knots can result in new endoscopic knots: A geometric review. J Am Coll Surg. 2007;205(5):717-23.

21. Hassinger SM, Wongworawat MD, Hechanova JW. Biomechanical characteristics of 10 arthroscopic knots. Arthroscopy. 2006;22(8):827-32.

22. Hasson HM. Suture loop techniques to facilitate microsurgical and laparoscopic procedures. J Reprod Med. 1987;32:765-7.

23. Heermann JB. Tensile strength and knot security of surgical suture materials. Am J Surg. 1971;37:209-17.

24. Holmlund DE. Knot properties of surgical suture materials. Acta Chir Scand. 1974;140:355-62.

25. Hughes PJ, Hagan RP, Fisher AC, Holt EM, Frostick SP. The kinematics and kinetics of slipknots for arthroscopic—Bankart Repair. Am J Sports Med. 2001;29:738-45.

26. Ilahi OA, Younas SA, Alexander J, Noble PC. Cyclic testing of arthroscopic knot security. Arthroscopy. 2004;20:62-8.

27. Kadirkamanathan SS, Shelton JC, Hepworth CC, Laufer JG, Swain CP. A comparison of the strength of knots tied by hand and at laparoscopy. J Am Coll Surg. 1996;182(1):46-54.

28. Karabacak RO, Shabgahi B, Biberoglu KÖ. A new practical knot technique for use in laparoscopy. Endoscopy. 1992;24:805.

29. Kim SH, Ha KI, Kim JS. Significance of the internal locking mechanism for loop security enhancement in the arthroscopic. Arthroscopy. 2001;17:850-5.

30. Kim SH, Ha KI. The SMC knot-a new slip knot with locking mechanism. Arthroscopy. 2000;16:563-5.

31. Kim SH, Yoo JC, Wang JH, Choi KW, Bae TS, Lee CY. Arthroscopic sliding knot: How many additional half-hitches are really needed? Arthroscopy. 2005;21(4): 405-11.

32. Kuniholm JF, Buckner GD, Nifong W, Orrico M. Automated knot tying for fixation in minimally invasive, robot-assisted cardiac surgery. J Biomech Eng. 2005;127:1001-8.

33. Lee TQ, Matsuura PA, Fogolin RP, Lin A, Kim D, McMahon PJ. Arthroscopic suture tying: A comparison of knot types and suture materials. Arthroscopy. 2001;17:348-52.

34. Lieurance RK, Pflaster DS, Abbott D, Nottage WM. Failure characteristics of various arthroscopically tied knots. Clin Orthop Relat Res. 2003;408:311-8.

35. Lo I. (2008). Essential principles of tying secure arthroscopic knots. [online] Available from https://www.vumedi.com/video/essential-principles-of-tying-secure-arthroscopic-knots/ [Last accessed May, 2024].

36. Lo IK, Burkhart SS, Athanasiou K. Abrasion resistance two types of nonabsorbable braided suture. Arthroscopy. 2004;20:407-13.

37. Lo IK, Burkhart SS, Chan KC, Athanasiou K. Arthroscopic knots: Determining the optimal balance of loop security and knot security. Arthroscopy. 2004;20(5):489-502.

38. Loutzenheiser TD, Harryman DT II, Yung SW, France M, Sidles JA. Optimizing arthroscopic knots. Arthroscopy. 1995;11:199-206.

39. Loutzenheiser TD, Harryman DT II, Ziegler DW, Yung SW. Optimizing arthroscopic knots using braided or monofilament suture. Arthroscopy. 1998;14:57-65.

40. Luks FI, Deprest J, Brosens I, Lerut T. Extracorporeal surgical knot. J Am Coll Surg. 1994;179:220-2.

41. Marrero MA, Corfman RS. Laparoscopic use of sutures. Clin Obstet Gynecol. 1991;34:387-94.

42. Meng MV, Stoller ML. Laparoscopic intracorporeal square-to-slip knot. Urology. 2002;59:932-3.

43. Mishra DK, Cannon Jr WD, Lucas DJ, Belzer JP. Elongation of arthroscopically tied knots. Am J Sports Med. 1997; 25:113-7.

44. Mishra RK (Ed). Textbook of Practical Laparoscopic Surgery. New Delhi: Jaypee Brothers Medical Publishers (P) Ltd.; 2007. pp. 104-23.

45. Ng JWT, Yeung B. Simple, instrument-assisted technique for tying a slip knot: A note of caution. ANZJ Surg. 2004;74:270-1.

46. Nottage WM, Lieurance RK. Arthroscopic knot tying techniques. Arthroscopy. 1999;15:515-21.

47. Pattas M, Theodorou D, Lagoudianakis E, Filis K, Menenakos E, Leandros E. Easy loop knot: A simple and safe extracorporeal knot. Am J Surg. 2006;191:821-2.

48. Perez Carro L, Garcia MS. Totally intra-articular arthroscopic knot: Push and twist technique. Arthroscopy. 1999;15:106-9.

49. Pier A, Thevissen P, Eikel M, Götz F. Laparoskopische Naht—und Knüpftechniken. Chirurg. 1994;65:473-83.

50. Prepageran N, Raman R. Hangman's knot in securing bypass tubes in endonasal dacryocystorhinostomy. Rhinology. 2002;40:95-100.

51. Pritchard C. (1999). Aspects of the Life and Work of Peter Guthrie Tait. [online] Available from https://clerkmaxwellfoundation.org/PritchardTaitBooklet.pdf [Last accessed May, 2024].

52. Puñal Rodríguez JA. Reliable double-component knots for laparoscopic surgery. Br J Surg. 1998;85:16-9.

53. Richmond JC. A comparison of ultrasonic suture welding and traditional knot tying. Am J Sports Med. 2001;29:297-9.

54. Sharp HT, Dorsey JH, Chovan JD, Holtz PM. A simple modification to add strength to the Roeder knot. J Am Assoc Gynecol Laparosc. 1996;3(2):305-7.

55. Sharp HT, Dorsey JH, Chovan JD, Holtz PM. The effect of knot geometry on the strength of laparoscopic slip knots. Obstet Gynecol. 1996;88(3):408-11.

56. Sharp HT, Dorsey JH. The 4-S modification of the Roeder knot: How to tie it. Obstet Gynecol. 1997;90(6):1004-6.

57. Shettko DL, Frisbie DD, Hendrickson DA. A comparison of knot security of commonly used hand-tied laparoscopic slipknots. Vet Surg. 2004;33(5):521-4.

58. Shimi SM, Lirici MM, Vander Velpen G, Cuschieri A. Comparative study of the holding strength of slipknots using absorbable and nonabsorbable ligature materials. Surg Endosc. 1994;8:1285-91.

59. Snyder JS. Technique of arthroscopic rotator cuff repair using implantable 4-mm revo suture anchors, suture shuttle relays, and no.2 nonabsorbable mattress sutures. Orthop Clin North Am. 1997;28:267-75.

60. Soper NJ, Hunter JG. Suturing and knot tying in laparoscopy. Surg Clin N Am. 1992;72:1139-52.

61. Tait PG (Ed). Listing's topologie (Introductory address to the Edinburgh mathematical Society, November 9, 1883). Scientific Papers Vol II. UK: Cambridge University Press; 1900. pp. 85-98.

62. Tait PG (Ed). On knots. Scientific papers Vol I. UK: Cambridge University Press; 1898. pp. 237-317.

63. Tera H, Aberg C. Tensile strength of twelve types of knots employed in surgery, using different suture materials. Acta Chir Scand. 1976;142:1-7.

64. Thal R. Knotless suture anchor. Clin Orthop. 2001;390: 42-51.

65. Trimbos JB, Van Rijssel EJ, Klopper PJ. Performance of sliding knots in monofilament and multifilament suture material. Obstet Gynecol. 1986;68(3):425-30.

66. Trimbos JB. Security of various knots commonly used in surgical practice. Obstet Gynecol. 1984;64(2):274-80.

67. Trostle SS, Hendrickson DK, Franke C. The effects of ethylene oxide and gas-plasma sterilization on failure strength and failure mode of pre-tied monofilament ligature loops. Vet Surg. 2002;31(3):281-4.

68. Udwadia TE. Operative technique for laparoscopic cholecystectomy. In: Kriplani A, Bhatia P, Prasad A, Govil D, Garg HP (Eds). Comprehensive Laparoscopic Surgery. New Delhi: Sagar Printers; 2007. pp. 40-51.

69. Van Rijssel EJ, Trimbos JB, Booster MH. Mechanical performance of square knots and sliding knots in surgery: A comparative study. Am J Obstet Gynecol. 1990;162: 93-7.

70. Weston PV. A new clinch knot. Obstet Gynecol. 1991;78:144-7.

71. Yiannakopoulos CK, Hiotus I, Antonogiannakis E. The triad knot: A new sliding self-locking knot. Arthroscopy. 2005;21:899.c1-3.

Roeder's Knot

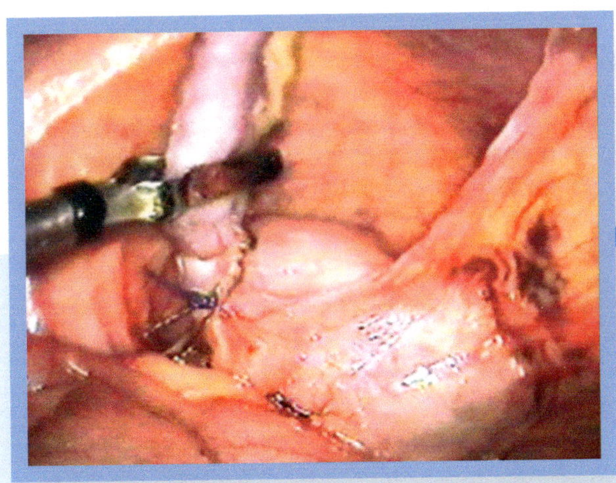

◼ INTRODUCTION

In the intricate world of laparoscopic surgery, where precision and efficiency are paramount, the laparoscopic Roeder's knot stands out as a pinnacle of surgical innovation. Developed to enhance the safety and reliability of knot tying in minimally invasive procedures, this knot has become a cornerstone in the repertoire of skilled laparoscopic surgeons. This chapter delves into the laparoscopic Roeder's knot, exploring its origins, methodology, benefits, and the profound impact it has had on laparoscopic surgery.

◼ ORIGINS OF THE ROEDER'S KNOT

The Roeder's knot, originally conceptualized for use in conventional surgery, was adapted for laparoscopic procedures to address the unique challenges posed by minimally invasive techniques. Named after its inventor, this knot was designed to provide a secure and reliable means of suturing that could be executed efficiently within the constrained spaces and limited visibility of laparoscopic environments.

◼ TECHNIQUE BEHIND THE KNOT

The laparoscopic Roeder's knot is a slip knot that is pretied outside the body and then introduced into the abdominal cavity through a cannula. This method involves the following key steps:

- *Pretying the knot:* The surgeon creates a loop with the suture material and wraps the free end around the loop several times. The number of wraps depends on the suture material and the required knot security.
- *Introducing the knot:* Using a specialized knot pusher, the pretied knot is gently advanced into the abdominal cavity through one of the laparoscopic ports.
- *Securing the tissue:* The ends of the suture are manipulated to encircle the tissue that needs to be sutured. The knot is then tightened by pulling on one end of the suture, while the other end is held in place.
- *Final adjustments:* The surgeon makes final adjustments to ensure the knot is securely tightened and positioned correctly, providing the necessary tension to approximate the tissue edges without compromising tissue integrity.

◼ ADVANTAGES OF THE ROEDER'S KNOT

The laparoscopic Roeder's knot offers several significant advantages over traditional knot-tying techniques in laparoscopic surgery:

- *Efficiency:* This method reduces the time required to securely tie sutures, a critical factor in minimizing operative time and reducing patient exposure to anesthesia.
- *Reliability:* The Roeder's knot is known for its strong and reliable knot security, reducing the risk of knot failure and postoperative complications.
- *Versatility:* Suitable for a wide range of laparoscopic procedures, this knot can be used in various tissues and settings, enhancing the surgeon's ability to adapt to different surgical scenarios.

◼ TRAINING AND MASTERY

Mastering the laparoscopic Roeder's knot requires practice and a thorough understanding of its mechanics. Simulation training, alongside expert guidance, provides an effective platform for surgeons to develop the dexterity and confidence needed to execute this technique proficiently.

◼ IMPACT ON LAPAROSCOPIC SURGERY

The introduction of the laparoscopic Roeder's knot has had a profound impact on the field of minimally invasive surgery. By offering a combination of efficiency, reliability, and versatility, this knotting technique has contributed to the advancement of laparoscopic surgery, enabling surgeons to perform complex procedures with enhanced precision and safety.

The laparoscopic Roeder's knot embodies the continuous evolution of surgical techniques toward greater precision, safety, and efficiency. As laparoscopic surgery progresses, the mastery of such advanced knotting techniques will remain essential for surgeons striving to provide the highest standard of care for their patients. The Roeder's knot, with its blend of simplicity and effectiveness, serves as a testament to the ingenuity and skill that define the art and science of modern surgery. The advanced laparoscopic procedures require surgeon to master suturing. The Roeder's knot is widely used in laparoscopic surgery for extracorporeal tying. The extracorporeal knots are tied and drawn externally and then slipped down by a knot pusher to the intended target and then locked by traction on the standing part against the knot pusher. However, it is significantly weaker than extracorporeally tied knots with several throws. The ability to reapproximate tissues laparoscopically utilizing suturing techniques is an essential skill for all the minimal access surgeon. Although knot tying in open surgery is easily learned and performed by surgeons, knot tying becomes both challenging and frustrating when performed laparoscopically.

Roeder's knot is preferred for the following:
- Ligature of large vessels and tubular structures in continuity with or without needle.
- Ligature of tubular structure with free end with the help of loop.
- Approximation of edges of defects with the needle, where the force required for approximation is substantial.
- Transfixation of large vascular pedicles.
- Suturing in areas of limited access where the working space for intracorporeal suturing is restricted.

Each step of Roeder's knot configuration and shaping should be carefully followed to avoid inadvertent locking of knot before slipping it down to desired target.

■ EQUIPMENT AND INSTRUMENTATION

Suture

Although pretied loops **(Fig. 1)** are available in the market, but surgeon should learn how to tie the extracorporeal knot.

Pretied loop can be used for any free structure such as appendix, but for continuous structure such as cystic duct, surgeon has to perform extracorporeal knotting intraoperatively.

Knot Pusher

For extracorporeal knotting, knot pushers are used. These knot pushers are of either closed jaw or of open jaw type **(Figs. 2 and 3)**.

Closed-jaw plastic or stainless steel knot pusher should be used for sliding the knot after configuration. The following rules should be followed for safe ligature of extracorporeal knot.
- The length of suture for free structure should be minimum 75 cm.
- The length of suture for continuous structure should be minimum 90 cm to 1.5 m and the gauge should be 2/0 or greater.

- The thread should be visible, pliable, and hold the knot securely.
- For any ligature material, the holding force of any surgical slip knot varies directly with its caliber.
- The holding and tensile strength of extracorporeal slip knot depends on the type of ligature material used.

Suture Material

Absorbable Sutures
- Catgut—poor gliding ability
- Vicryl—good maneuverability

Nonabsorbable Sutures
- Prolene—good gliding ability, but memory of thread makes it tedious to work inside the abdominal cavity.
- Ethibond—good maneuverability, less memory than prolene.

A single chromic catgut, vicryl, or prolene can be used for multiple Roeder's knots, which are economically viable for routine use in developing countries. Roeder's knot tied with polyamide are less secure than knots tied with Dacron, lactomer, and polydioxanone. Catgut should be used dry and knot should be tied immediately otherwise it will swell and sliding of knot will be difficult. The Roeder's knot is one of the oldest knot used in minimal access surgery and initially it was used with catgut.

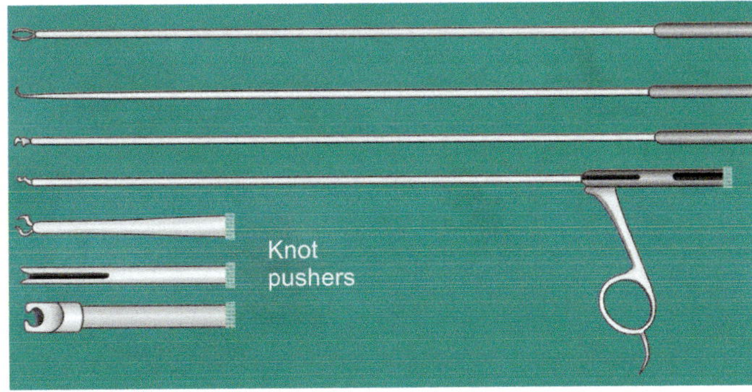

Fig. 2: Laparoscopic knot pusher.

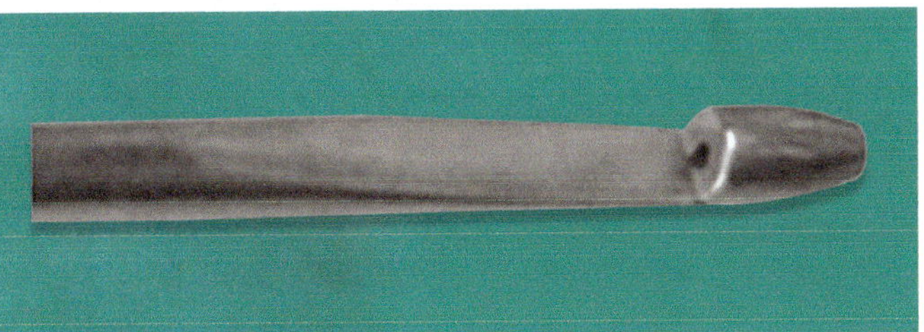

Fig. 3: Knot pusher.

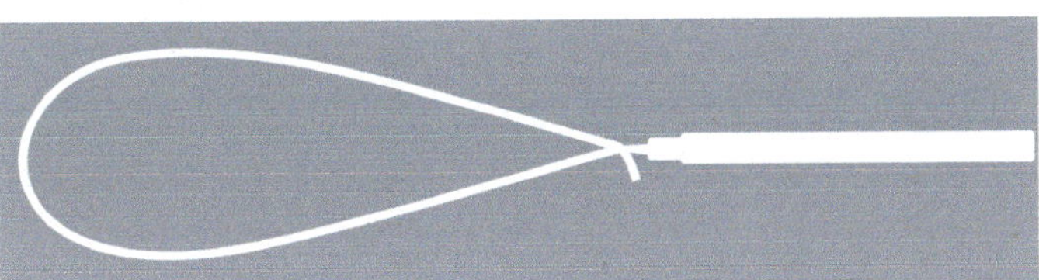

Fig. 1: Pretied loop.

TASK ANALYSIS OF EXTRACORPOREAL KNOT FOR FREE STRUCTURE

- The suture length for the extracorporeal knot in free structures is 75 cm.
- Hold the Bhandarkar knot pusher in your left hand and pass 2 cm of suture through the eye at the tail end of the Bhandarkar knot pusher using your right hand.
- Reverse feed the knot pusher into the 3 mm reducer; this reverse feeding step is crucial.
- After the reducer is inserted, pull the thread out from the eye at the tail end of the knot pusher. The role of this eye is solely to safely guide the suture through the reducer.
- Now, pass the other end of the suture through the eye at the head end using your right hand.
- Request your assistant's finger to help you tie the extracorporeal slip knot.
- There are three types of extracorporeal knots: (1) Roader's knot, (2) Meltzer's knot, and (3) Mishra's knot, each with distinct configurations.
- The Roader's knot configuration is 1:3:1—1 hitch, 3 consecutive winds, and 1 half-knot lock. It is secure for structures up to 8 mm in diameter.
- Adjust the loop's diameter to 6 cm by gently sliding it using your right hand's finger and thumb.
- Hide the knot and its loop under the reducer.
- Now, introduce the knot pusher and the reducer through either a 5 or 10 mm port. If using a 10-mm port, add an additional 5 mm reducer to prevent gas leakage.
- Introduce an atraumatic grasper from the contralateral port.
- Ensure the loop of the knot is positioned near the free structure.
- Insert the free structure's tip into the loop using the atraumatic grasper.
- Feed the knot pusher and loop behind the structure, similar to placing a garland around someone's neck.
- Slide the knot to the desired location by stabilizing the knot pusher with your left hand and pulling the suture with your right hand.
- Perform this process gently to ensure the structure remains unaware of the tying. Avoid exerting any undue pressure on the tubular structure being ligated.
- After tightening the knot three times consecutively, remove the knot pusher and 3 mm reducer. Introduce hook scissors from the same port and cut the suture, leaving a 1 cm tail.
- The extracorporeal knot is highly secure, and a single knot is sufficient for ligating various tubular structures, including the appendix, fallopian tube, pieces of omentum, small pedunculated myomas, or paraovarian simple cysts.

TECHNIQUE AND STEPS

The gloved index finger of assistant may be used to make Roeder's knot **(Fig. 4)**.

Step 1

The left hand should be used to hold the right long limb and right hand to hold short left limb of suture **(Fig. 5)**.

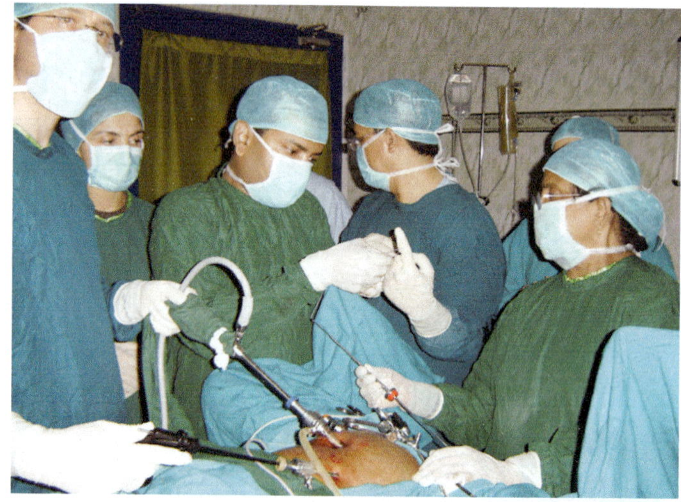

Fig. 4: Assistant finger is required to tie extracorporeal knot in operation theater.

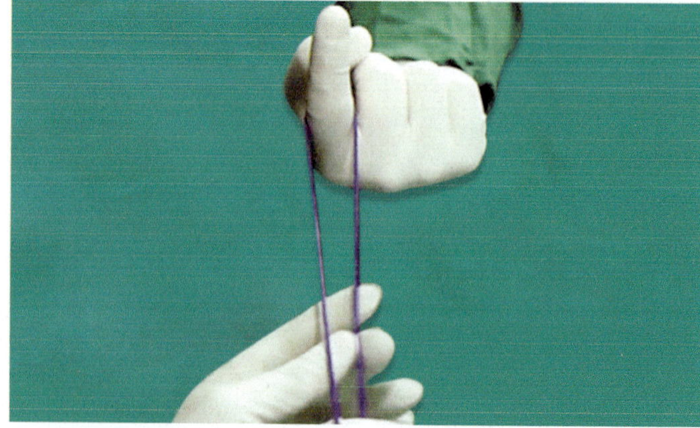

Fig. 5: Short limb is held in right hand and long limb in the left hand.

Step 2

The short limb of thread should be crossed over the long limb in such a way that short should be above the long **(Fig. 6)**.

Step 3

The intersection point of thread should be pinched by left hand index finger and thumb. Surgeon should keep sufficient length of short limb. Right hand will make necessary hitches and loops **(Fig. 7)**. The diameter of loop made this way should be minimum 4 cm.

Step 4

The short limb (working limb) should be passed in between the loop from below upward using thumb and middle finger of right hand **(Fig. 8)**.

Step 5

The short limb should be pulled from up by thumb and index finger of right hand to make first hitch **(Fig. 9)**.

Step 6

The short limb should be passed to encircle the whole loop from below upward using thumb and middle finger of right hand **(Fig. 10)**.

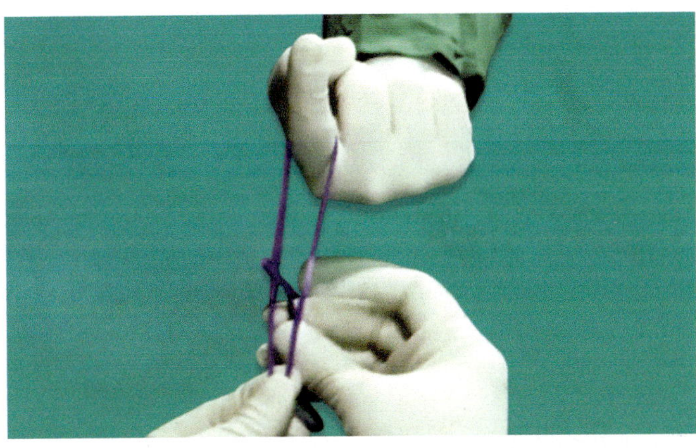

Fig. 8: Short limb is passed in the loop.

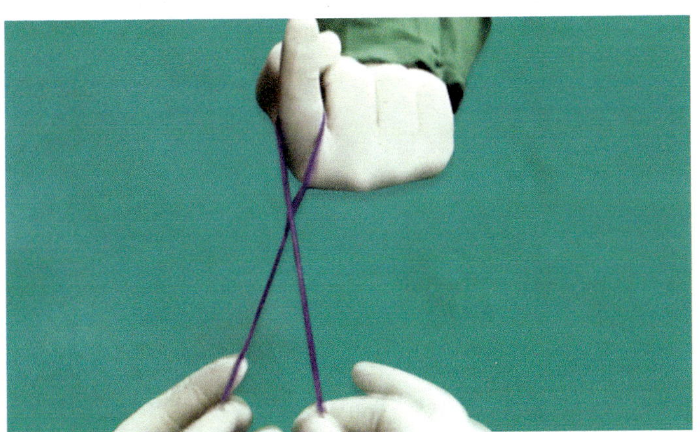

Fig. 6: Short limb is crossed over long limb.

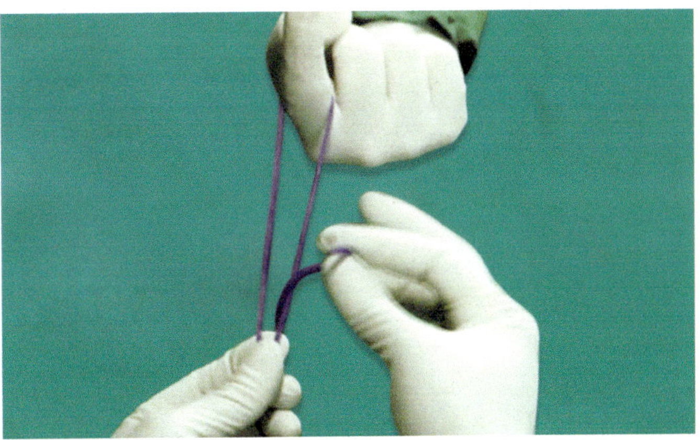

Fig. 9: Short limb is pulled from up.

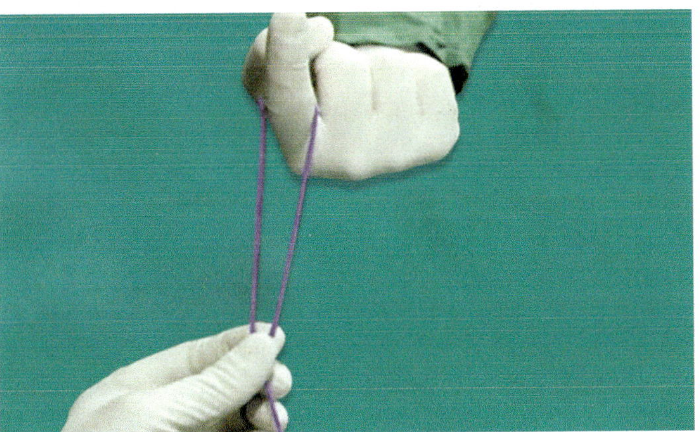

Fig. 7: Intersection point is held.

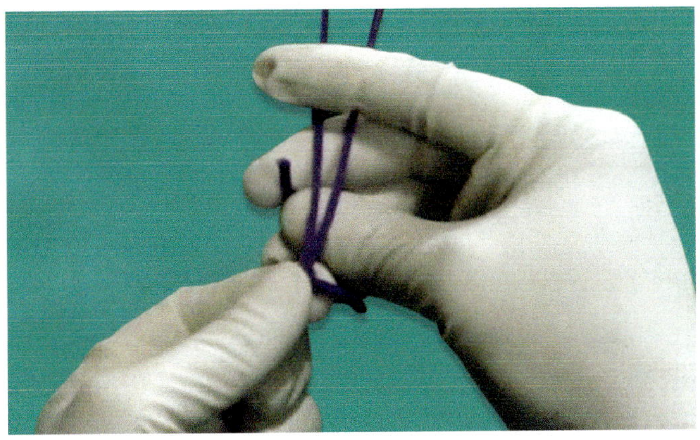

Fig. 10: Loop is encircled by short limb.

Step 7

The short limb should be pulled from up by index finger and thumb of right hand to make first wind (**Fig. 11**).

Step 8

Steps 6 and 7 should be repeated to make second wind (**Fig. 12**).

Step 9

Steps 6 and 7 should be repeated to make third wind (**Fig. 13**).

Step 10

After making three winds, short limb should be passed inside the loop from below upward using index finger and thumb of right hand (**Fig. 14**).

Step 11

Once short limb projects up, it should be pushed down by thumb inside the loop to make half locking knot (**Fig. 15**).

Step 12

The tail end should be pulled from below to tighten the half locking knot (**Fig. 16**).

Step 13

Once the knot is configured properly, it should be checked by sliding over the long limb (**Figs. 17 and 18**).

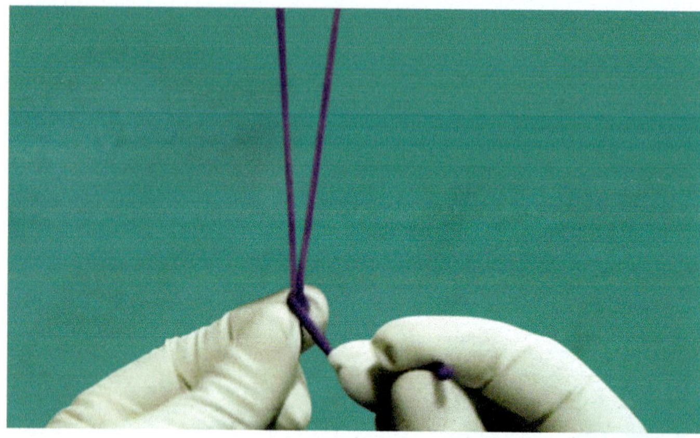

Fig. 13: Third wind is made.

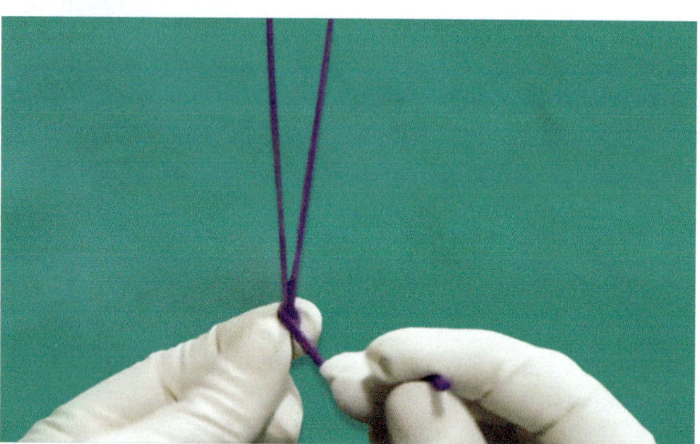

Fig. 11: First wind is made.

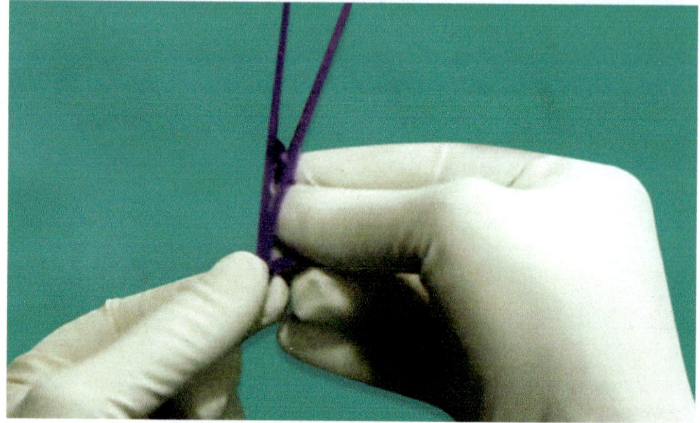

Fig. 14: Short limb is passed in the loop.

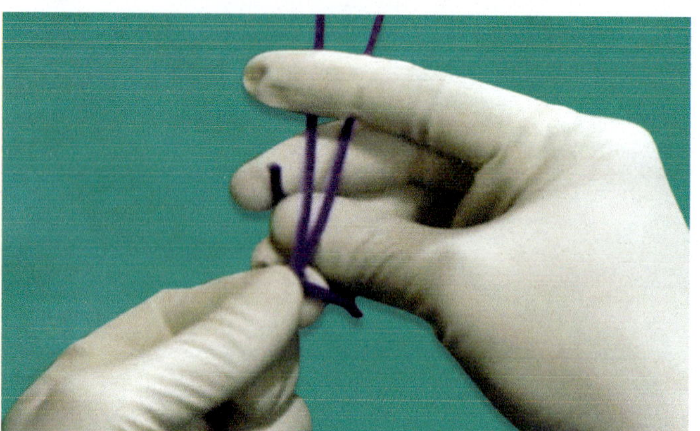

Fig. 12: Second wind is made.

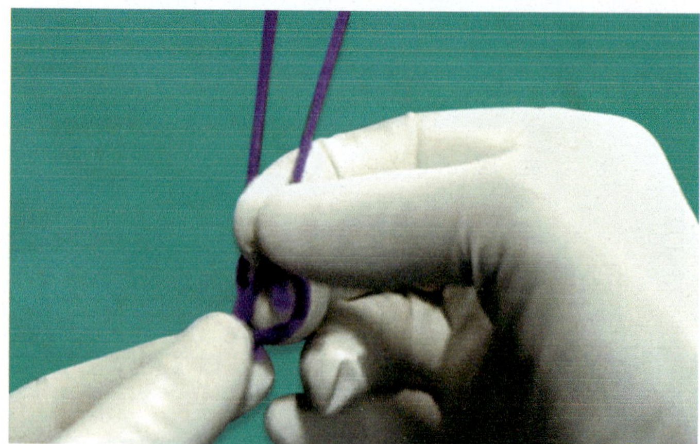

Fig. 15: Half knot is made.

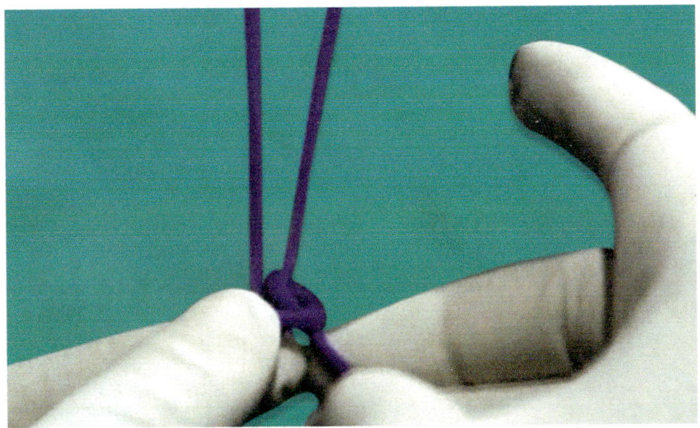

Fig. 16: Half knot is tightened.

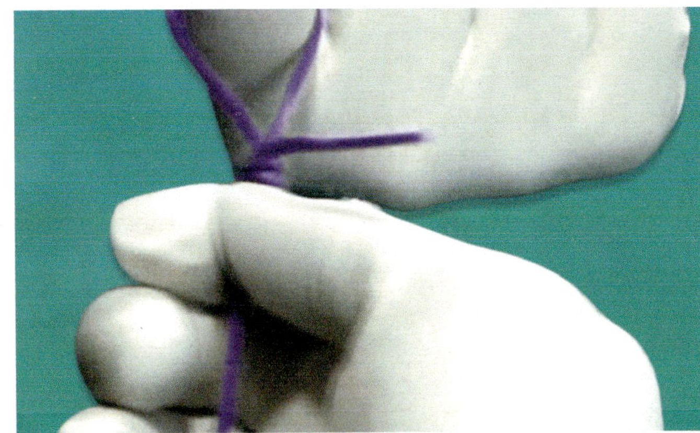

Fig. 17: Sliding action is checked.

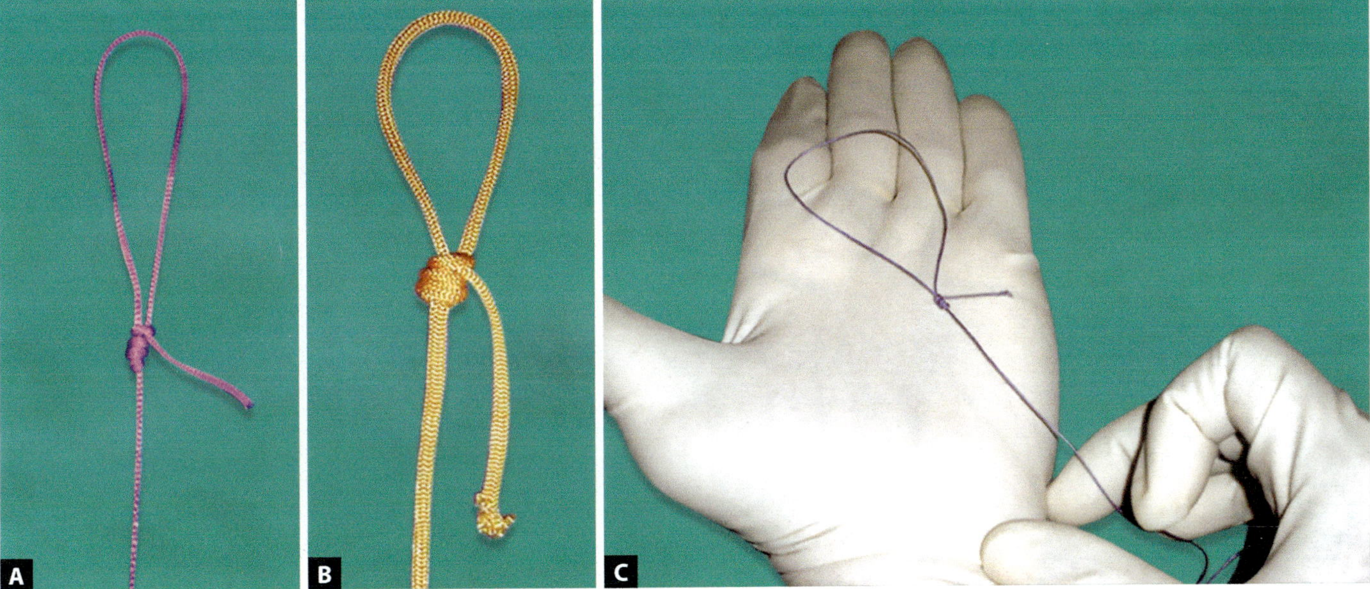

Figs. 18A to C: Roeder's knot is ready.

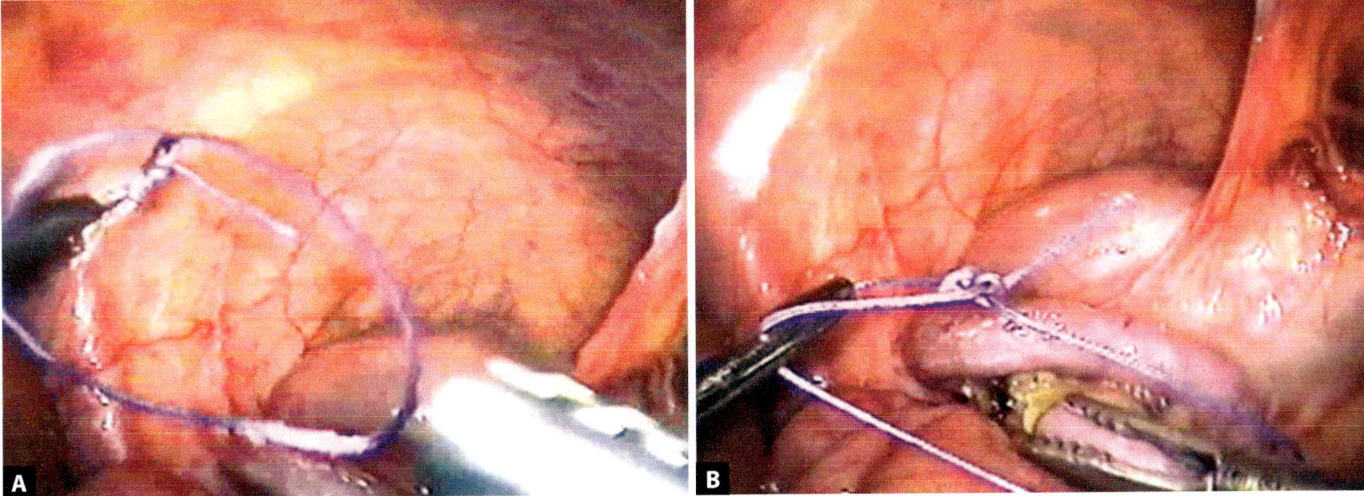

Figs. 19A and B

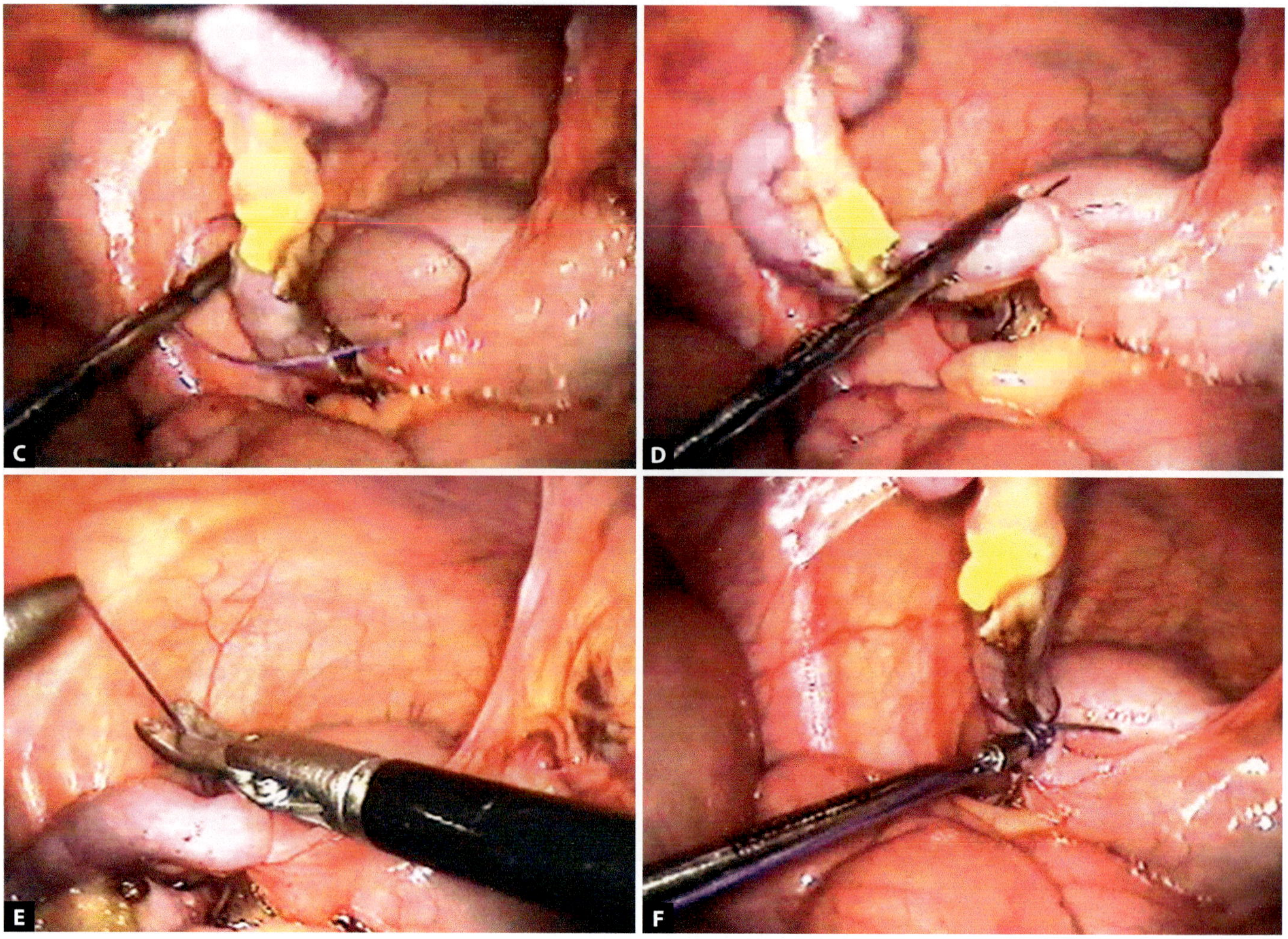

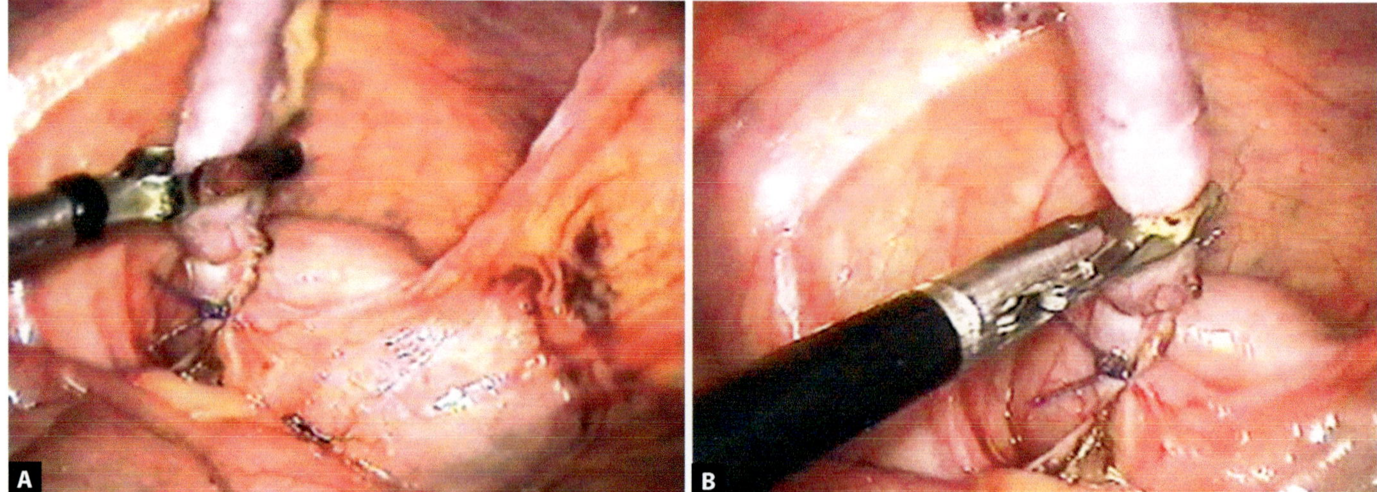

Figs. 19A to F: Tying Roeder's knot over appendix.

Figs. 20A and B: Roeder's knot for appendicectomy.

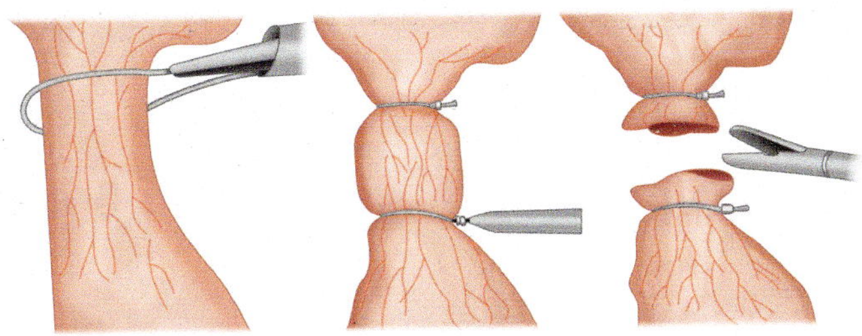

Fig. 21: Extracorporeal knot can be used in case of adhesion with omentum.

CLINICAL APPLICATION

- *Roeder's knot for free structure like appendix (**Figs. 19A to F**):* Two endoloop sutures are passed in sequence through one of the 5 mm ports and pushed around the base of appendix on top of each other at a distance of 3–5 mm. A third endoloop suture can be applied 6 mm distal to the second suture so that surgeon will cut between second and third (**Figs. 20A and B**).
- Roeder's knot for continuous structure like omentum adhered to anterior abdominal wall (**Fig. 21**).

CONCLUSION

Laparoscopic suturing and knotting is a skill that requires a great deal of practice. The Roeder's knot is widely used in laparoscopic surgery for extracorporeal tying. It is one of the first primitive knots used in endoscopic surgery. This knot is also available commercially as a pretied loop. We have revised the method of proper tying step-by-step, which is easy to practice and cost-effective, especially in cost-conscious, developing countries. Properly tied Roeder's knot gives us an ideal stitch which can be used to tie ductal structures and pedicles with correct tension which resists reverse slippage.

Roeder's knot can be remembered as 1:3:1.

BIBLIOGRAPHY

1. Chen MH, Khalil H (Eds). Laparoscopic Suturing Techniques for Surgeons. Oxford: Oxford University Press; 2022.
2. Choi E, Kim DY. The Use of Biodegradable Sutures in Laparoscopic Surgery. J Biomed Mat. 2024;15(3):438-45.
3. Fernandez R, Martin CJ. Ergonomics in Laparoscopic Suturing: Minimizing Surgeon Fatigue. J Ergonomics Surg. 2023;17(3):145-54.
4. Gomez R, Lee T. Evolution of Suturing Techniques in Laparoscopic Surgery. J Minim Invasive Surg. 2021;28(2):123-32.
5. Gupta S, Mehra R. Barriers to Learning Laparoscopic Suturing: A Survey of Surgical Residents. Education Surg. 2023;47(1):55-62.
6. Harper D, Lombardi A. Adapting Traditional Suturing Techniques for Laparoscopic Applications. Surg Techniques Rev. 2021;35(4):320-8.
7. Kumar V, Saxena AK (Eds). Advanced Techniques in Laparoscopic Surgery. Berlin: Springer; 2020.
8. Lavelle JF, Sinclair MF. Automated Suturing Devices in Laparoscopic Surgery: A Comparative Analysis. Technol Surg. 2020;22(6):789-98.
9. Lee J, Kim S. Innovations in Laparoscopic Suturing Instruments. Int J Med Robot. 2022;18(1):e2210.
10. Mendez C, Gupta A (Eds). Laparoscopic Suturing: Mastery Through Technique and Practice. London: Elsevier Health Sciences; 2023.
11. Mishra RK (Ed). Textbook of Laparoscopy for Surgeons and Gynecologists, 4th edition. New Delhi: Jaypee Brothers Medical Publishers (P) Ltd.; 2021. pp. 900.
12. Morrison T, Jacobs LR. Teaching Laparoscopic Suturing: The Role of Simulation in Medical Schools. Med Teacher. 2021;43(7):778-84.
13. Nguyen L, Ho CP. Impact of Suture Materials on Laparoscopic Knot Reliability. Mat Surg. 2024;9(2):200-10.
14. O'Reilly MP, Saunders BH. Virtual Reality Training for Laparoscopic Surgery. Cambridge: Cambridge University Press; 2022.
15. Patel R, Thompson J. The Role of Simulation in Learning Laparoscopic Suturing and Knotting. Med Education Online. 2021;26:1857289.
16. Rodriguez A, Davis SS. Robotic-Assisted Laparoscopic Knot Tying: Methods and Efficiency. Surg Innov. 2019;26(4):459-66.
17. Shimi SM, Lirici MM, Vander Velpen G, Cuschieri A. Comparative study of holding strength of slipknot using absorbable and nonabsorbable ligature materials. Surg Endosc. 1994;11:1285-91.
18. Smith JA, Patel VR (Eds). Principles of Laparoscopic Suturing and Knotting. New York: Springer; 2023.
19. Surgical Knots and Suturing Techniques. (2024). Available from https://en.wikipedia.org/wiki/Surgical_knot.
20. Sharp HT, Dorsey JH, Chovan, PM, Holtz PM. The Effect of Knot Geometry on the Strength of Laparoscopic Slip Knots. Obstet Gynecol. 1996;88(3):408-11.
21. Wang Y, Thompson C. Innovations in Knot Tying Techniques for Minimally Invasive Surgery. Innov Surg. 2022;18(4):250-60.
22. Williams NE, Tan JL. Comparative Study of Knot Security in Laparoscopic Surgery. J Surg Res. 2022;245:217-23.
23. Zimmerman KA, Patel ND. Laparoscopic Knotting: A Visual Guide for Surgeons. Philadelphia: Lippincott Williams & Wilkins; 2022.

Meltzer's knot

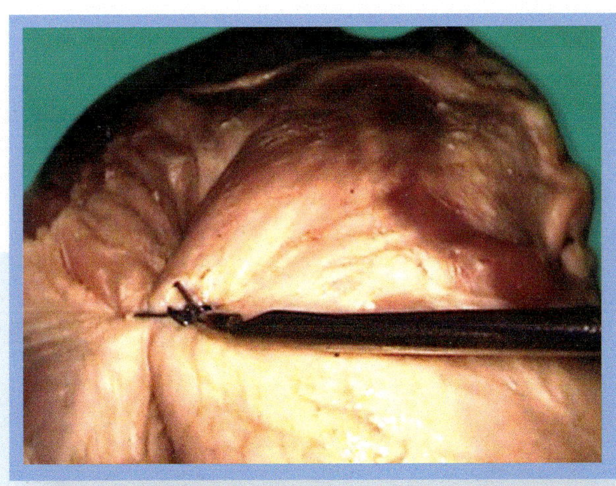

■ INTRODUCTION

Today, endoscopic surgery is rapidly becoming a popular alternative to traditional procedures for a variety of diseases. Most of the endoscopic procedures may require the utilization of laparoscopic suturing at one point or the other. Laparoscopic suturing aids the surgeon in approximating tissues and control of hemostasis. Endoscopic suturing is technically challenging and is a major source of discouragement for many aspiring endoscopic surgeons and even the young endoscopic surgeons. However, it is a popular saying in endoscopic surgery that there is no future without suture. The ability to suture laparoscopically opens the door to perform more complex surgical procedures. The implication is that many operations that have traditionally been performed at laparotomy may now be accomplished laparoscopically.

In the works of Champion et al. and Nduka CC et al., the importance of laparoscopic suturing and the need for the aspiring endoscopic surgeons to appropriately learn the art could not have been more succinctly discussed.

Meltzer's knot is a type of extracorporeal knot which was first described by Meltzer, a prominent endoscopic surgeon in 1991 Tubingen, Germany. It is basically a modification of Roeder's knot; hence, many authorities also refer to Meltzer's knot as a modified Roeder's knot. Meltzer's knot is much stronger than the original Roeder's knot. Meltzer recommended use of polydioxanone suture (PDS) for tying the Meltzer's knot because of the ease with which the knot can be slipped into the body cavity because holding and tensile characteristics of the extracorporeal slip knots depend on the type of ligature material used and the type of knot applied.

In terms of its application and usefulness in extracorporeal suturing, Meltzer's knot has superseded Roeder's knot because it is much stronger than the original Roeder's knot. Meltzer's knot basically has three components:
1. Two hitches
2. Three winds
3. Two half locking hitches. It can be also described as:
   a. Double initial half knot
   b. Three and a half round turns over the limbs of the loop
   c. Double second half knot
   d. Careful stacking of turns between the knots
   e. Sliding in position by push rod

This can readily be remembered by the mnemonic 2:3:2 (compared with 1:3:1 of Roeder's knot). Various techniques and steps of making the Meltzer's knot (and other modifications) and other extracorporeal knots have been described at various points in time. However, the choice will depend on the skill of the surgeon and the clinical situation at hand.

■ APPLICATION OF MELTZER'S KNOT

Presently, Meltzer's knot is used by many surgeons to tie free structures, especially within the abdominal cavity. For example, Meltzer's knot is quite popular for ligating the base of the vermiform appendix after the mesoappendix has been excised. Meltzer's knot is also very useful in tying the medial end of the cystic duct during cholecystectomy and to fix the cystic duct drainage cannula after transcystic clearance of ductal stones. The Meltzer's knot is also useful in tying vascular pedicles as it can be pushed down unto a pedicle, for example, for suturing uterine artery pedicle and large infundibulopelvic ligament. It can also be used with great advantage for reconstructing the uterus after myomectomy and for colposuspension. In general, extracorporeal knots are preferred during ligature in continuity of large vessels, suturing in areas of limited access where the working space is restricted and in the approximation of edges of defects, where the force required to approximate the edges is substantial.

■ ADVANTAGES OF MELTZER'S KNOT

- Meltzer's knot gives a much secured knot and thus reduces the chances of risks of slipped ligature compared to Roeder's knot.
- In good hands, it reduces the overall operation time because it obviates the need for complex maneuvers of intracorporeal knots and yet it offers a very stable knot.
- Meltzer's knot can be used with confidence even with slippery material such PDS; because of more hitches, it is more secure.

■ DISADVANTAGES OF MELTZER'S KNOT

- Meltzer's knot has more hitches and half knots and overload large amount of suture that is pushed through the needle tract.
- Suture can get fractured by some knot pushers.
- It may cause low-volume air leak as the suture passes through the trocar.

- The knot pusher may become dislodged from the suture during transit into the abdominal cavity.
- There has to be a wide range of sutures as some sutures do not slide well.
- It requires close cooperation between the surgeon and assistance and this may lead to a tedious and more time-consuming surgery.
- It is difficult to loosen if the surgeon wants to modify the tension on a ligated tissue.

■ STEPS OF MELTZER'S KNOT

Method of Making Extracorporeal Meltzer's Pretied Loop for Free Structure Like Appendix

Figures 1 to 10 deal with the abovementioned method as follows.

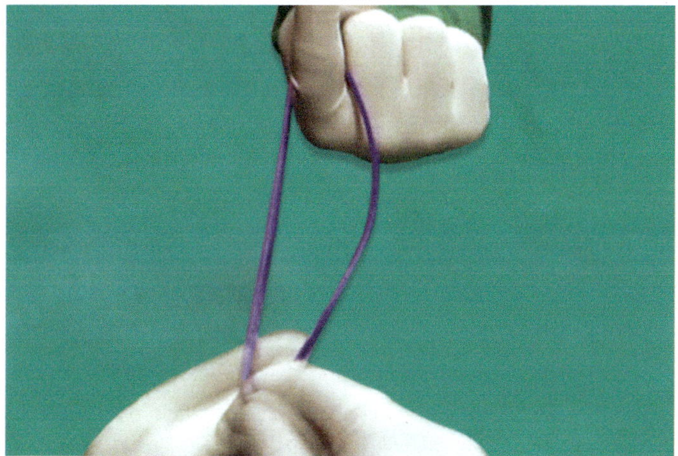

Fig. 1: The shorter limb on the right hand over the longer limb on the left hand of the surgeon.

Method of Making Extracorporeal Meltzer's Knot for Continuous Structure

Intra-abdominal Component of Extracorporeal Meltzer's Knot

See **Figures 11 to 18**.

■ CLINICAL APPLICATION

Appendicectomy by Meltzer's knot are described through **Figures 19 and 20**.

TASK ANALYSIS OF EXTRACORPOREAL KNOT FOR CONTINUOUS STRUCTURE

- The length of suture for extracorporeal knot in continuous structures is 90 cm.
- Before commencing the extracorporeal knot for continuous structures, create a surgical window by dissecting the tissue plane at the desired ligation site.
- Secure one end of the 90 cm suture with the Maryland instrument. Feed and conceal one third of the Maryland and suture within the 5 mm reducer. Then, introduce both the Maryland and suture simultaneously through a 10 mm port.
- Introduce an atraumatic grasper through another 5 mm port.
- Guide the suture through the surgical window and have it grasped by the atraumatic grasper.
- The camera operator plays a pivotal role here. Ensure the light cable is directed to the right and illuminates the target area, showcasing the tip of the Maryland instrument to the surgeon.

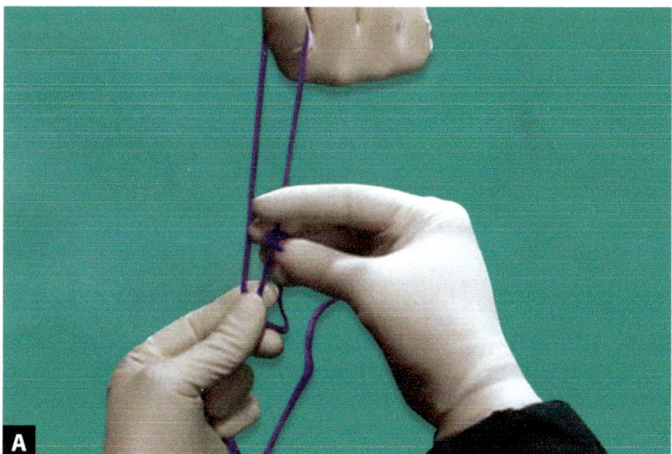
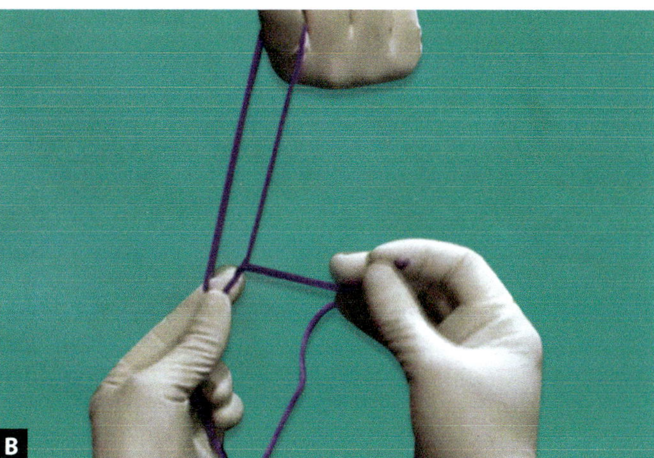

Figs. 2A and B: The first hitch is being taken on long-standing thread by passing the tail end between the two limbs from below upward.

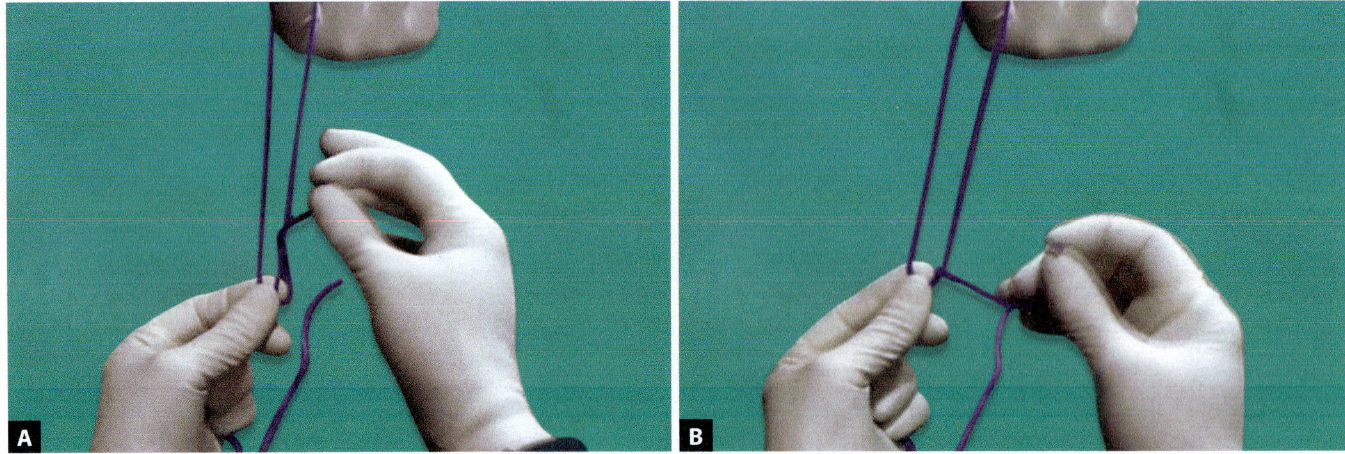

Figs. 3A and B: The second hitch being taken by passing the tail under the right limb and pulling the tail to the right.

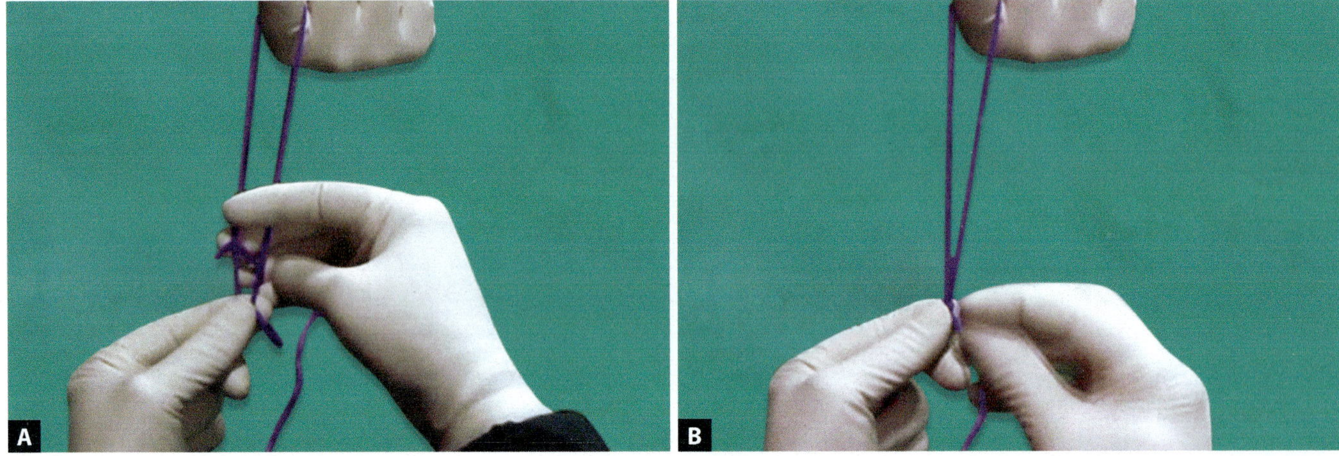

Figs. 4A and B: The first wrap is being taken by passing the tail end beneath both the limbs and the first wrap is being accomplished by turning around both limbs and completed by pulling the tail snug fit.

- Transfer the suture from the grasper back to the Maryland instrument.
- Feed the suture inside the abdominal cavity at least four times using the atraumatic grasper, bringing in a total of 20 cm of suture length inside the abdomen.
- Throughout the suture-feeding process, the camera operator should focus the telescope on the tip of the cannula.
- With each feeding, pull a minimum of 5 cm of suture inside.
- Once the suture feeding is complete, reposition the grasper between the suture loop and tissue.
- Use the Maryland instrument to guide the suture out, keeping the grasper in place between the loop and the tissue.

- While extracting the suture, ensure that the grasper remains steady between the suture to prevent tissue damage due to shearing.
- After the tail end of the suture is outside the reducer, instruct the assistant to place their finger on the washer of the reducer, between the two suture ends, to prevent gas leakage.
- Proceed to tie the extracorporeal knot and the assistant's finger should continue to cover the reducer to prevent gas leakage.
- You have the option to use any of the extracorporeal slip knots (Roader's, Meltzer's, or Mishra's knot) based on the diameter of the structure and the quality of your suture material.

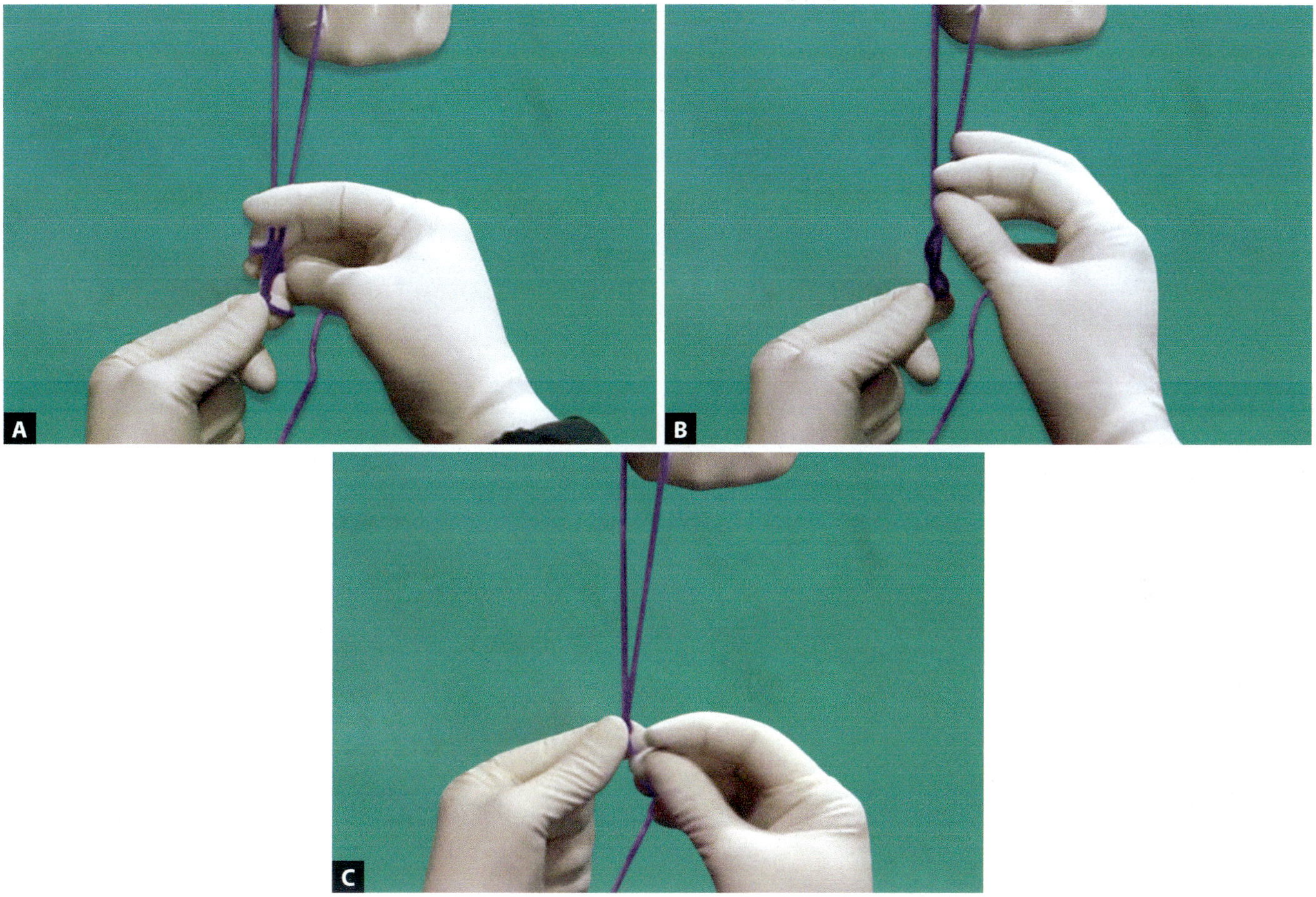

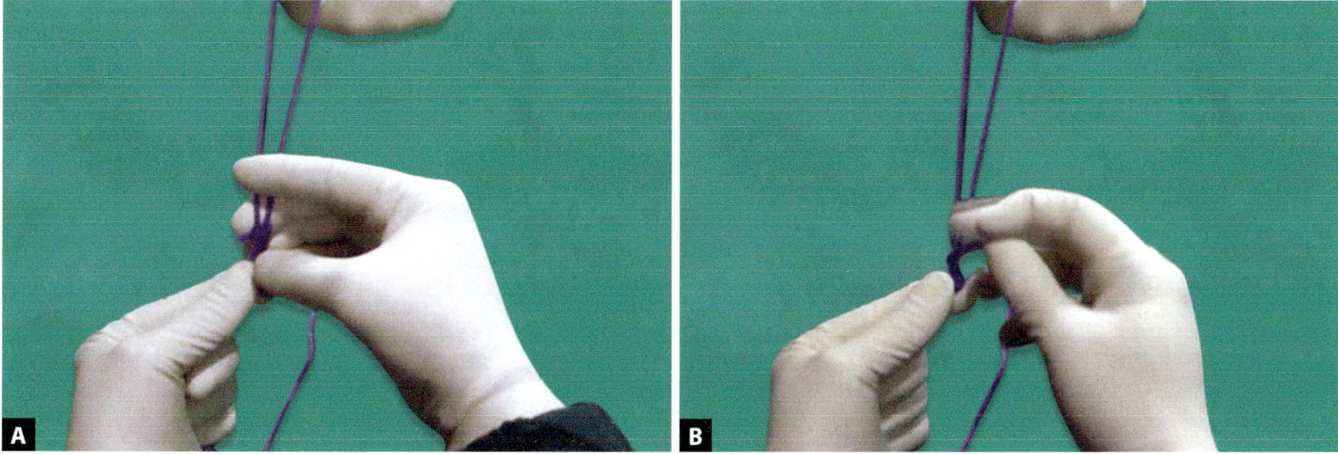

Figs. 5A to C: The second wrap is begun by passing the tail end beneath both limbs, turning around both limbs and then completed by pulling the tail end.

Figs. 6A and B: The third wrap begun by passing the tail end beneath both limbs, turning the tail end around both limbs and then completed by pulling the tail end.

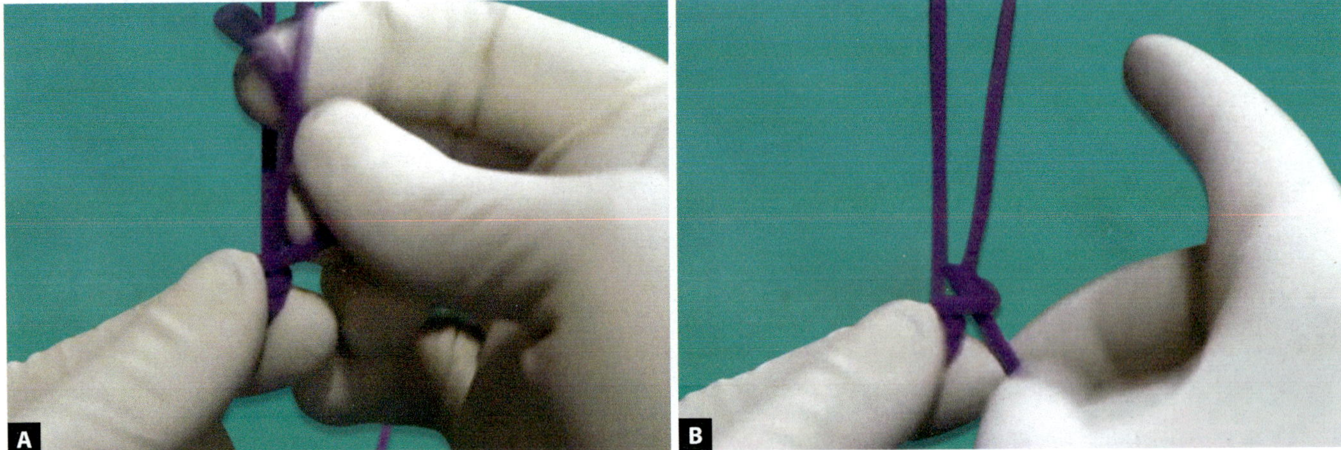

Figs. 7A and B: The first locking half knot is begun by passing the tail beneath the right limb and then passing the tail in a loop formed by the tail against the long limb and it is the then completed by pulling the tail to snugly fit the knot.

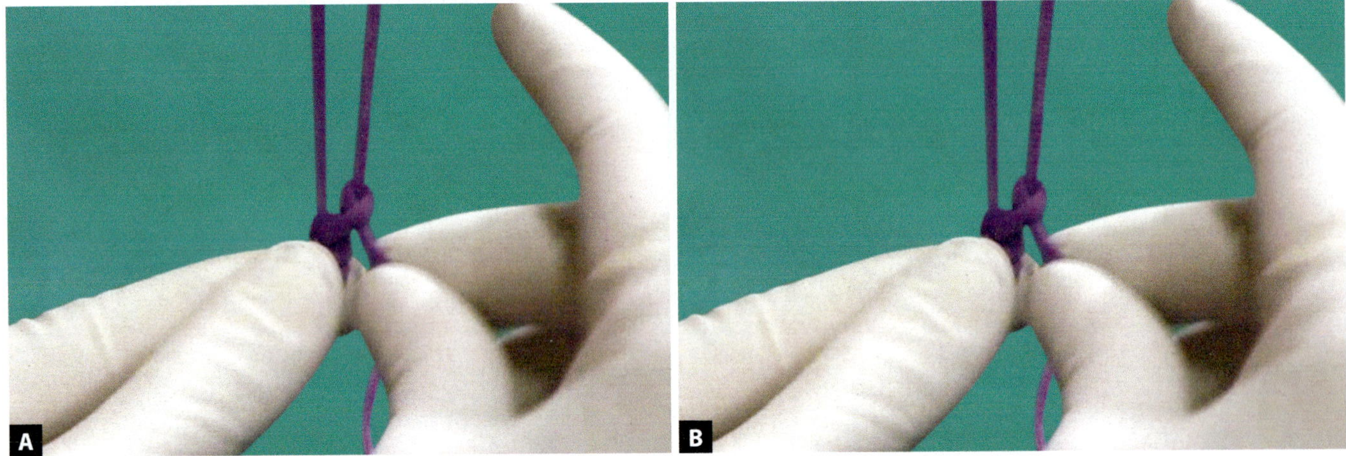

Figs. 8A and B: The second locking half knot is begun by passing the tail beneath the long limb and then passing the tail through the loop formed by the tail against the long limb and then finally completed by pulling the tail to snuggly fit the knot.

- Feed the suture from the head end of the Bhandarkar knot pusher and pull it out from the tail end of the knot pusher.
- Reverse feed the knot pusher into the 3 mm reducer.
- Introduce the knot pusher and reducer into the 5 mm reducer, having the assistant remove their finger from the reducer. Push the knot pusher into the abdomen under visual guidance.
- Push the knot pusher while pulling the suture to shorten the loop.
- Position the tip of the knot pusher where you intend to tie the knot.
- The knot will naturally slide to the desired location where you want to tie it, aligning with the tip of the knot pusher.

- The pushing of the knot pusher and pulling of the suture should be done delicately to ensure the structure remains unaware of the ligation process.
- After tightening the knot three times consecutively, retract the knot pusher and 3 mm reducer. Introduce hook scissors from the same port and cut the suture, leaving a 1 cm tail.
- Extracorporeal knots are robust, and one knot is adequate for securing continuous structures such as the cystic duct, cystic artery, renal artery, and splenic artery.

■ DISCUSSION

The significance of extracorporeal knots, particularly Meltzer's knot, cannot be overstated. Many complications

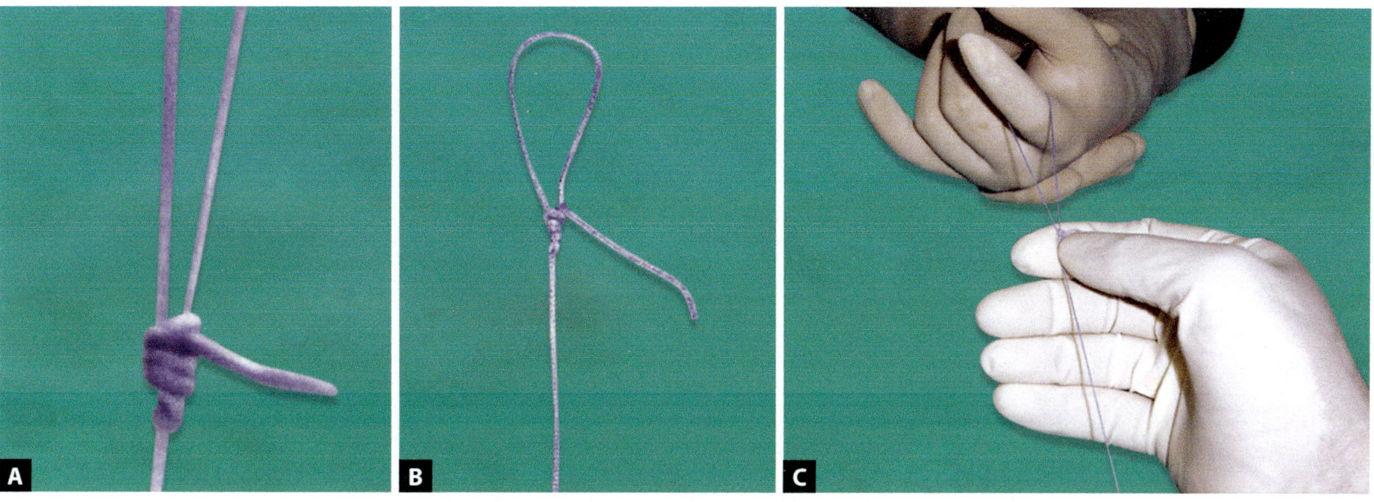

Figs. 9A to C: Pretied loop of Meltzer's knot.

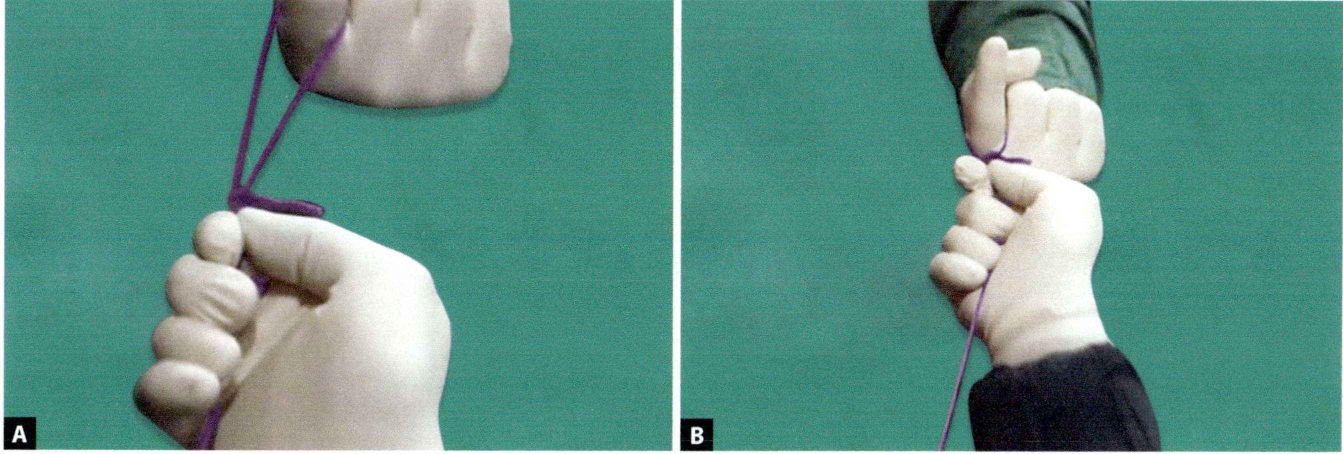

Figs. 10A and B: The completed Meltzer's knot is being slipped gently toward the desired point with the help of knot pusher until the knot gets to the point.

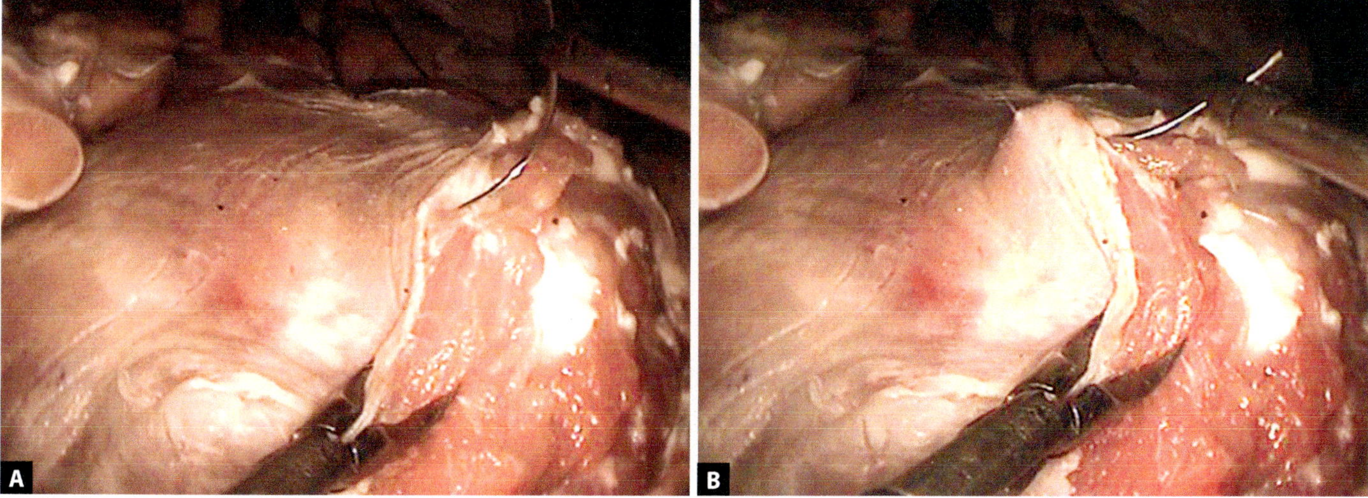

Figs. 11A and B: Passing a suture with a needle through the tissue in order to prepare an extracorporeal Meltzer's knot with needle.

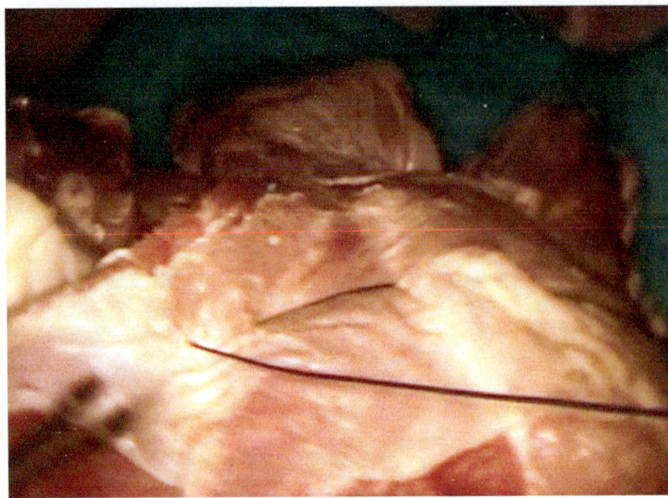

Fig. 12: The suture is being pulled outside the body through cannula in order to prepare the Meltzer's knot.

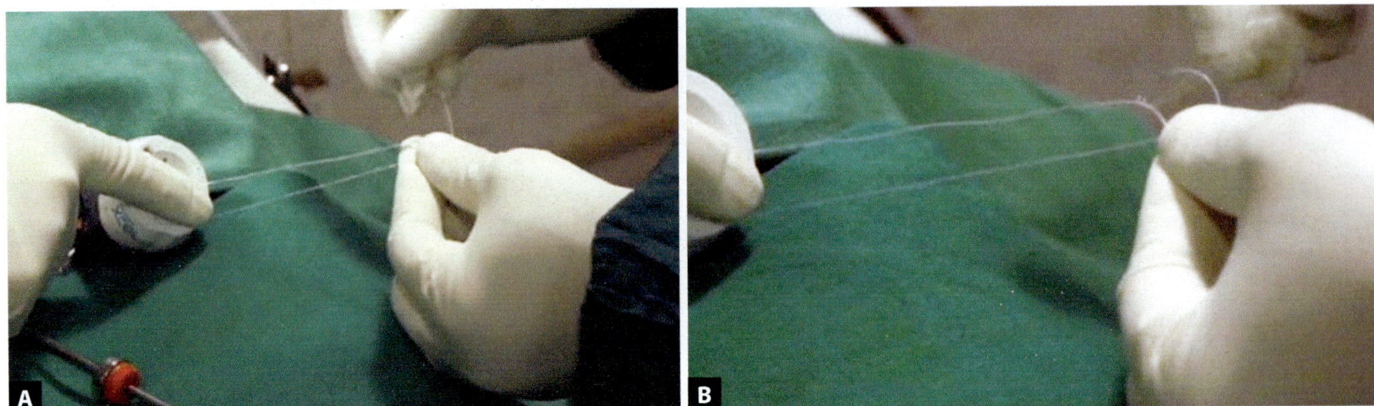

Figs. 13A and B: The assistant finger should be kept in between the thread in such a way the gas should not leak and it should help the surgeon to make the knot and the Meltzer's knot is tied same way as pretied loop.

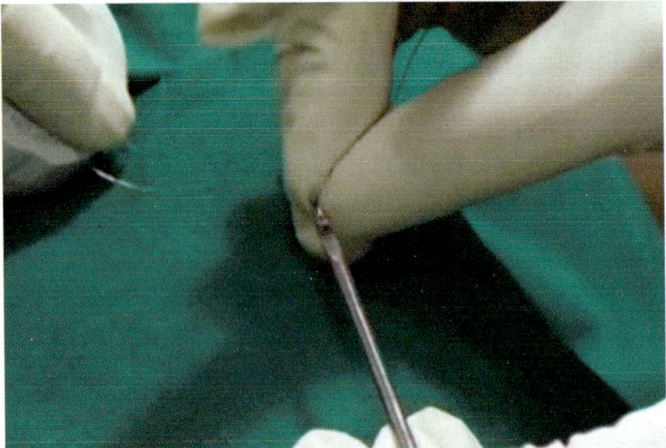

Fig. 14: Once the Meltzer's knot is ready, the standing end of the suture is reverse loaded over knot pusher.

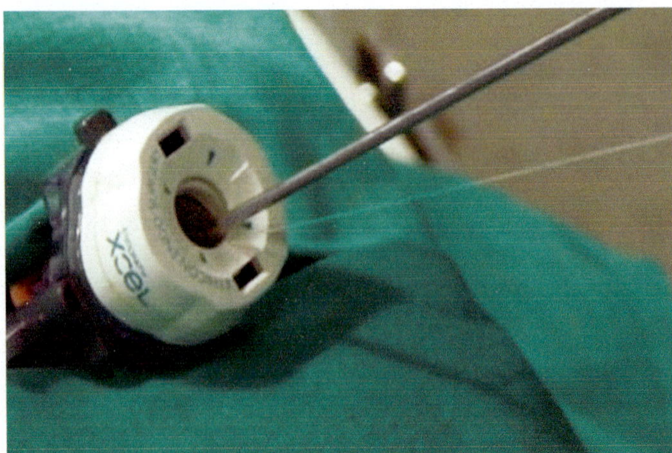

Fig. 15: The knot is pushed inside the abdominal cavity with the help of knot pusher.

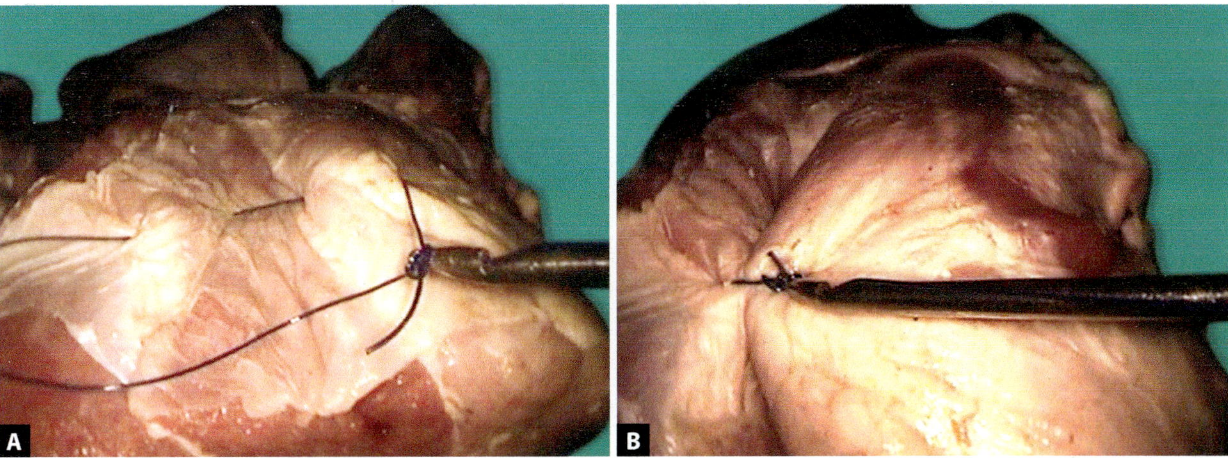

Figs. 16A and B: The suture is being pushed in with the aid of the knot pusher until the knot is applied to the point desired to be sutured or ligated.

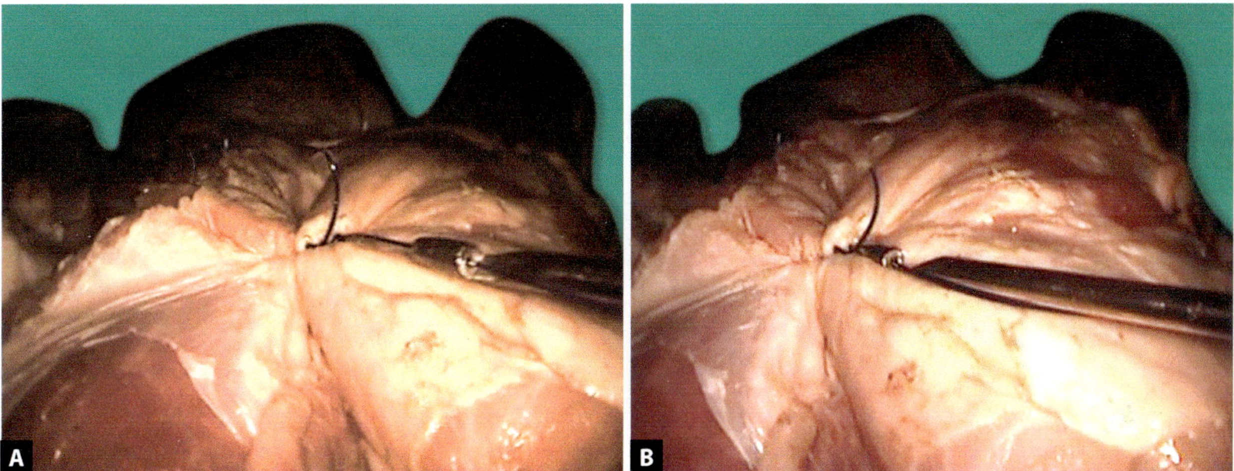

Figs. 17A and B: The knot pusher is being withdrawn slightly and pushed down again in order to tighten the knot. This process is repeated about three to four times until the knot is snugged with the tissue.

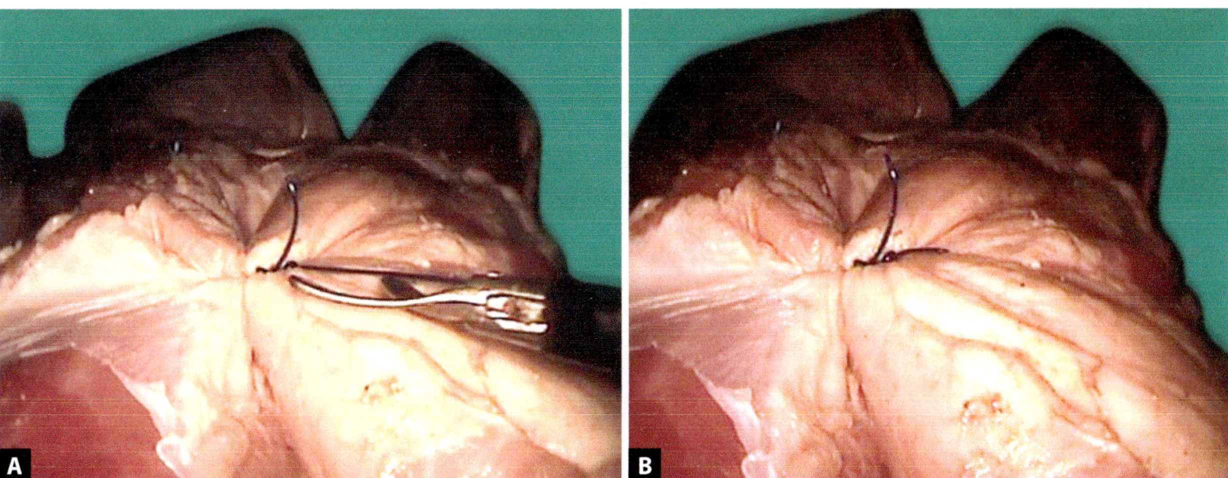

Figs. 18A and B: The scissors is introduced from the same port and suture is cut leaving 1-cm long suture.

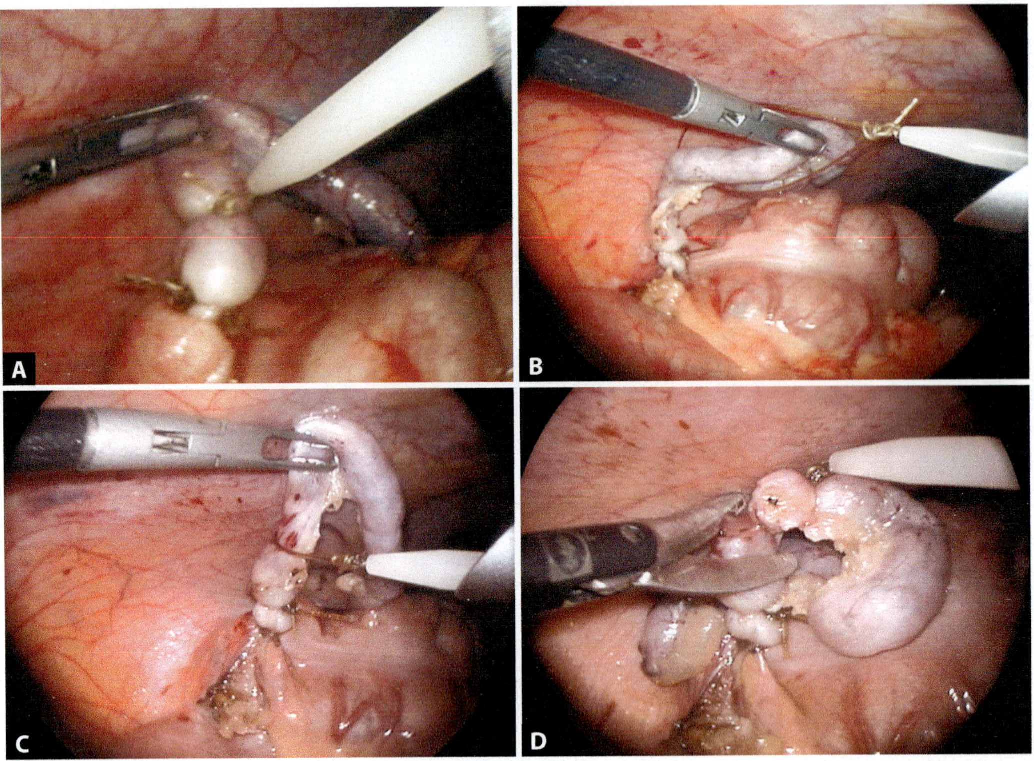

Figs. 19A to D: Pretied loop of Meltzer's knots used for appendicectomy.

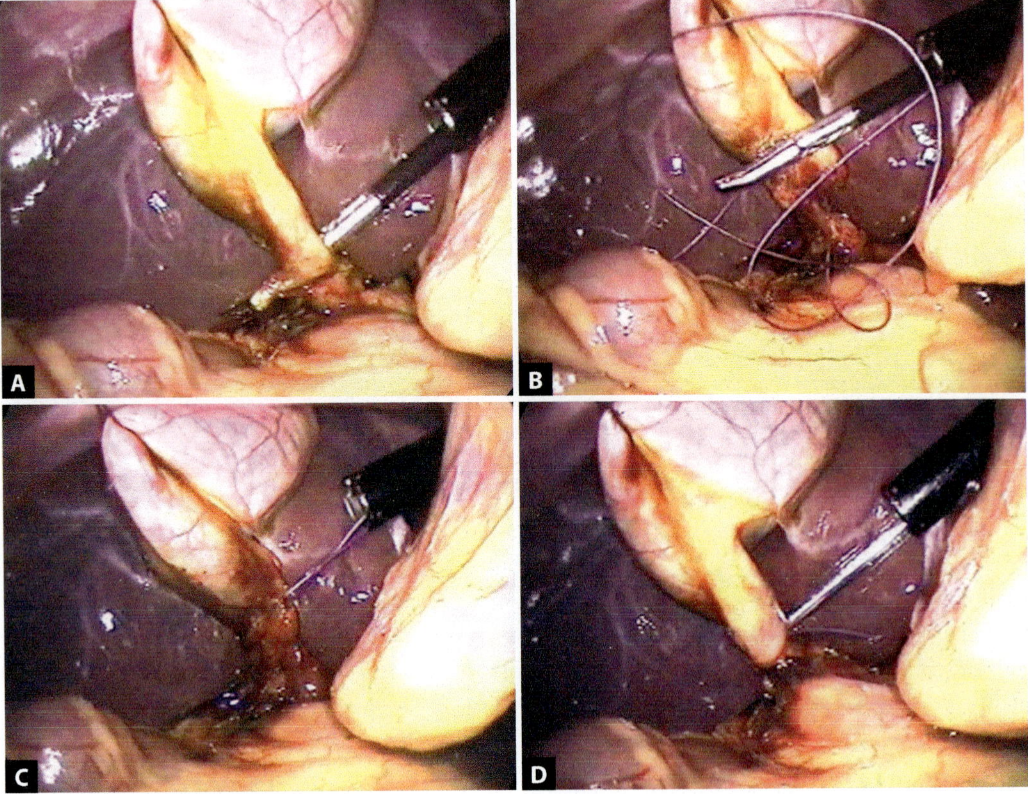

Figs. 20A to D: Extracorporeal Meltzer's knot for continuous structure applied over cystic duct.

in laparoscopic surgery are often linked to inadequate suturing techniques during endoscopic procedures. The adoption of Meltzer's knot has played a vital role in reducing the occurrence of ligature slippage and other associated complications. Meltzer's knot is now generally preferred over the Roeder's knot due to its increased number of wraps and initial and locking hitches. Compared to Roeder's knot, Meltzer's knot offers a more secure tie.

Meltzer's knot, being an extracorporeal knot, is pushed onto the pedicle using a knot pusher, while the remaining suture end is used for countertraction. This method allows the knot to slide down smoothly, reducing the loop around the pedicle as the knot is tightened. During the final tightening phase, the tip of the knot pusher, along with the knot, should be in direct contact with the tissue, while traction is applied to the remaining suture end. These characteristics make Meltzer's knot particularly well-suited for monofilament sutures such as PDS, nylon, or monocryl as they minimize complications such as knot locking.

However, when using braided sutures such as vicryl, this knot may not slide easily and there is a risk of premature knot locking. Additionally, because the slipknot involves the suture passing through the tissue as the knot is pushed toward the pedicle, there is a greater "sawing" effect on the tissue, making premature locking more likely with multifilament sutures compared to monofilament ones.

Meltzer's knot is a highly robust sliding knot that can be mastered with practice. One of its primary advantages is that it requires only one passage of the knot pusher, minimizing issues with potential loss of pneumoperitoneum (the gas used to create a working space during laparoscopic surgery).

Because it can be pushed onto a pedicle, Meltzer's knot is suitable for tying vascular pedicles, making it the preferred choice for securing uterine artery pedicles and large infundibulopelvic ligaments. It is also valuable for reconstituting the uterus after myomectomy. However, due to its strength, it can be challenging to loosen if tension modification is necessary, as in colposuspension.

Given the security of Meltzer's knot, it finds relevance in various procedures such as appendicectomy, cholecystectomy, splenectomy, etc. Therefore, aspiring laparoscopic surgeons should receive thorough training in laparoscopic suturing techniques. The use of extracorporeal knots offers numerous advantages over intracorporeal techniques. Training programs should emphasize extracorporeal suturing techniques early in laparoscopic surgical training, allowing surgeons to develop this skill over time. Various objective assessment programs can help surgeons gauge their proficiency in endoscopic suturing techniques. Institutions should also have regular evaluation and appraisal programs to enhance the performance of laparoscopic surgeons.

■ RECOMMENDATIONS

- Implement an objective structured training program to train and assess laparoscopic surgeons, ensuring they meet specific criteria for laparoscopic suturing techniques before performing complex procedures.
- Establish programs for continuous training and retraining of laparoscopic surgeons to enhance their skills.
- Emphasize the use of endotrainers for skill development.
- Encourage participation in workshops, conferences, and seminars to learn new suturing techniques and improve practice.
- Younger surgeons should seek opportunities for attachments and postings with senior colleagues and regularly update their libraries with modern books on laparoscopic surgery.

■ CONCLUSION

The skilled laparoscopic surgeon should be proficient in laparoscopic suturing and knotting, as it is crucial for performing advanced, complex procedures with precision and safety while minimizing complications. Proficiency in endosuturing provides confidence in reconstructing vital organs, repairing inadvertent injuries, or controlling bleeding when other methods are not suitable. Therefore, it is essential for laparoscopic surgeons to receive adequate training in the art of laparoscopic suturing techniques, including Meltzer's extracorporeal knot. This will significantly enhance the overall performance of laparoscopic surgeons and contribute to the reduction of morbidity and mortality associated with laparoscopic surgery.

■ BIBLIOGRAPHY

1. Al Falloiji M. Making loops in laparoscopic surgery state of the art. Surg Laparosc Endosc. 1993;3:477-81.
2. Bhatia P, John SJ, Deed JPS (Eds). Step by Step Art of Endosuturing. New Delhi: Jaypee Brothers Medical Publishers (P) Ltd.; 2007. pp. 109-40.
3. Champion JK, Hunter J, Trus T, Laycock W. Teaching basic video skills as an aid in laparoscopic suturing. Surg Endosc. 1996;10:23-35.
4. Chen MH, Khalil H (Eds). Laparoscopic Suturing Techniques for Surgeons. Oxford: Oxford University Press; 2022.

5. Choi E, Kim DY. The Use of Biodegradable Sutures in Laparoscopic Surgery. J Biomed Mat. 2024;15(3):438-45.

6. Chou D, Elkington N, Shukla-Kulkarni A, Hashim E. Sliding knots. In: Jain N (Ed). State of the Art Atlas and Textbook of Laparoscopic Suturing. New Delhi: Jaypee Brothers Medical Publishers (P) Ltd.; 2006. pp. 45-53.

7. Chua HB. A tripod device for an extracorporeal slip knot (Roeder's knot). J R Coll Surg Edin. 1997;42:403-6.

8. Dunsmore RC. Laparoscopic intracorporeal square-to-slip knot. J Am Coll Surg. 1995;180:689-99.

9. Fernandez R, Martin CJ. Ergonomics in Laparoscopic Suturing: Minimizing Surgeon Fatigue. J Ergonomics Surg. 2023;17(3):145-54.

10. Gomez R, Lee T. Evolution of Suturing Techniques in Laparoscopic Surgery. J Minim Invasive Sur. 2021;28(2):123-32.

11. Gupta S, Mehra R. Barriers to Learning Laparoscopic Suturing: A Survey of Surgical Residents. Education Surg. 2023;47(1):55-62.

12. Harper D, Lombardi A. Adapting Traditional Suturing Techniques for Laparoscopic Applications. Surg Techniques Rev. 2021;35(4):320-8.

13. Karabacak RO, Shabgahi B, Biberoglu KO. A new practical knot technique for use in laparoscopic endoscopy. Endoscopy. 1992;24:805-8.

14. Kumar V, Saxena AK (Eds). Advanced Techniques in Laparoscopic Surgery. Berlin: Springer; 2020.

15. Lavelle JF, Sinclair MF. Automated Suturing Devices in Laparoscopic Surgery: A Comparative Analysis. Technol Surg. 2020;22(6):789-98.

16. Lee J, Kim S. Innovations in Laparoscopic Suturing Instruments. Int J Med Robot. 2022;18(1):e2210.

17. Luks FI, Deprest J, Brosens I, Lerut T. Extracorporeal surgical knot. J Am Coll Surg. 1994;179(2):220-2.

18. Meltzer A, Schurr MO, Lirici MM, Klemm B, Stockel D, Buess G. Future trends in endoscopic surgery. Endosc Surg Allied Technol. 1994;2:76-82.

19. Mendez C, Gupta A. Laparoscopic Suturing: Mastery Through Technique and Practice. London: Elsevier Health Sciences; 2023.

20. Mishra RK (Ed). Textbook of Practical Laparoscopic Surgery. New Delhi: Jaypee Brothers Medical Publishers (P) Ltd.; 2008.

21. Mishra RK (Ed). Two Port Technique for Laparoscopic Cholecystectomy. India: The Hindu, Online edition of India's National Newspaper; 2006.

22. Mishra RK, (2007). Textbook of Practical Laparoscopic Surgery. Jaypee Brothers Medical Publishers, New Delhi, pp. 104-23.

23. Morrison T, Jacobs LR. Teaching Laparoscopic Suturing: The Role of Simulation in Medical Schools. Med Teacher. 2021;43(7):778-84.

24. Mishra RK (Ed). Textbook of Laparoscopy for Surgeons and Gynecologists, 4th edition. New Delhi: Jaypee Brothers Medical Publishers (P) Ltd.; 2021. pp. 900.

25. Nathanson LK. Laparoscopic appendicectomy. Hosp Update. 1992;18:580-5.

26. Nduka CC, Darzi A. Teaching laparoscopic surgery: Training courses are popular and valuable (letter). Br Med J. 1994;308:1435.

27. Nguyen L, Ho CP. Impact of Suture Materials on Laparoscopic Knot Reliability. Mat Surg. 2024;9(2): 200-10.

28. Novira Y, Horchani A. The pre-looped intracorporeal knot: a new technique for knot tying in laparoscopic surgery. J Urol. 2001;166;195-7.

29. O'Reilly MP, Saunders BH. Virtual Reality Training for Laparoscopic Surgery. Cambridge: Cambridge University Press; 2022.

30. Palanivelu C (Ed). Textbook of Surgical Laparoscopy. New Delhi: Jaypee Brothers Medical Publishers (P) Ltd.; 2002.

31. Palanivelu C (Ed). The Art of Laparoscopic Surgery. New Delhi: Jaypee Brothers Medical Publishers (P) Ltd.; 2007.

32. Patel R, Thompson J. The Role of Simulation in Learning Laparoscopic Suturing and Knotting. Med Education Online. 2021;26:1857289.

33. Rodriguez A, Davis SS. Robotic-Assisted Laparoscopic Knot Tying: Methods and Efficiency. Surg Innov. 2019;26(4):459-66.

34. Sharp HT, Dorsey JH, Chovan JD, Holtz PM. A simple modification to add strength to the Roeder knot. J Am Asssoc Gynecol Laparosc. 1996;3:305-7.

35. Sharp HT, Dorsey JH, Chovan JD, Holtz PM. The effect of knot geometry on the strength of laparoscopic slip knots. Obstet Gynecol. 1996;88:408-11.

36. Shimi SM, Lirici MM, Vander Velpen G, Cuschieri A. Comparative study of holding strength of slipknot using absorbable and nonabsorbable ligature materials. Surg Endosc. 1994;11:1285-91.

37. Smith JA, Patel VR (Eds). Principles of Laparoscopic Suturing and Knotting. New York: Springer; 2023.

38. Soper NJ, Hunter JG. Suturing and knot tying in laparoscopic surgery. Surg Clin N Am. 1992;72:1139-52.

39. Surgical Knots and Suturing Techniques. (2024). Available from https://en.wikipedia.org/wiki/Surgical_knot.

40. Trimbos JB, Van Aissel EJC, Klooper PJ. Performance of sliding knots in monofilament and multifilament suture materials. Obstet Gynecol. 1986;68:425-30.

41. Trimbos JB. Security of various knots commonly used in surgical practice. Obstet Gynecol. 1984;64:274-80.

42. Wang Y, Thompson C. Innovations in Knot Tying Techniques for Minimally Invasive Surgery. Innov Surg. 2022;18(4): 250-60.

43. Williams NE, Tan JL. Comparative Study of Knot Security in Laparoscopic Surgery. J Surg Res. 2020;245:217-23.

44. Zimmerman KA, Patel ND. Laparoscopic Knotting: A Visual Guide for Surgeons. Philadelphia: Lippincott Williams & Wilkins; 2022.

Mishra's Knot

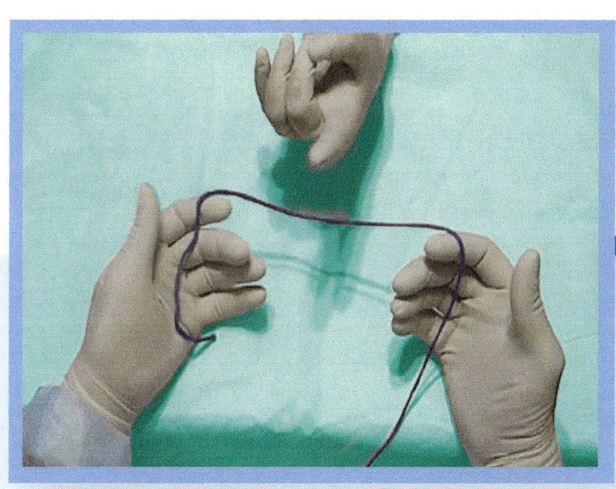

INTRODUCTION

The demand for laparoscopic surgery continues to grow due to its many benefits for patients. However, success in this field is inextricably linked to exceptional suturing skills. Surgeons must navigate the unique challenges of laparoscopic suturing to ensure optimal patient outcomes, reduced complications, and increased efficiency in the operating room. Investing in the development and mastery of suturing skills is not just a requirement but a commitment to excellence in laparoscopic surgery, ultimately benefiting both surgeons and their patients.

CHALLENGES OF SUTURING IN LAPAROSCOPY

Performing sutures in laparoscopic surgery presents unique challenges:

- *Limited space:* The confined space within the abdomen or pelvis can make suturing intricate and challenging. Surgeons must adapt to working in this restricted environment.
- *Instrument dexterity:* Laparoscopic instruments have limited degrees of freedom compared to a surgeon's hand. Precise movements and manipulation are required to perform sutures effectively.
- *Knot tying:* Tying knots in laparoscopy can be more challenging than in open surgery. Surgeons must master intracorporeal knot-tying techniques to ensure secure closures.

IMPACT OF GOOD SUTURING SKILLS

- *Enhanced patient outcomes:* Accurate suturing leads to fewer postoperative complications, reduced pain, and faster recovery times for patients. A well-sutured incision site minimizes the risk of infection and herniation.
- *Reduced operating time:* Surgeons with advanced suturing skills can complete procedures more efficiently, reducing the overall duration of surgery. This can be crucial for both patient's safety and surgeon's comfort.
- *Versatility:* Proficient suturing skills allow surgeons to tackle a broader range of laparoscopic procedures, increasing their versatility and the scope of their practice.
- *Minimized conversion rate:* Good suturing skills can prevent the need for conversion to open surgery due to complications arising from inadequate suturing, saving both time and resources.

MISHRA'S KNOT

In the world of laparoscopic surgery, where precision and safety are paramount, every technique and tool plays a vital role. Among these, Mishra's knot stands out as a silent hero, revolutionizing the way surgeons secure sutures in minimally invasive procedures. Developed by the innovative Dr RK Mishra, this knot has become a cornerstone in laparoscopic surgery, offering enhanced security, flexibility, and versatility.

GENESIS OF MISHRA'S KNOT

Dr RK Mishra, a pioneer in the field of laparoscopic surgery, recognized the need for a secure and efficient knot that could be seamlessly incorporated into minimally invasive procedures. Thus, Mishra's knot was born, a knot designed to address the unique challenges posed by laparoscopy.

ANATOMY OF MISHRA'S KNOT

Mishra's knot is a seven-throw knot characterized by its exceptional strength and reliability. Its configuration is simple yet highly effective: One hitch, one wind, and one lock are followed by two additional sets of one wind and one lock. This distinctive structure ensures that the knot remains securely tied even in the face of tension and movement.

ROLE OF MISHRA'S KNOT IN LAPAROSCOPIC SURGERY

Mishra's knot plays a crucial role in laparoscopic surgery across various domains:

- *Security in ligations:* Mishra's knot offers unparalleled security in ligating structures within the abdominal cavity. Its unique configuration ensures that it can withstand the dynamic environment of laparoscopy, where movements are precise but can be quite rigorous.
- *Versatility:* One of the key strengths of Mishra's knot is its versatility. It can be employed for ligating structures of varying sizes, from delicate tubular structures to more substantial vessels. This adaptability makes it a go-to choice for laparoscopic surgeons.
- *Reduced risk of slippage:* Mishra's knot's multiple throws and locks significantly reduce the risk of knot slippage, a concern that plagues traditional knots in laparoscopy. This enhances patient safety and minimizes the need for knot adjustments during surgery.

- *Minimized tissue trauma:* The knot's design ensures that it does not create excessive trauma to the surrounding tissues during tightening, reducing the risk of tissue damage, bleeding, and postoperative complications.
- *Time efficiency:* Mishra's knot is quick to tie, saving precious minutes in the operating room. Its simplicity allows for efficient knot placement and ensures that surgery proceeds smoothly.
- *Wide applicability:* Mishra's knot is not limited to specific procedures; it can be employed in a range of laparoscopic surgeries, from cholecystectomy to myomectomy, and appendicectomy to tubal ligation. This versatility adds to its appeal among laparoscopic surgeons.

TASK ANALYSIS OF EXTRACORPOREAL MISHRA'S KNOT

- The length of suture used in the extracorporeal knot for free structure should be a minimum of 75 cm.
- Take the Bhandarkar knot pusher in left hand and pass 2 cm suture through the eye in the tail end of the Bhandarkar knot pusher by the right hand.
- The knot pusher is now reversely fed in the 3 mm reducer. Reverse feeding is important.
- Once the reducer is fed, the thread is pulled out from the eye of the tail of the knot pusher. The job of the eye in the tail is just to pass the suture safely from the reducer.
- Now, the other end of the suture is passed through the eye of the head end using the right hand.
- Ask the assistant for a finger and the extracorporeal slip knot is tied.
- The configuration of Mishra's knot is 1-1-1-1-1-1-1: One hitch, 1 wind, 1 lock, 2nd wind, 2nd lock, again 3rd wind, and the final lock. It is the most secure knot among the three for the structure up to 18 mm tubular structure.
- Make the diameter of the loop 6 cm by sliding the loop by the right hand's finger and thumb.

- After that, hide the knot and its loop under the reducer.
- Now, the knot pusher and the reducer are introduced through the 5 mm or 10 mm port. If it is introduced through the 10-mm port, additional 5 mm reducer should be introduced over 3 mm reducer to prevent the leakage of the gas.
- An atraumatic grasper should also be introduced from the contralateral port.
- The loop of the knot should go near the free structure.
- The atraumatic grasper should be introduced in the loop and after that it should hold the tip of the free structure over which you want to tie.
- Now, the knot pusher should go to feed the loop behind the structure. The same way our hands go behind when we put garland on someone's neck.
- The knot, now, can be slid to the desired place where you want to tie the knot by establishing the knot pusher with left hand and pulling the suture with the right hand.
- It should be done in such a fashion that the structure should not know that it is getting tied. Any traction of pulling and pushing should never be exerted over the tubular structure that you are ligating.
- After tightening the knot consecutively three times, the knot pusher and 3 mm reducer are pulled and hook scissors are introduced from the same port and the suture is cut leaving 1 cm tail.

Proficiency in Mishra's knot tying is a valuable skill for laparoscopic surgeons. Training programs and workshops are available to help surgeons master this technique. The step-by-step guidance provided in these programs ensures that surgeons can confidently integrate Mishra's knot into their practice, ultimately benefiting their patients.

STEP BY STEP DESCRIPTION OF MISHRA'S KNOT

Step-by-step description of Mishra's knot has been given in **Figures 1A to X**.

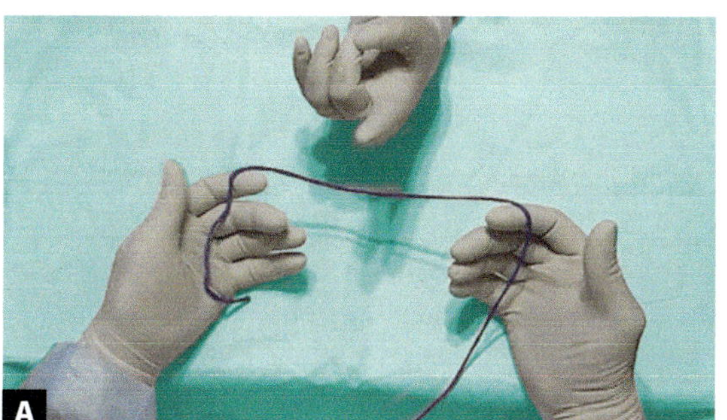
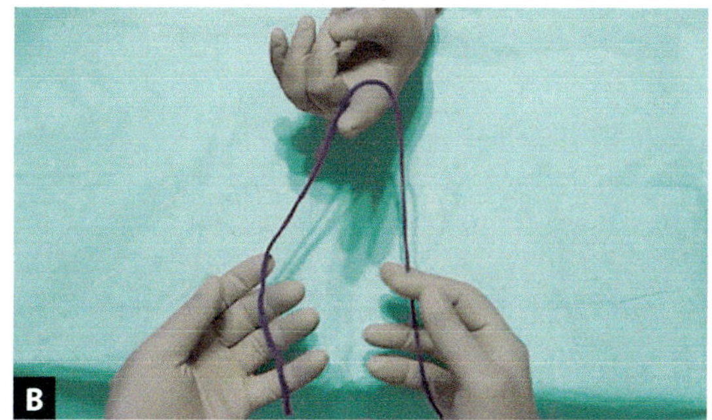

Figs. 1A and B

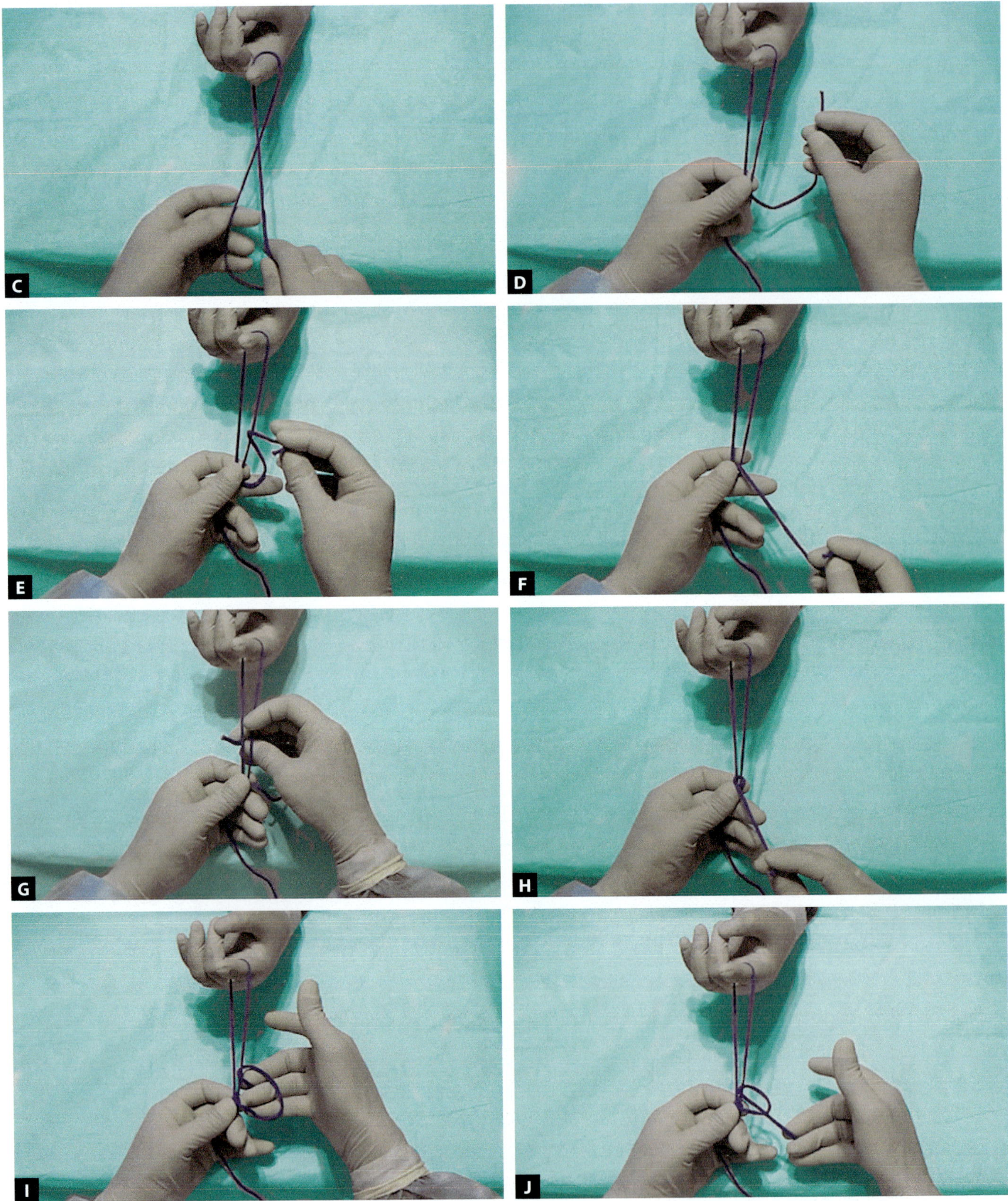

Figs. 1C to J

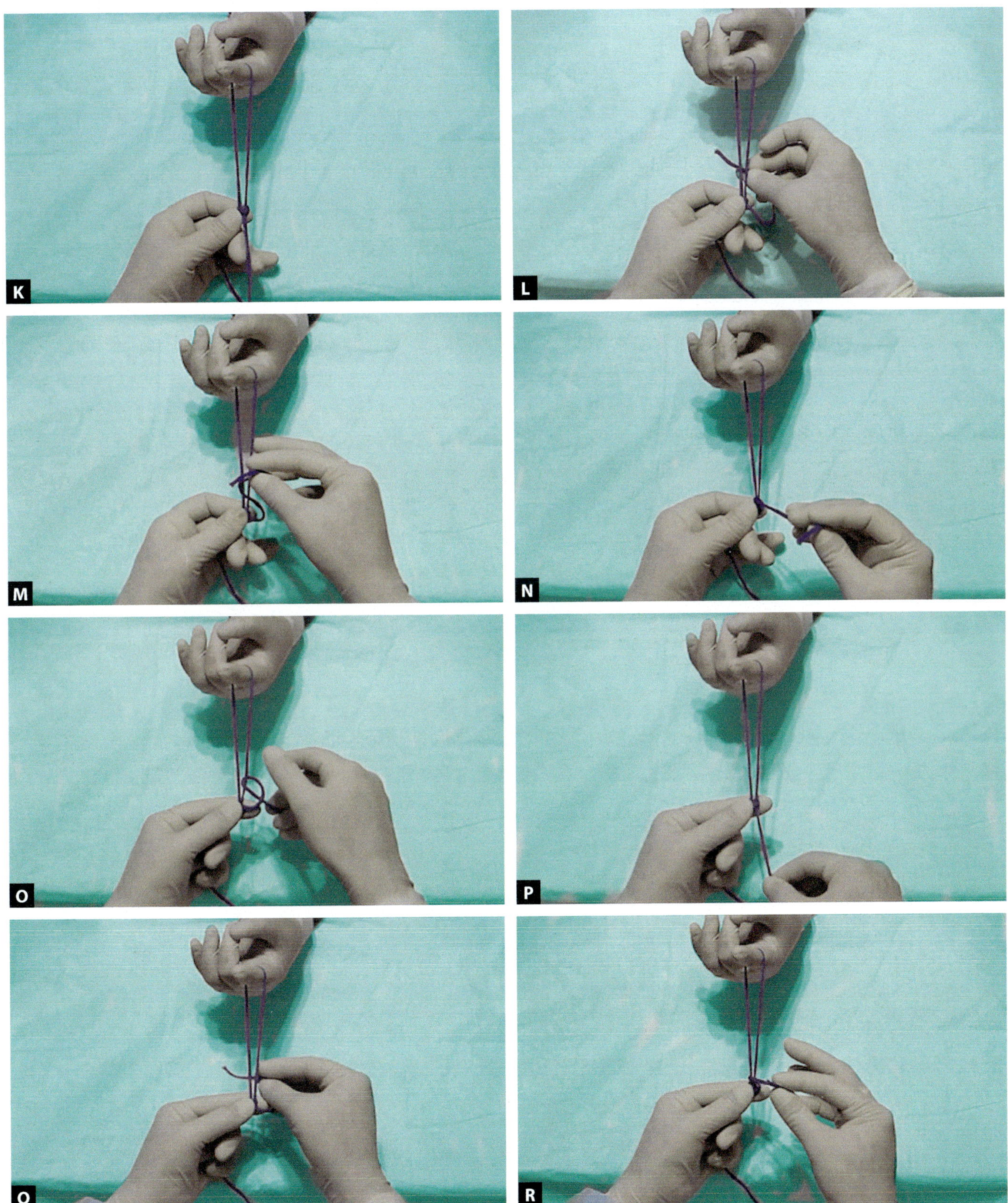

Figs. 1K to R

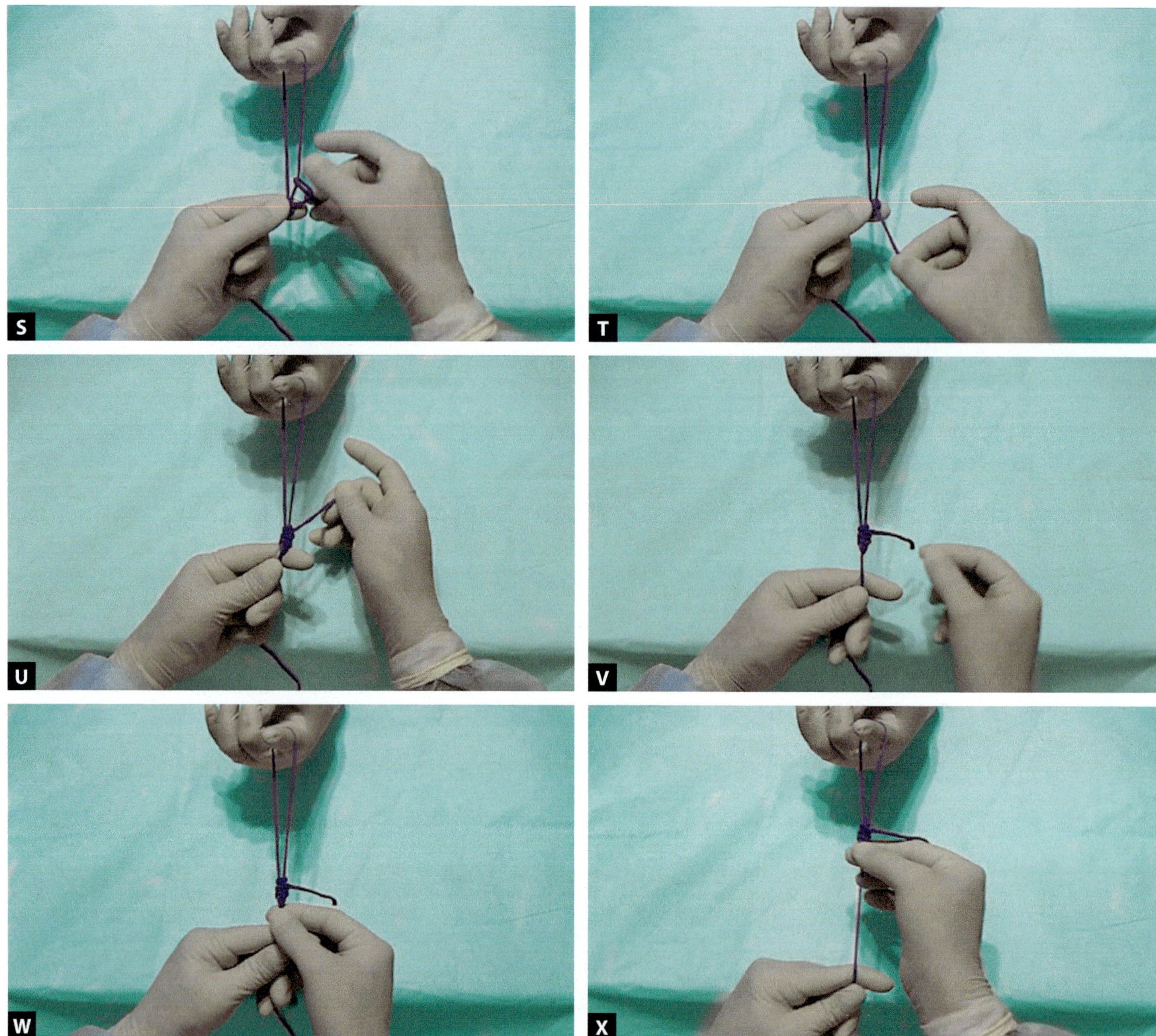

Figs. 1A to X: (A) Ask the assistant for a finger; (B) Encircle suture around figure keeping short arm to the left and long to right; (C) Cross the hand and bring left shorter end of thread over right; (D) Pinch both the threads by left index finger and thumb and hold shorter end with right hand; (E) Take a single hitch by passing shorter thread from below up in between the thread; (F) Tighten the first hitch and pinch it by left hand index finger and thumb; (G) Take first wind by short end (encircle around both the thread) by right hand; (H) Tighten the first wind and pinch it with left hand index figure and thumb; (I) Take a first half knot by right hand on right side of limb; (J) Tighten the first half knot by pulling short limb; (K) Pinch first half knot by left index figure and thumb; (L) Take second wind by encircling shorter thread around the limb by right hand; (M) Tighten the second wind by pulling the shorter end by right hand; (N) Pinch the second wind by left hand index figure and thumb; (O) Take a first half knot by right hand on right side of limb; (P) Pinch second half knot by left index figure and thumb; (Q) Take third wind by encircling shorter thread around the limb by right hand; (R) Pinch the third wind by left hand index figure and thumb; (S) Take third and final half knot by right hand on right side of limb; (T) Tighten the third and final half knot by pulling short limb; (U) Check if the winds are stacked properly; (V) Ensure winds are not over ridden or elongated; (W) Slide the knot over longer limb using right hand index finger; (X) If knots are sliding that means the knot is properly tied.

Mastering the techniques of knotting and suturing is an essential skill for laparoscopic surgeons, gynecologists, and urologists. Proficiency in knotting is indispensable for anyone aiming to perform advanced surgical procedures. Prof. Mishra's "Mishra Knot", introduced in the World Journal of Laparoscopic Surgery in 2007, has since become a widely adopted technique by hundreds of surgeons globally.

■ CONCLUSION

In conclusion, a surgeon's knot emerged as the optimal choice, offering a harmonious balance between loop security and knot security within the tested knot configurations. Conversely, a sliding knot without half-hitches on alternating posts (RHAPs) displayed poor loop security and knot security, making it an unsuitable choice for use.

However, the addition of three RHAPs resulted in improved knot security for all tested sliding knots, along with enhanced loop security for most of these knots. This addition effectively bolstered the knot security of all sliding knots, making them adequately resistant to predicted in vivo loads.

Furthermore, Mishra's knot was found to be one of the most secure and safe extracorporeal knots in laparoscopy. Its applicability extends to all continuous tubular structures of up to 22 mm in diameter. This technique's simplicity, ease of execution, and rapidity render it highly desirable for use. Notably, it can be applied with any suture material of any size.

In summary, this chapter emphasizes the importance of knot security in laparoscopic surgery and highlights the crucial role of techniques such as Mishra's knot in ensuring patient safety and surgical success. As the field of laparoscopic surgery continues to evolve, mastering advanced knot-tying techniques remains an essential skill for both experienced and aspiring laparoscopic surgeons.

■ BIBLIOGRAPHY

1. Akindele RA, Fasanu AO, Mondal SC, Komolafe JO, Mishra RK. Comparing extracorporeal knots in laparoscopy using knot and loop securities. World J Laparos Surgery. 2014;7(1):28-32.
2. Burkhat SS, Wirth MA, Simonich M, Salem D, Lanctot D, Athanasiou K. Knot security in simple sliding knots and its relationship to rotator cuff repair: How secure must the knot be? Arthroscopy. 2000;16(2):202-7.
3. Chan KC, Burkhart SS. Arthroscopic knot tying. In: McGinty J, Burkhat S, Jackson R, et al. (Eds). Philadelphia: Lippincott, Williams and Wilkins; 2004.
4. Chen MH, Khalil H. Laparoscopic Suturing Techniques for Surgeons. Oxford: Oxford University Press; 2022.
5. Choi E, Kim DY. The Use of Biodegradable Sutures in Laparoscopic Surgery. J Biomed Mat. 2024;15(3):438-45.
6. Comparison of Laparoscopic Traditional and Knotless Sutures." ClinicalTrials.gov, National Library of Medicine, May 26, 2020. Available from: https://classic.clinicaltrials.gov/ct2/show/NCT04401306.
7. Croce E, Olmi S. Intracorporeal knottying and suturing techniques in laparoscopic surgery: Technical details. JSLS. 2000;4(1):17-22.
8. Fernandez R, Martin CJ. Ergonomics in Laparoscopic Suturing: Minimizing Surgeon Fatigue. J Ergonomics Surg. 2023;17(3):145-54.
9. Gomez R, Lee T. Evolution of Suturing Techniques in Laparoscopic Surgery. J Minim Invasive Surg. 2021;28(2):123-32.
10. Gupta S, Mehra R. Barriers to Learning Laparoscopic Suturing: A Survey of Surgical Residents. Education Surg. 2023;47(1):55-62.
11. Hage JJ. How capsizing, flipping and flyping of traditional knots can result in new endoscopic knots: a geometric review. J Am Coll Surg. 2007;205(5):717-23.
12. Harper D, Lombardi A. Adapting Traditional Suturing Techniques for Laparoscopic Applications. Surg Techniques Rev. 2021;35(4):320-8.
13. Kim SH, Ha KI. The SMC knot: A new slip knot with locking mechanism. Arthroscopy. 2000;16(5):563-5.
14. Kumar V, Saxena AK. Advanced Techniques in Laparoscopic Surgery. Berlin: Springer; 2020.
15. Lavelle JF, Sinclair MF. Automated Suturing Devices in Laparoscopic Surgery: A Comparative Analysis. Techno Surg. 2020;22(6):789-98.
16. Lee J, Kim S. Innovations in Laparoscopic Suturing Instruments. Int J Med Robot. 2022;18(1):e2210
17. Lieurance RK, Pflaster DS, Abbott D, Nottage WM. Failure characteristics of various arthroscopically tied knots. Clin Orthop Relat Res. 2003;408:311-8.
18. Mendez C, Gupta A. Laparoscopic Suturing: Mastery Through Technique and Practice. London: Elsevier Health Sciences; 2023.
19. Minimally Invasive Gynecologic Surgery Utilizing the Artsential Articulating Laparoscopic Instruments." ClinicalTrials.gov, National Library of Medicine, Feb 12, 2021. Available from: https://classic.clinicaltrials.gov/ct2/show/NCT04401306.

20. Mishra RK. Textbook of Laparoscopy for Surgeons and Gynecologists, 4th edition. New Delhi: Jaypee Brothers Medical Publishers (P) Ltd; 2021.

21. Morrison T, Jacobs LR. Teaching Laparoscopic Suturing: The Role of Simulation in Medical Schools. Medical Teacher. 2021;43(7):778-84.

22. Nguyen L, Ho CP. Impact of Suture Materials on Laparoscopic Knot Reliability. Materials in Surgery. 2024;9(2):200-10.

23. Nottage WM, Lieurance RK. Current concepts: Arthroscopic knot tying. Arthroscopy. 1999;15:515-21.

24. O'Reilly MP, Saunders BH. Virtual Reality Training for Laparoscopic Surgery. Cambridge: Cambridge University Press; 2022.

25. Patel R, Thompson J. The Role of Simulation in Learning Laparoscopic Suturing and Knotting. Medical Education Online. 2021;26:1857289.

26. Rodriguez A, Davis SS. Robotic-Assisted Laparoscopic Knot Tying: Methods and Efficiency. Surg Innov. 2019;26(4):459-66.

27. Sami Walid M, Heaton RL. Laparoscopy-to-laparotomy quotient in obstetrics and gynecology residency programs. Arch Gynecol Obstet. 2011;283(5):1027-31.

28. Shimi SM, Lirig M, Vander-Velpen G, Cusehieri A. Comparative study of holding strength of slipknot using absorbable and nonabsorbable ligature materials. Surg Endosc. 1994;11:1285-91.

29. Smith JA, Patel VR (Eds). Principles of Laparoscopic Suturing and Knotting. New York: Springer; 2023.

30. Stephen W, Eubanks ES, Lee L, Swanstrom MD, Soper NJ. Mastery Of Endoscopic and Laparoscopic Surgery. 2nd edition. Lippincott Williams, Wilkins; 2004.

31. Wang Y, Thompson C. Innovations in Knot Tying Techniques for Minimally Invasive Surgery. Innovations in Surgery. 2022;18(4): 250-60.

32. Westerbring–van der Putten EP, Goossens RHM, Jakimowicz JJ, Dankelman J. Haptics in minimally invasive surgery: A review. Minim Invasive Ther. 2008;17(1): 3-16.

33. Weston PV. A new clinch knot. Obstet Gynecol. 1991;78(1):144-7.

34. Williams NE, Tan JL. Comparative Study of Knot Security in Laparoscopic Surgery. J Surg Res. 2020;245:217-23.

35. Zimmerman KA, Patel ND. Laparoscopic Knotting: A Visual Guide for Surgeons. Philadelphia: Lippincott Williams & Wilkins; 2022.

Tayside Knot

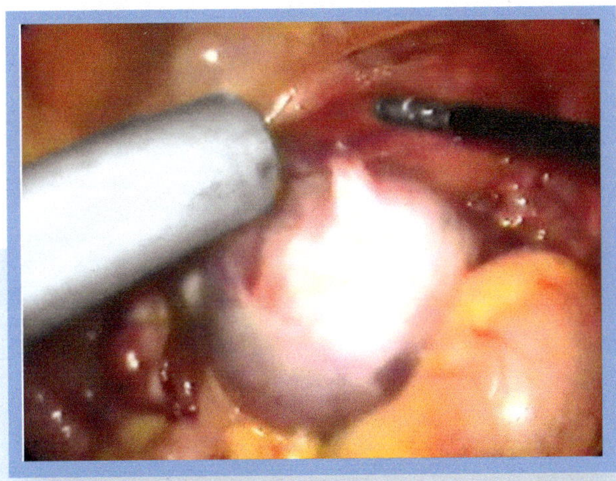

INTRODUCTION

Just like in open surgery, the surgeon must skillfully make precise cuts and skillfully bring tissues together. This process is crucial for ensuring effective hemostasis, and in this context, the art of proficient surgical knotting becomes paramount.

Historically, the Tayside knot derives its name from the Tay River, situated in Great Britain. It was collaboratively developed by two prominent British universities, namely Edinburgh and Aberdeen. Given that both institutions are located on the same side of the Tay River, the knot is commonly referred to as the Tayside knot. Its inception was influenced by the Fisherman utility knot, a well-known knot among the residents of Scotland's east coast.

Just as Meltzer's knot is an offshoot of the Roeder knot, so is the Tayside knot a further modification of the Meltzer's knot. Although quite secure when applied, it is an infrequently used knot in laparoscopic surgery **(Fig. 1)**.

APPLICATION

The Tayside knot finds valuable application in the ligation of substantial vessels, including but not limited to the azygos vein, splenic artery vein, and the inferior mesenteric vein. These critical anatomical structures require a high level of knot security during surgical procedures. For optimal results, it is recommended to use braided sutures of size 2-0 or larger, as well as Dacron material.

ADVANTAGES

The advantages of the Tayside knot are as follows.
- Employed for the secure ligation of critical structures such as large arteries and veins, the Tayside knot offers a level of resistance to reverse slippage akin to that of a surgeon's knot.
- It is tissue-friendly due to the knot's unique configuration, which ensures that the knot's bulk does not press against the tissue being secured. Consequently, it minimizes trauma and reduces the likelihood of recurrent bleeding.
- This extracorporeal knot is user-friendly, making it particularly accessible for less-experienced laparoscopic surgeons. This stands in contrast to the more intricate nature of intracorporeal suturing techniques.
- In terms of cost-effectiveness, the Tayside knot proves economical when compared to other methods used for achieving hemostasis, which often necessitate the use of expensive equipment.

DISADVANTAGES

The disadvantages of Tayside knot are as follows.
- It is a relatively complex knot compared to other modes of extracorporeal knotting. It, therefore, demands more effort by young laparoscopic surgeons.
- It is selective in the choice of suture materials. It is found to be at its best with braided sutures.

TYING A TAYSIDE KNOT

Tying a Tayside knot is displayed in **Figures 2 to 7**.

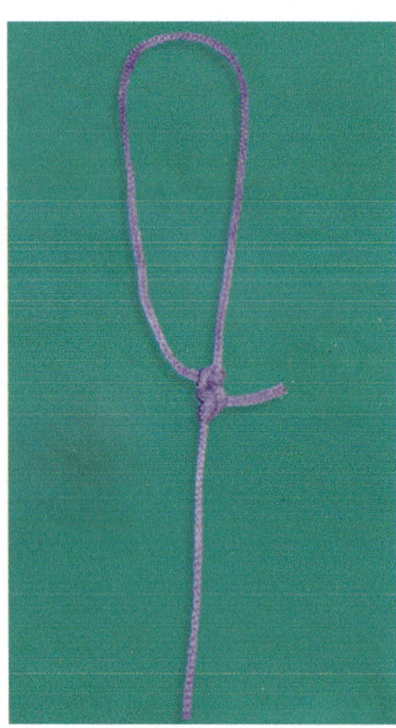

Fig. 1: Tayside knot.

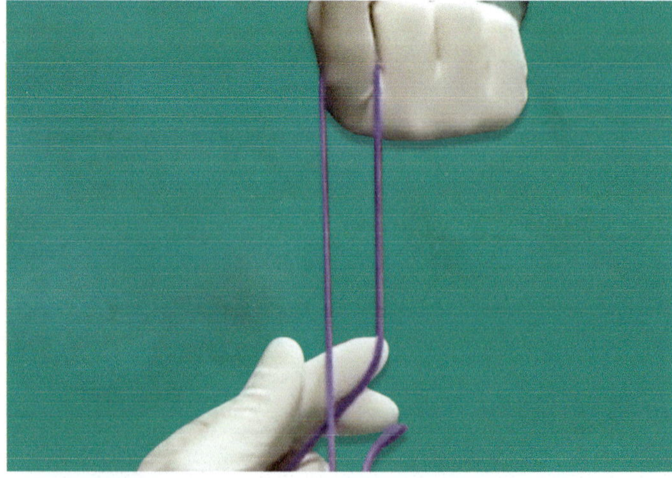

Fig. 2: Standing end in the left hand and working end in the right hand.

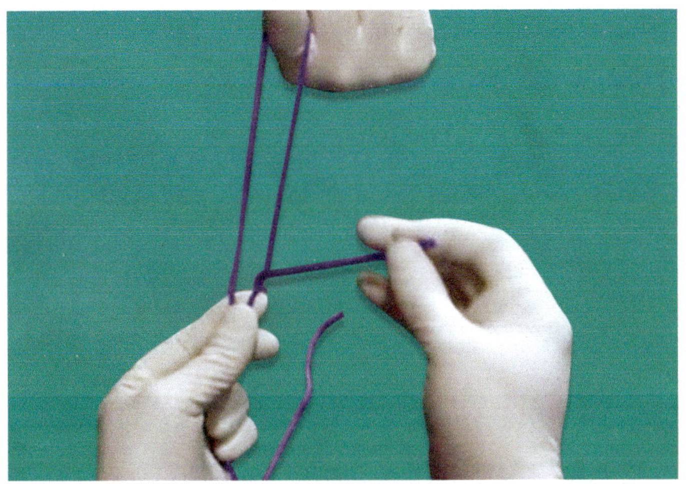

Fig. 3: A single hitch is taken first.

■ CLINICAL APPLICATION

The application method for the extracorporeal Tayside knot when dealing with continuous structures closely mirrors that of Roeder's and Meltzer's knots. Here is a step-by-step breakdown:

1. *Prepare a lengthy ligature:* Begin with a long piece of ligature, typically ranging from 90 to 150 cm. This length is necessary to allow for the threading of a pusher onto the ligature, which will then be passed into the abdominal cavity, wrapped around the continuous structure to be ligated, brought back out, and still leave sufficient length for knot tying.

2. *Introduce the ligature into the abdomen:* Initially, the ligature is inserted into the abdominal cavity. It will be used to encircle and ligate the continuous structure.

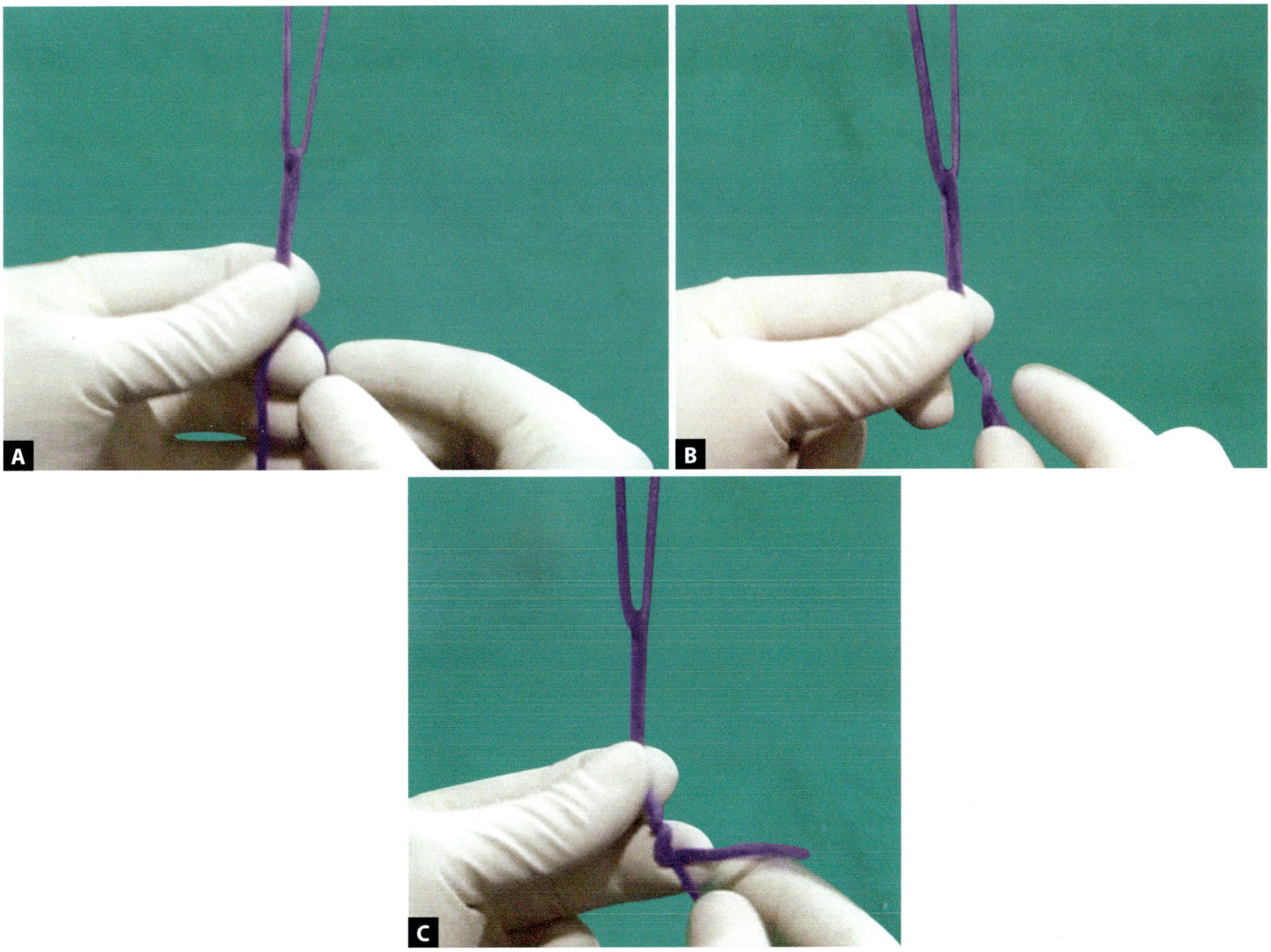

Figs. 4A to C: Four and a half rounds are taken approximately 1 cm below the first hitch over long-standing limb of thread.

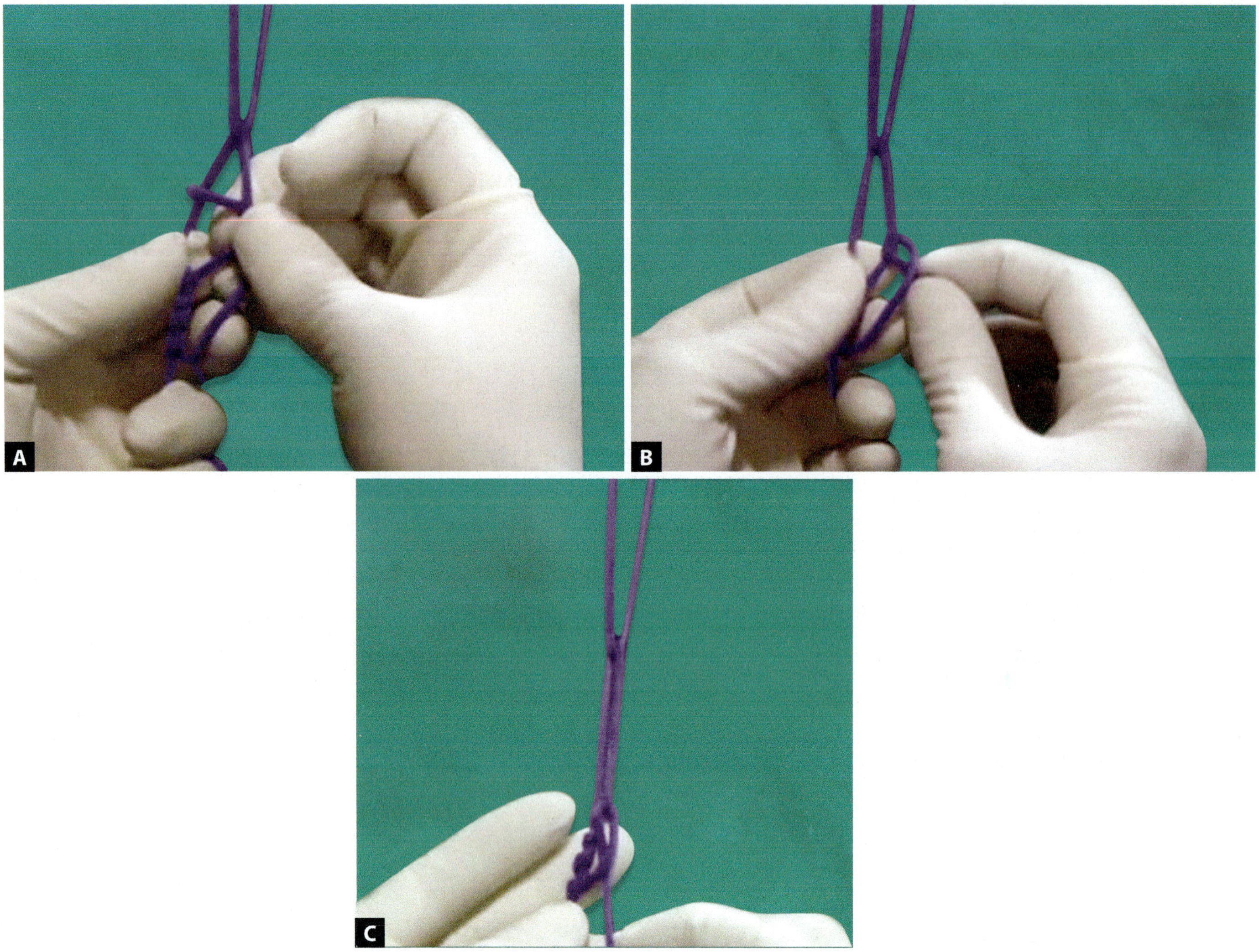

Figs. 5A to C: A locking hitch is made by passing the tail through the second and third loops.

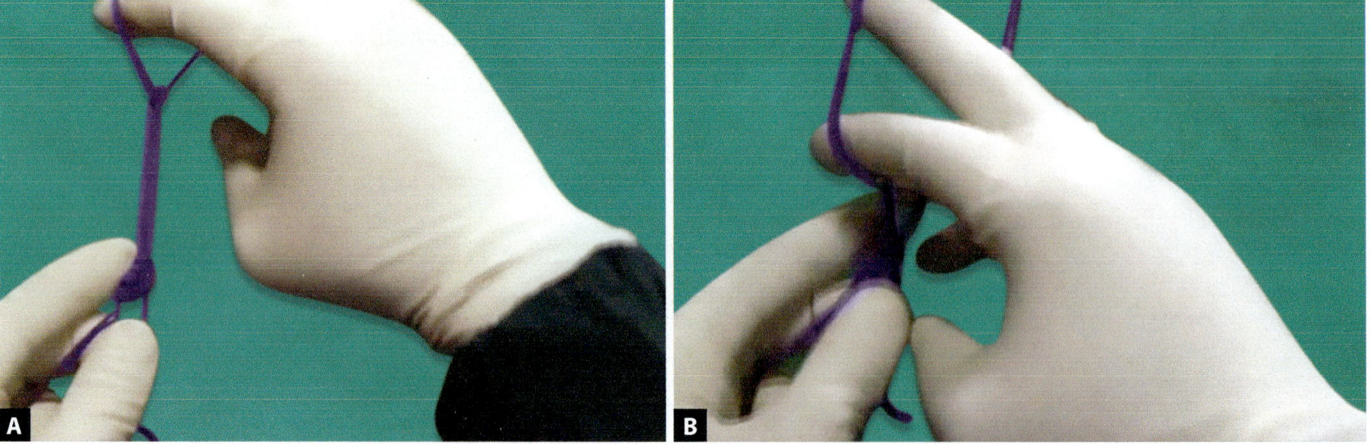

Figs. 6A and B: Finally, the first hitch is brought closer to the locking hitch by spreading the first loop.

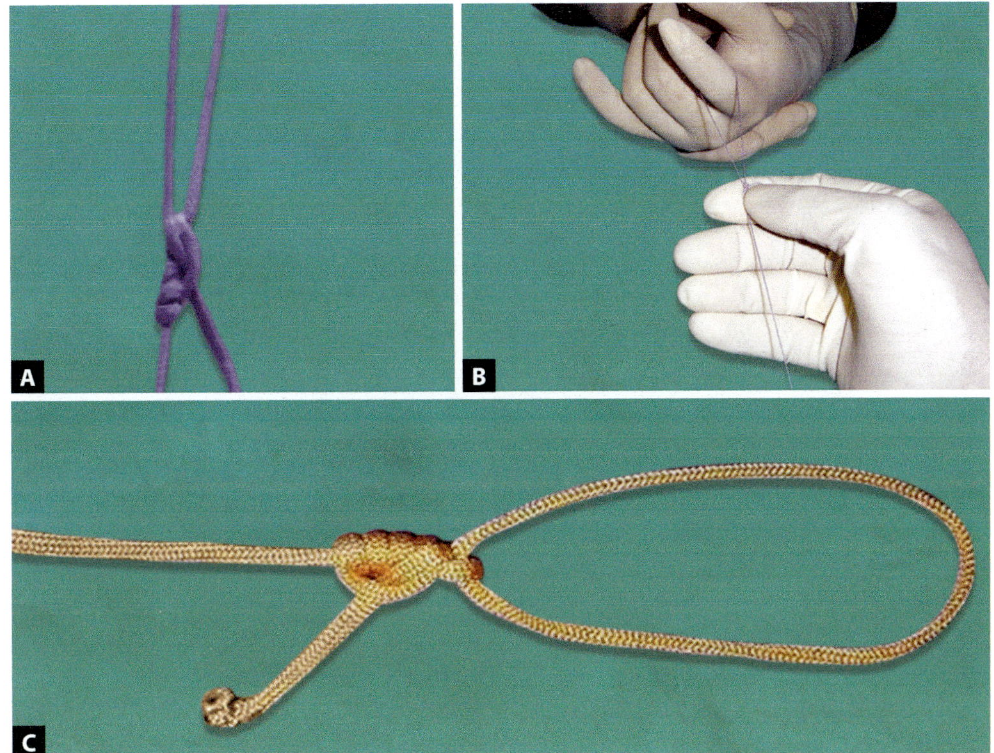

Figs. 7A to C: The knot is stacked properly and the extra tail (if any) is cut. Once the knot is configured properly, it should be checked by sliding over the long thread.

3. *Thread the push rod:* Thread a push rod onto a segment of the ligature material. This push rod is typically about 1.5 m long and assists in smoothly maneuvering the ligature around the target structure.
4. *Secure the ligature's end:* The end of the ligature that emerges from the tapered end (the end without the push rod) is carefully grasped using an atraumatic endoscopic grasper.

This method enables precise handling and secure ligation of continuous structures within the abdominal cavity, and it follows a similar approach to applying Roeder's and Meltzer's knots.

The grasper and suture material are then passed into an introducer tube. The introducer tube is then passed through an 11 mm cannula. The grasper and ligature are extended into the cavity and passed to one side and behind the structure to be ligated. A second grasper is introduced through a second port to grasp the ligature from the other side of the structure. The first grasper releases the ligature and takes it back from the second in front of the structure. The first grasper and ligature are withdrawn from the abdomen through the introducer tube while the

second is used to protect the structure from the shearing effect of the suture. An external slip knot is tied externally. The knot tied is determined by the size of the vessel to be controlled and the material in use. The knot is pushed into the abdomen by the push rod and positioned prior to tightening. The rod is withdrawn a little and scissors are introduced to cut the suture. A suture with a needle can also be used to initiate a Tayside knot, which can be used to do interrupted suturing of tissues; for example, to suture the uterus after myomectomy **(Figs. 8 to 11)**.

■ DISCUSSION

The art of suturing plays a pivotal role in surgery and forms a fundamental component of surgical training. In open surgery, where binocular vision is utilized, acquiring this skill is relatively straightforward. However, in minimal access surgery, it becomes considerably more challenging and demands a great deal of patience. This is primarily due to the monocular vision inherent in minimal access surgery, in contrast to the binocular vision available in open surgery. Moreover, the surgeon lacks the natural tactile feedback of tissue while suturing; instead, suturing

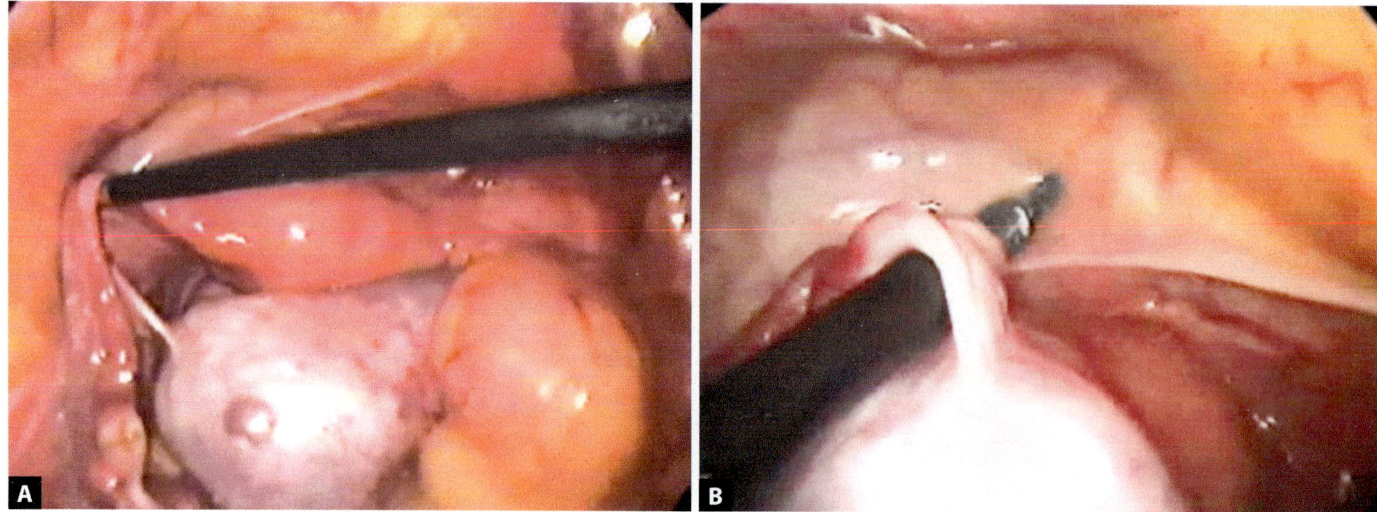

Figs. 8A and B: A window is created behind ovarian ligament and suture is passed though that window with the help of Maryland dissector.

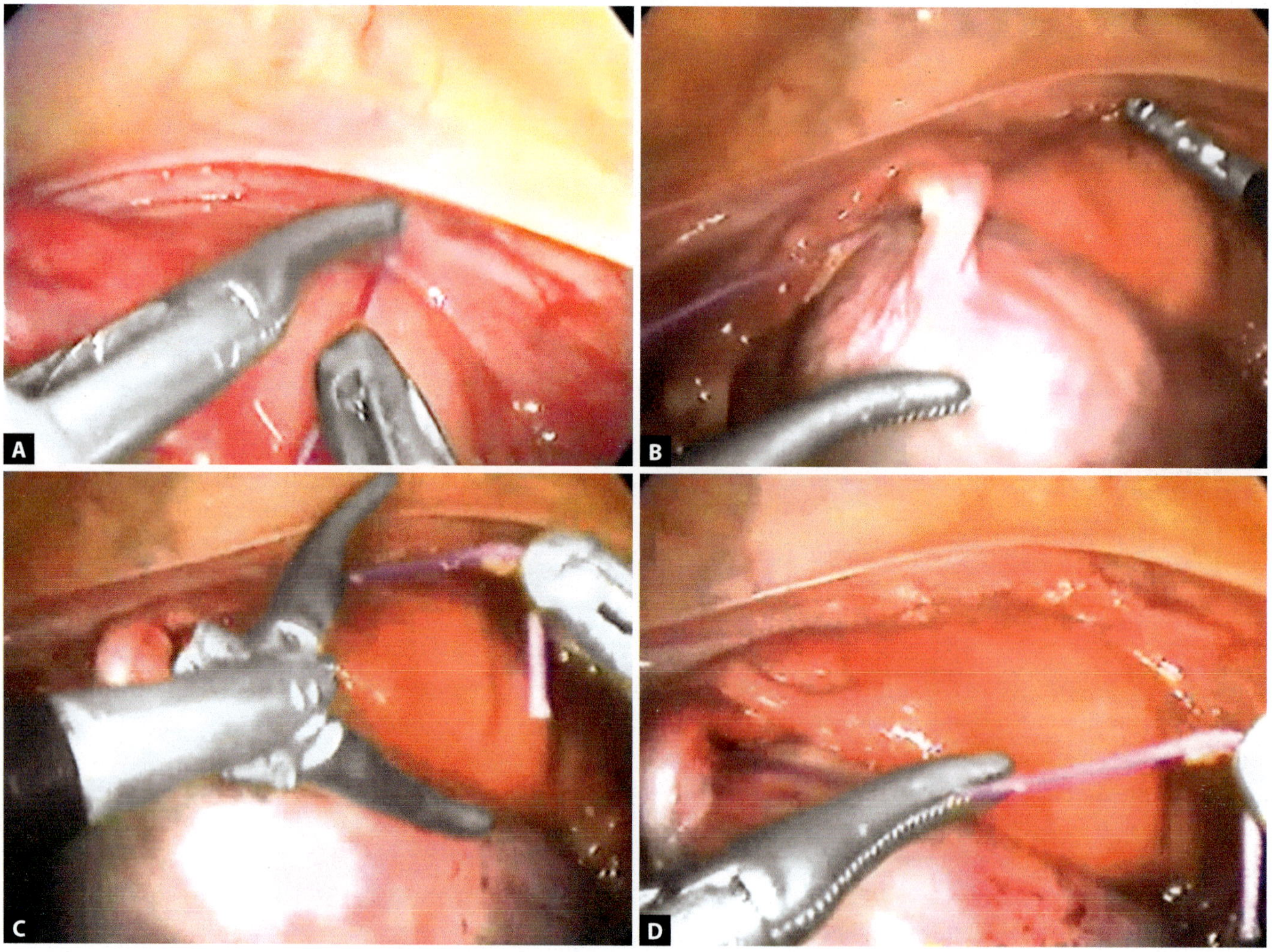

Figs. 9A to D: The suture tip is held by another grasper and Maryland is withdrawn from the window. The tip of suture is again transferred to same Maryland once it is pulled out from the window.

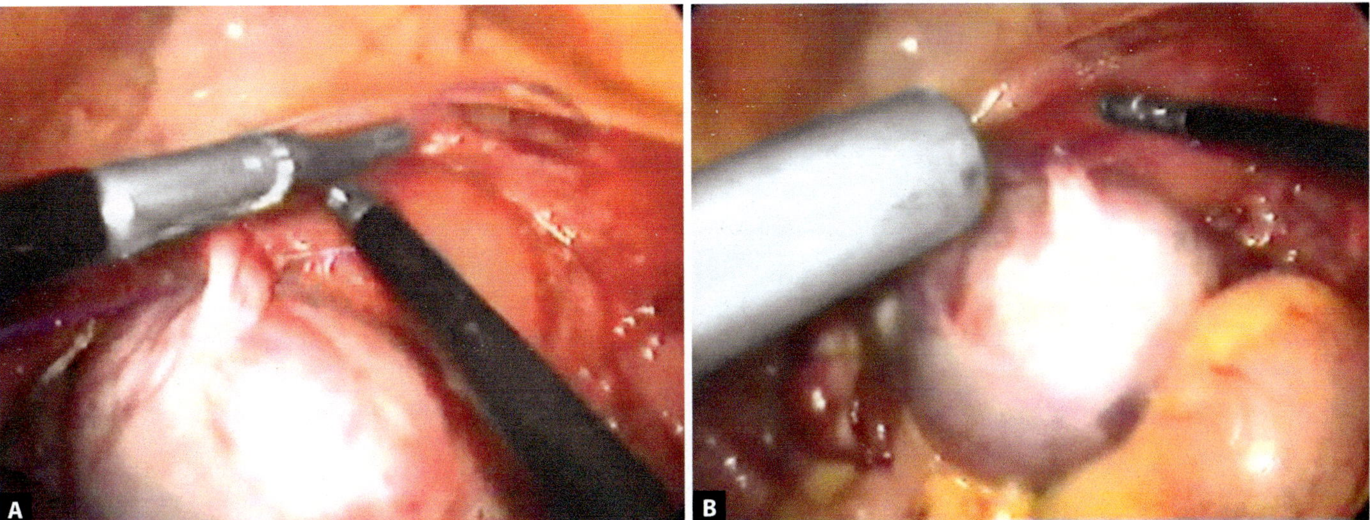

Figs. 10A and B: The working end of the suture is pulled outside to tie the Tayside knot. It is important to keep one grasper behind the structure in between the loop while pulling the suture out to support the suture, so that there should not be any traction while pulling the suture out.

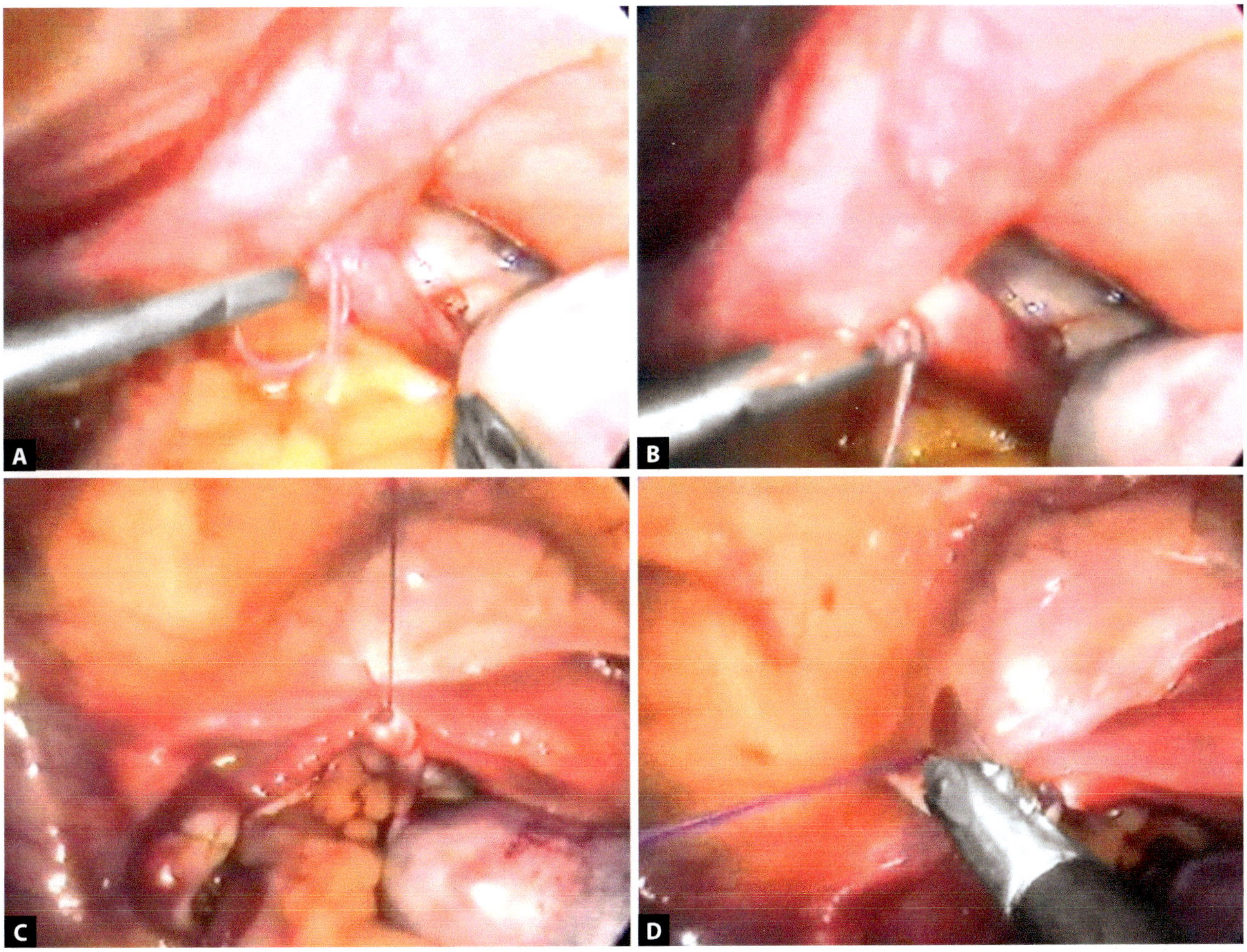

Figs. 11A to D: The knot is pushed through the knot pusher and nicely tied around the ovarian ligament. The scissors are used and oophorectomy is completed.

is executed using elongated instruments while observing the surgical field and activities on a monitor. Consequently, many laparoscopic surgeons find it more convenient to rely on preprepared tools for tissue approximation. Nonetheless, these alternatives can never fully replace the time-tested traditional method of suturing.

Extracorporeal knotting serves as a bridge between these suturing approaches. It is performed outside the body and involves the use of the surgeon's natural dexterity. The knot is subsequently introduced into the operative field with the assistance of a knot pusher. This technique demands the use of a well-established secure knot that is also gentle on tissues. The time-tested Tayside knot embodies all these qualities of an ideal extracorporeal knot.

When applied to tissue, the Tayside knot firmly secures itself without compromising the tissue integrity. The significance of secure knotting becomes especially paramount when dealing with vital structures like large arteries and veins, as knot slippage in such cases can have catastrophic consequences. Additionally, the Tayside knot is tissue-friendly, as the bulk of the knot does not exert pressure on the secured tissue. This stands in contrast to most other extracorporeal knots where the bulk of the knot rests on the tissue, potentially causing more trauma and increasing the risk of recurrent bleeding. Notably, the Tayside knot has proven to be effective in procedures like two-port needlescopic cholecystectomy.

While vascular clipping with staplers is a convenient practice, easier to apply and less time-consuming, it presents a significant drawback in terms of cost-effectiveness. For example, applying a set of vascular clips during an operation such as a splenectomy can cost around $250. Furthermore, the applicators for these clips are relatively expensive and require regular replacement. In an era marked by economic challenges, especially in developing countries, this expense may not be readily affordable.

CONCLUSION AND RECOMMENDATIONS

The Tayside knot stands out for its affordability, security, and tissue-friendliness. These last two attributes make it superior to other methods of extracorporeal knotting, especially when delicate structures like major blood vessels are involved. These advantages more than make up for the somewhat more intricate maneuvering required during its execution. It is somewhat ironic that such an effective knotting technique is often underutilized.

As a result, we strongly recommend its adoption by all laparoscopic surgeons, especially those practicing in developing countries.

The Tayside knot has proven to be a valuable tool in laparoscopic surgery due to its affordability, security, and tissue-friendliness. It is particularly effective for ligating delicate structures such as major blood vessels, where secure knotting is crucial to prevent catastrophic consequences. Despite its somewhat complex technique, the benefits of the Tayside knot far outweigh the challenges, making it an excellent option for achieving hemostasis in minimally invasive procedures. Given its advantages over other extracorporeal knotting methods, especially in terms of minimizing trauma and cost-effectiveness, it is recommended that laparoscopic surgeons, particularly those in developing countries, adopt the Tayside knot in their practice to enhance surgical outcomes and patient safety.

BIBLIOGRAPHY

1. Bhaatia P, John SJ, Deed JPS. Extracorporeal knot tying. Art of Endosuturing. New Delhi: Jaypee Brothers Medical Publishers (P) Ltd; 2003. pp. 111-3.
2. Chen MH, Khalil H. Laparoscopic Suturing Techniques for Surgeons. Oxford: Oxford University Press; 2022.
3. Choi E, Kim DY. The Use of Biodegradable Sutures in Laparoscopic Surgery. Journal of Biomedical Materials. 2024;15(3):438-45.
4. Fernandez R, Martin CJ. Ergonomics in Laparoscopic Suturing: Minimizing Surgeon Fatigue. Journal of Ergonomics in Surgery. 2023;17(3):145-54.
5. Gomez R, Lee T. Evolution of Suturing Techniques in Laparoscopic Surgery. J Minim Invasive Surg. 2021;28(2):123-32.
6. Gupta S, Mehra R. Barriers to Learning Laparoscopic Suturing: A Survey of Surgical Residents. Education in Surgery. 2023;47(1):55-62.
7. Harper D, Lombardi A. Adapting Traditional Suturing Techniques for Laparoscopic Applications. Surgical Techniques Review. 2021;35(4):320-8.
8. Kumar V, Saxena AK. Advanced Techniques in Laparoscopic Surgery. Berlin: Springer; 2020.
9. Lavelle JF, Sinclair MF. Automated Suturing Devices in Laparoscopic Surgery: A Comparative Analysis. Technology in Surgery. 2020;22(6):789-98.
10. Lee J, Kim S. Innovations in laparoscopic suturing instruments. Int J Med Robot Comput Assist Surg. 2022; 18(1), e2210.
11. Lee KW, Poon CM, Leung KF, Lee DWH CW, Ko CW. Two-port needlescopic cholecystectomy: Prospective study of 100 cases. Hong Kong Med J. 2005;11(1):30-5.

12. Mendez C, Gupta A. Laparoscopic Suturing: Mastery Through Technique and Practice. London: Elsevier Health Sciences; 2023.

13. Mishra RK. Laparoscopic tissue approximation techniques. Textbook of Practical Laparoscopic Surgery. New Delhi: Jaypee Brothers Medical Publishers (P) Ltd; 2009. pp. 111-3.

14. Mishra RK. Textbook of Laparoscopy for Surgeons and Gynecologists, 4th edition. New Delhi: Jaypee Brothers Medical Publishers (P) Ltd; 2021.

15. Morrison T, Jacobs LR. Teaching Laparoscopic Suturing: The Role of Simulation in Medical Schools. Medical Teacher. 2021;43(7):778-84.

16. Nguyen L, Ho CP. Impact of Suture Materials on Laparoscopic Knot Reliability. Materials in Surgery. 2024;9(2):200-10.

17. O'Reilly MP, Saunders BH. Virtual Reality Training for Laparoscopic Surgery. Cambridge: Cambridge University Press; 2022.

18. Patel R, Thompson J. The Role of Simulation in Learning Laparoscopic Suturing and Knotting. Medical Education Online. 2021;26:1857289.

19. Patsalos C, Karanas D, Seavropoulos M, Tierris I, Bablekos G, Nicolaou I, et al. The relationship between five kinds of laparoscopic knots and five types of suture materials and histological findings in tissues: An experimental study on rabbits. Surg Laparosc Endosc Percutan Tech. 2003;13(3).

20. Rodriguez A, Davis SS. Robotic-Assisted Laparoscopic Knot Tying: Methods and Efficiency. Surgical Innovation. 2019;26(4):459-66.

21. Shimi SM, Lirici M, Vander Velpen G, Cushieri A. Holding and tensile characteristics of extracorporeal slipknots. Surg Endosc. 1994;8(12):1285-91.

22. Shimi SM, Lirig M, Vander-Velpen G, Cusehieri A. Comparative study of holding strength of slipknot using absorbable and nonabsorbable ligature materials. Surg Endosc. 1994;11:1285-91.

23. Smith JA, Patel VR (Eds). Principles of Laparoscopic Suturing and Knotting. New York: Springer; 2023.

24. Surgical Knots and Suturing Techniques. (2024). [online] Available from https://en.wikipedia.org/wiki/Surgical_knot [last accessed........].

25. Tok K, Roon C, Lee K, Leong H. Operative cholecyctectomy. J Laparoendosc Adv Surg Tech. 2006;16(3).

26. Wang Y, Thompson C. Innovations in Knot Tying Techniques for Minimally Invasive Surgery. Innovations in Surgery. 2022;18(4): 250-60.

27. Williams NE, Tan JL. Comparative Study of Knot Security in Laparoscopic Surgery. J Surg Res. 2020;245:217-23.

28. Zimmerman KA, Patel ND. Laparoscopic Knotting: A Visual Guide for Surgeons. Philadelphia: Lippincott Williams & Wilkins; 2022.

Weston Knot

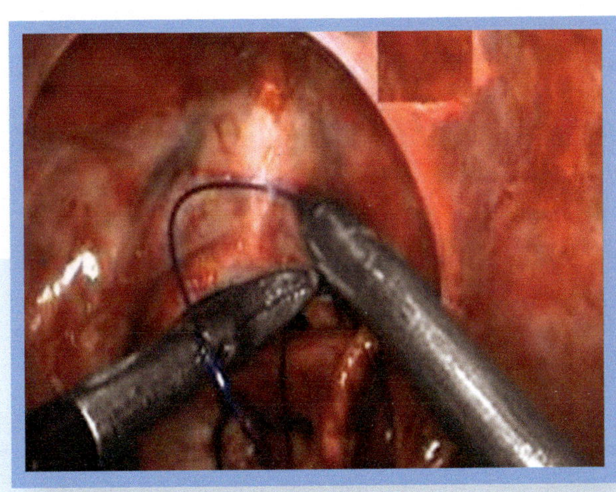

INTRODUCTION

Laparoscopy represents a modern surgical technique that offers various methods for tissue approximation, including extracorporeal and intracorporeal knots, surgical glues (tissue adhesive), clips, staplers, and laser welding. Despite the recent advancements in tissue approximation, the skill of laparoscopic knot tying is likely to remain essential for general surgeons and gynecologists when performing suturing.

The use of knots in human history dates back to primitive times when they were employed for trapping animals and crafting weapons. Today's laparoscopic knots essentially evolved from techniques used by seamen, fishermen, weavers, and executioners.

Ever since the introduction of endoscopes, surgeons have been continually searching for improved and stronger materials and methods for knot tying.

One such knot is the Weston knot, introduced by Peter V Weston. It is a sliding extracorporeal knot, specifically a highly efficient slip knot. Notably, it is the simplest of all sliding knots, allowing for quick execution as it can be easily slid down without the need for a knot pusher. The Weston knot finds utility in ligating pedicles, especially in situations where access is limited. It readily secures with monofilament materials and takes less time to tie compared to numerous square knots.

In the dynamic field of laparoscopic surgery, where innovation and precision play pivotal roles, the laparoscopic Weston knot emerges as a quintessential technique for surgeons. This specialized knot, tailored for the challenges and intricacies of minimally invasive procedures, represents a blend of tradition and innovation in surgical suturing. This chapter explores the laparoscopic Weston knot, its methodology, advantages, and its indispensable role in enhancing surgical outcomes in laparoscopic operations.

WESTON KNOT

The Weston knot, traditionally known for its application in various surgical disciplines, has been adeptly adapted for laparoscopic use. This adaptation reflects a commitment to achieving secure suturing in the limited-access environment of laparoscopic surgery. The knot's design allows for efficient execution and reliable stability—critical factors in the success of minimally invasive surgical procedures.

TECHNIQUE OF THE LAPAROSCOPIC WESTON KNOT

The laparoscopic Weston knot is characterized by its unique tying method, designed to ensure knot security and tissue approximation with minimal tension. The technique involves the following steps:

1. *Suture placement:* Initially, the suture is placed through the tissue using laparoscopic instruments, ensuring accurate approximation of the tissue edges.
2. *Knot formation:* The surgeon forms the Weston knot outside the patient's body. This step involves creating a loop with the suture and then weaving the tail end through this loop in a specific pattern that enhances the knot's security once tightened.
3. *Transferring the knot:* Using a knot Maryland, the pretied Weston knot is carefully transferred down the suture and into the surgical site. It can even be transferred without any knot pusher. The surgeon then tightens the knot by pulling on the suture ends, ensuring the desired tension and tissue approximation.
4. *Securing the knot:* Additional throws may be added to secure the knot further, depending on the specific requirements of the surgical procedure and the tissue characteristics.

ADVANTAGES OF THE WESTON KNOT IN LAPAROSCOPIC SURGERY

The laparoscopic Weston knot offers several advantages that make it a preferred choice in many laparoscopic procedures:

- *Reliability:* Its unique structure provides a high level of security, reducing the risk of knot slippage or loosening postsurgery.
- *Efficiency:* The technique allows for quick execution, which is beneficial in reducing operative times and minimizing patient exposure to anesthesia.
- *Versatility:* It can be used in various surgical specialties, including general surgery, orthopedic, gynecology, and urology, demonstrating its adaptability to different tissues and operative needs.

CHALLENGES AND LEARNING CURVE

Mastering the laparoscopic Weston knot requires practice and a deep understanding of its mechanics. The limited tactile feedback in laparoscopic surgery demands that surgeons develop a keen sense of spatial awareness and manual dexterity. Training models and simulation-based learning play a crucial role in overcoming the learning curve associated with this technique.

The laparoscopic Weston knot signifies a confluence of surgical tradition and innovation, offering a reliable, efficient, and versatile solution for suturing in the constrained environment of laparoscopic surgery. As minimally invasive techniques continue to evolve, mastering such advanced knotting techniques will be paramount for surgeons aiming to optimize patient outcomes. The Weston knot stands as a testament to the ongoing advancements in surgical science, embodying the pursuit of excellence in patient care through innovation.

◾ APPLICATION

Due to its user-friendly nature as a sliding knot that eliminates the need for a knot pusher, the Weston knot finds application in challenging locations on resilient structures, not only in certain gynecologic laparoscopic procedures but also in selected ophthalmic and orthopedic surgeries.

◾ CHARACTERISTICS OF SUTURE MATERIAL

For the successful application of the Weston knot, a lengthy ligature measuring approximately 90 cm is necessary. This length is essential to enable the ligature to be passed into the abdominal cavity, encircle the targeted structure for ligation, and be brought out again, all while leaving enough length for the surgeon to effectively tie the knot.

The choice of suture material depends on the specific clinical situation.

Monofilament sutures such as polydioxanone (PDS), nylon, or Monocryl are preferred materials for this type of knot. These suture materials exhibit significantly lower slippage compared to catgut. Moreover, catgut, while effective, is highly reactive within the body and is gradually being replaced by these newer materials due to their reduced foreign body reaction.

On the other hand, braided sutures such as vicryl and silk are less commonly used for the sliding knot technique. This is because they are less likely to slide, which increases the risk of premature knot locking, potentially compromising the effectiveness of the knot.

◾ TASK ANALYSIS FOR WESTON KNOT

- Cutting suture 90 cm with Endoski needle which is proximal two thirds straight and distal and one third curved.
- Insert Maryland in the reducer.
- Hold the suture with Maryland at the tail end and pull it out through the reducer and then hold it near the needle and hide it in the reducer.
- Insert the Maryland with the reducer into the abdomen.
- Drop the needle over the tissue in such a way that the tip should be in the left and the tail in the right side.
- *Align the needle by the following three techniques*:
  - Pressing the needle by the upper jaw of the needle holder at the junction of one third and two thirds.
  - Holding the needle by the left hand at the curvature and pulling the suture up near the needle by the right hand.
  - Hang the needle by the left hand like a pendulum and go with the open jaw of the needle holder keeping the moving jaw to the left and dragging it to the right.
- Stabilize the tissue by the left hand and take a bite by keeping the needle at 90° angle to the tissue and rotating the tip of the needle to bring it to the other side.
- Bring the tip of the needle one third out and catch it with the left instrument, keeping the convex end toward the tissue.
- Guard the tissue by the needle holder, keeping the concave part of the instrument toward the tissue and pulling the needle by the left-hand instrument and feed the suture four times.
- Hold the suture by the needle holder as soon as the needle is out.
- The configuration of Weston knot is 1:1:1.
- Weston knot is a self-locking sliding knot, which has one hitch, one reverse hitch, and one final wrap and lock. The steps of Weston knot are:
  - *Step 1:* The index finger of the assistant may be used to make Weston knot. The left hand should be used to hold the short limb and the right hand for long limb of thread.
  - *Step 2:* The short limb of the thread is crossed over the long limb.
  - *Step 3:* The intersection point of thread should be pinched by left hand index finger and thumb. At the time of making intersection, surgeon should keep sufficient length of short limb to make it comfortable. It is important to remember that left hand is used only to hold the intersection point, while the right hand will make the necessary hitches and loops.
  - *Step 4:* The short limb is passed between the thread upward.

- *Step 5:* The short limb should be pulled from up by the right hand to make first hitch.
- *Step 6:* The short limb is placed toward the left side and is passed between the two limb upward to make a reverse hitch.
- *Step 7:* The short limb should encircle the thread from below upward and should be put in the first loop to lock it.
- Now, hide the knot in the reducer with or without Maryland and push the knot sliding downward to the desired place where you want to tie by keeping the suture in the left hand and pulling the suture with the right hand.
- After tightening the knot, you can take a final square knot to secure.
- Introduce the scissors from the right port and cut the suture.
- You can again reuse the same suture needle to tie another knot.
- Weston knot is used in gynecological surgeries and also in arthroscopic surgeries. It can be used in situations where suture slides smoothly and freely through tissue and the anchoring device.

■ STEPS

Definition of post limb and wrapping limb (Fig. 1):
- *Post limb:* The straight portion of the suture limb purely defined as the suture limb under the most tension.
- *Wrapping limb:* The free portion of the suture limb that wraps around the post limb.

Step 1

A single hitch has been performed **(Figs. 2A to C)**.

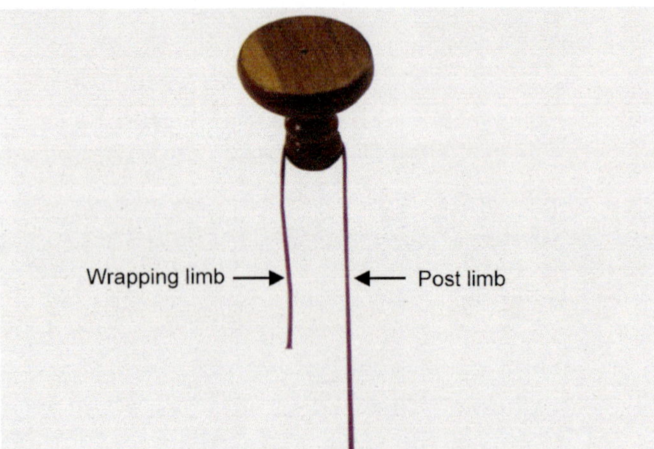

Fig. 1: Two limbs of the suture.

Step 2

The wrapping tail end wind over the strand of the suture in a clockwise direction passed over the top of only one strand from below upward **(Figs. 3A to C)**.

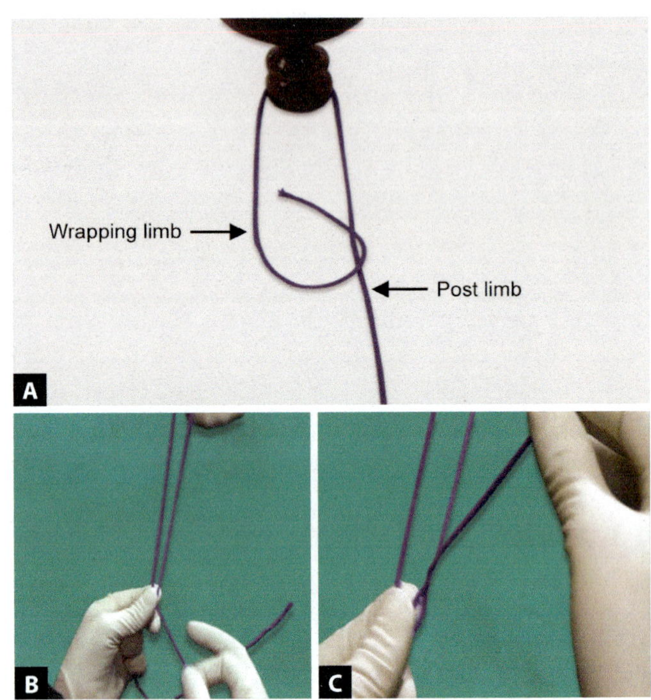

Figs. 2A to C: Single hitch.

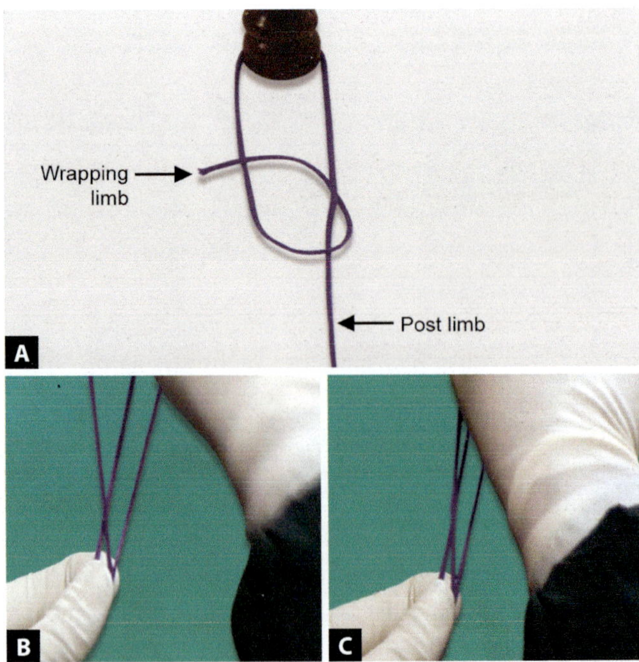

Figs. 3A to C: Wrapping limb wind over.

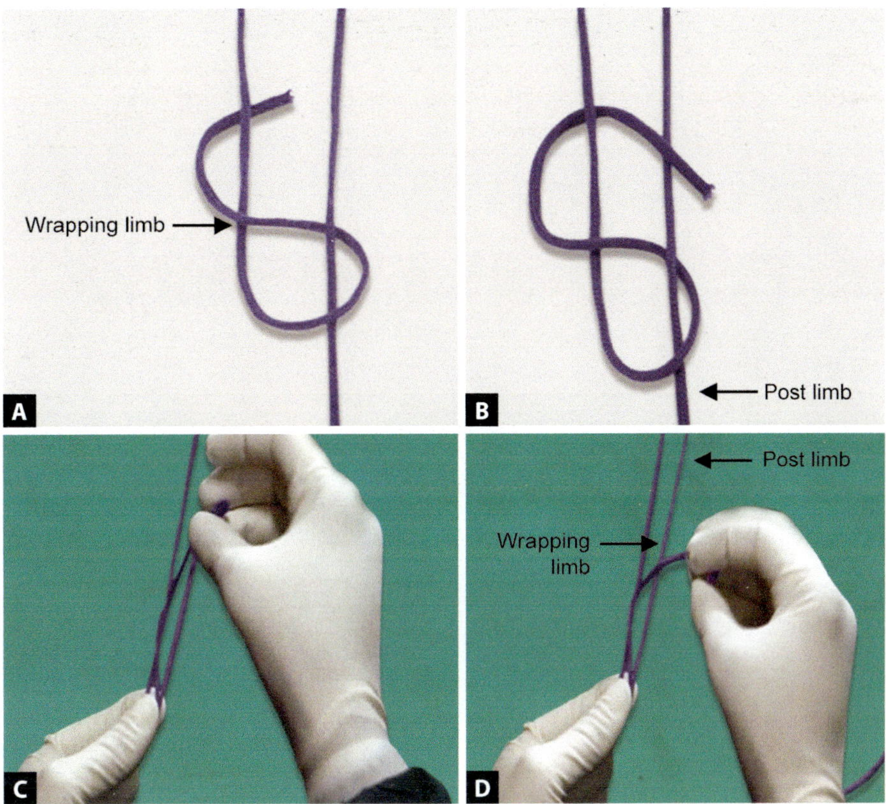

Figs. 4A to D: Threading between the strand.

Step 3

The tail end threaded between the two strands and brought to the top around the other strand **(Figs. 4A to D)**.

Step 4

The tail end is placed through the loop formed by the initial single hitch **(Figs. 5A to C)**.

Step 5

The final knot has a resemblance of figure of eight wrapped around a suture **(Figs. 6A to C)**.

Step 6

Weston knot is already formed; the tail of the knot should be long enough to allow easy knot tying **(Figs. 7A and B)**.

Step 7

The knot can often be slipped down through a port with a tugging motion on the post limb and pushed down slowly **(Figs. 8A to C)**.

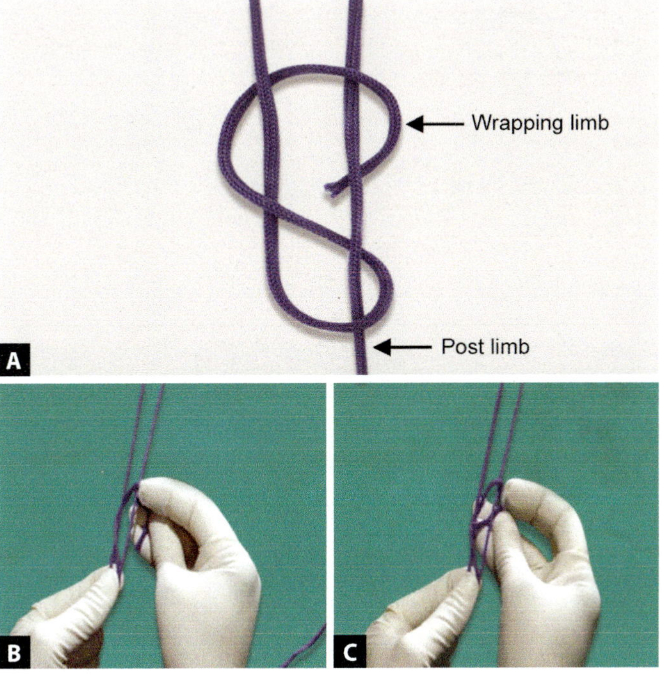

Figs. 5A to C: Loop formation.

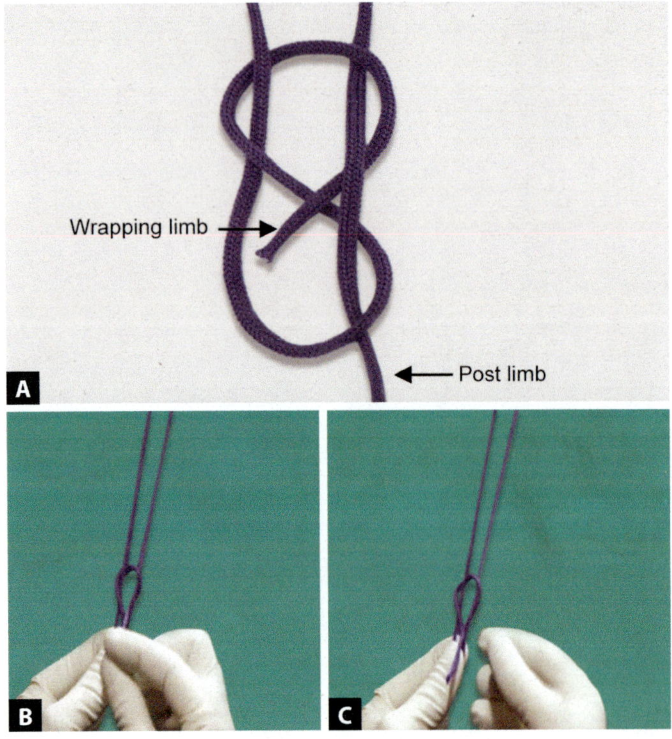

Figs. 6A to C: Figure of 8 formation.

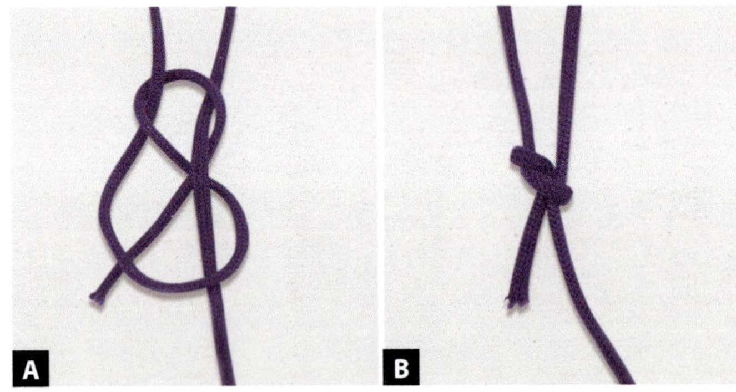

Figs. 7A and B: Formation of Weston knot.

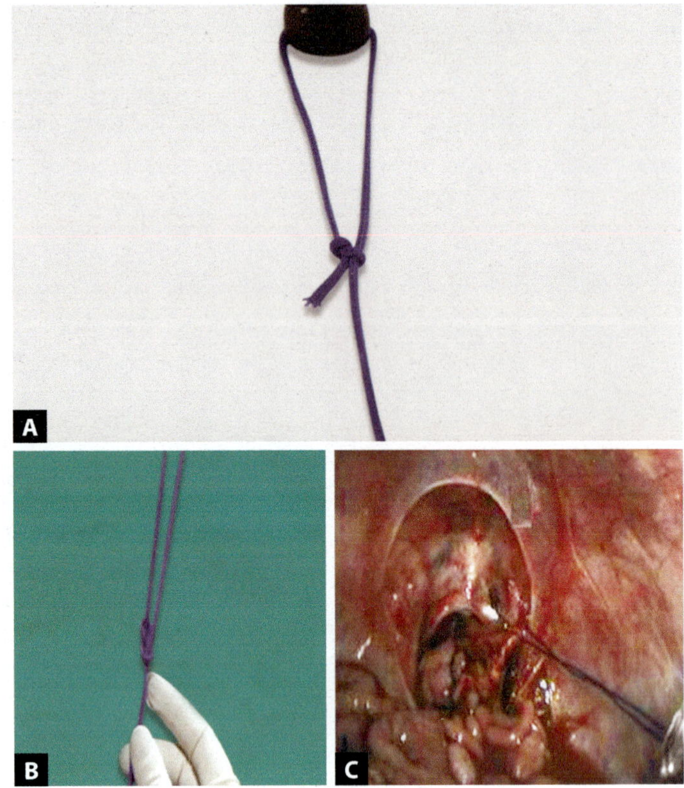

Figs. 8A to C: Slipping of the knot.

Step 8

Following the initial slipping of the knot, it is recommended to secure the knot before finalizing the tie. This locking step is essential to reduce the risk of knot loosening during the subsequent intracorporeal knot-tying process.

To accomplish this, one can employ a straightforward technique. Begin by bending the post limb of the suture. Then, while holding the post limb just above the knot, gently push it toward the knot itself. Simultaneously, apply counter tension by pulling the shorter end of the wrapping limb. This locking maneuver proves particularly beneficial when dealing with suspensory sutures in procedures like colposuspension **(Figs. 9A and B)**.

Step 9

Intracorporeal reinforcing knot **(Figs. 10A and B)**

■ ADVANTAGES

- Simple to use and can slipped down without a knot pusher
- Quick suture
- Suitable for suturing firm tissue while allowing the correction of excessive tension as cooper ligament in laparoscopic Burch suspension or crura of diaphragm during hiatus hernia repair.

■ DISADVANTAGES

- It is weak in strength and needs intracorporeal locking throw to prevent slipping back.

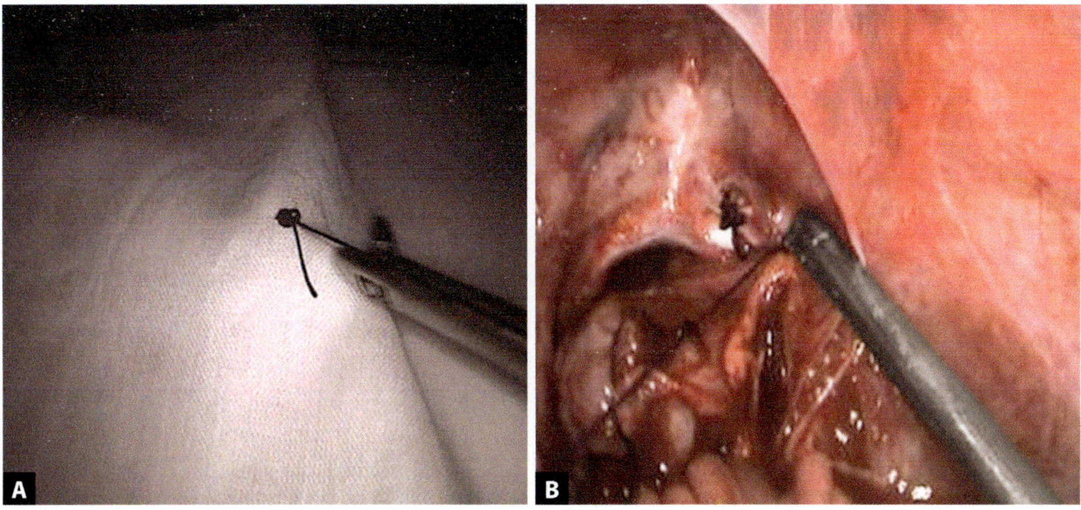

Figs. 9A and B: Knot locking.

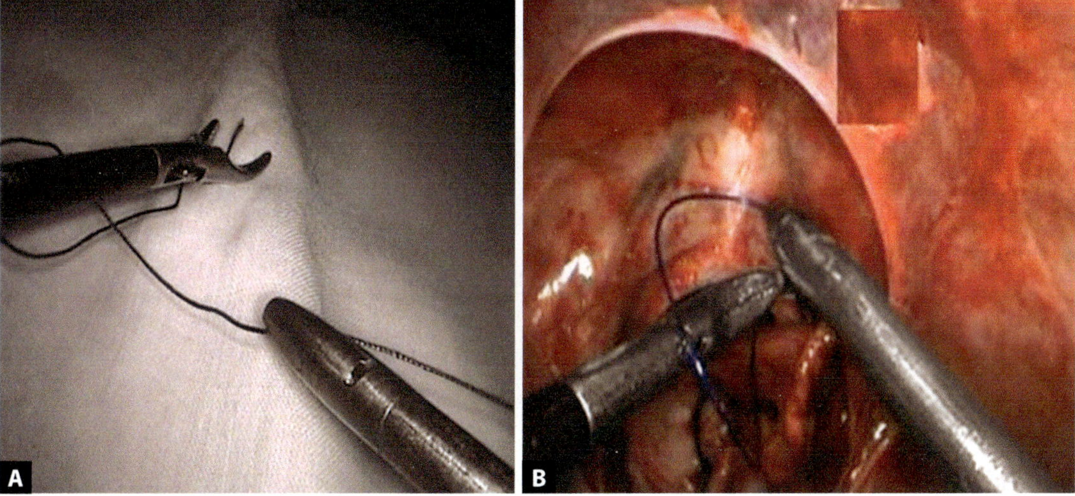

Figs. 10A and B: Reinforcement knot.

- The upward traction pulls on the pedicle (since used without the knot pusher), so it is unsuitable when tying delicate structures as vascular pedicle or bowel.
- Failure of knot tying can occur. This will results in loss of tissue apposition and will lead to clinical failure.

CLINICAL APPLICATIONS

Weston knot is favored in some gynecologic procedures such as laparoscopic colposuspension, laparoscopic pelvic floor repair, and closure of vaginal vault in total laparoscopic hysterectomy **(Figs. 11 and 12)**.

It is also used by ophthalmologist for post chamber operation. Orthopedic surgeon also uses it during orthoscopic surgeries of joint during arthroscopy.

RECOMMENDATION

- To use it in difficult places where intracorporeal suture is difficult to apply
- To apply it on tough structures where pulling force will not affect the tissue integrity because knot pusher is not used

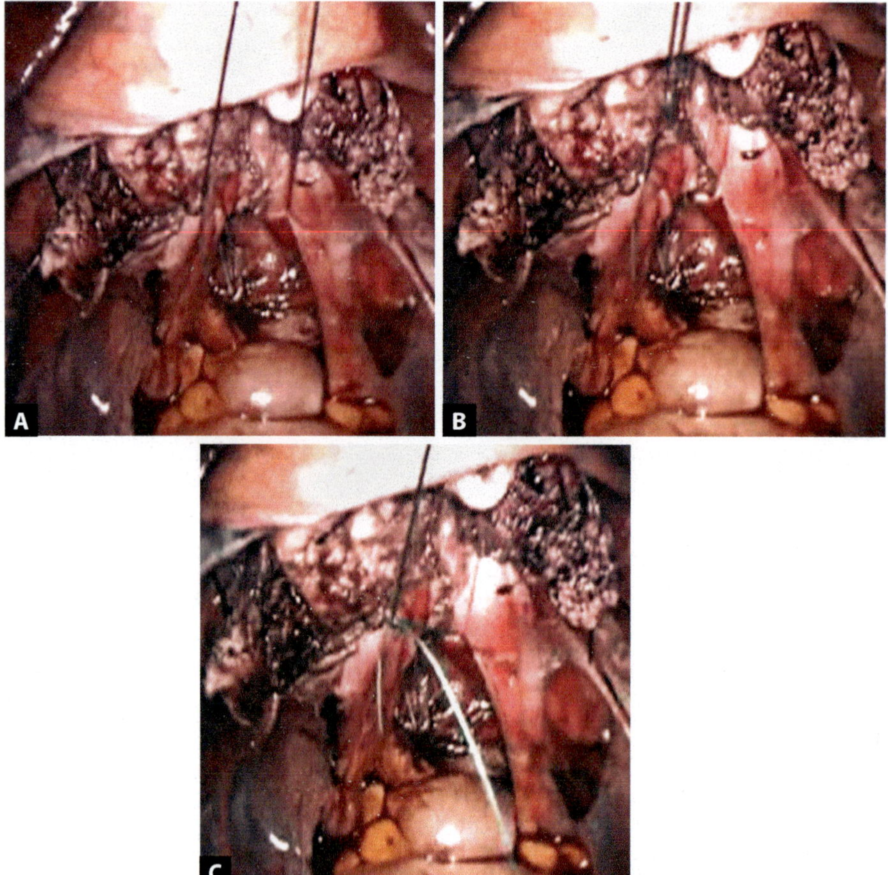

Figs. 11A to C: Uterosacral ligament.

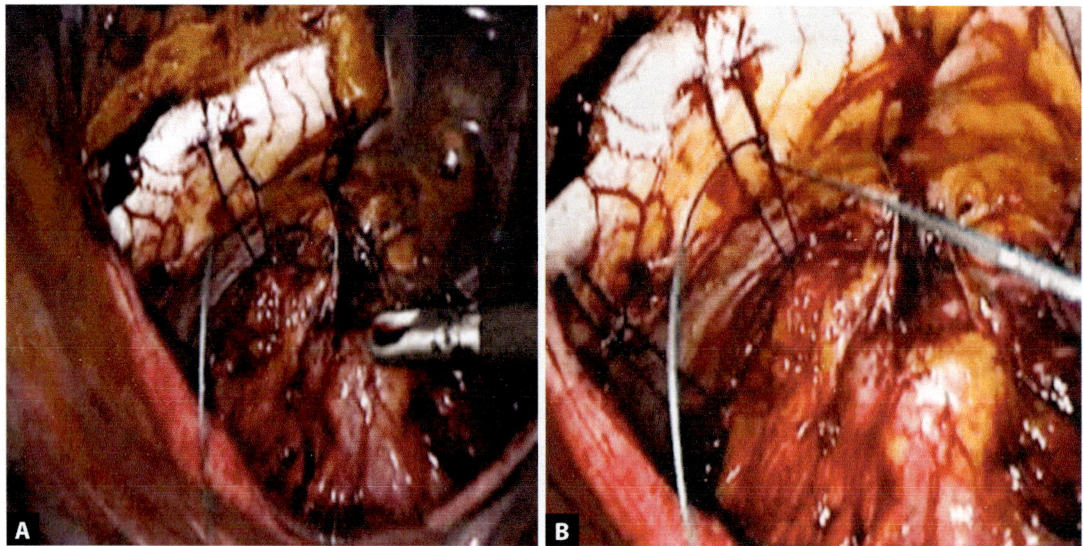

Figs. 12A and B: Colposuspension.

■ CONCLUSION

The Weston knot is an effective extracorporeal sliding suture that offers simplicity, quick execution, and easy manipulation, making it a preferred choice for various endoscopic surgeons. When coupled with high-quality sutures and skilled knot-tying techniques, it results in an optimal knot configuration. This combination, along with proficient surgical skills, leads to the anticipation of excellent clinical outcomes and high success rates.

■ BIBLIOGRAPHY

1. Chen MH, Khalil H (Eds). Laparoscopic Suturing Techniques for Surgeons. Oxford: Oxford University Press; 2022.
2. Choi E, Kim DY. The Use of Biodegradable Sutures in Laparoscopic Surgery. J Biomed Mat. 2024;15(3):438-45.
3. Cushieri A, Shimi SM, Vander Velpen G. Holding and tensile characteristics of extracorporeal slipknots. Surg Endosc. 1994;8(12): 1285-91.
4. Fernandez R, Martin CJ. Ergonomics in Laparoscopic Suturing: Minimizing Surgeon Fatigue. J Ergonomics Surg. 2023;17(3):145-54.
5. Gomez R, Lee T. Evolution of Suturing Techniques in Laparoscopic Surgery. J Minim Invasive Sur. 2021;28(2):123-32.
6. Gupta S, Mehra R. Barriers to Learning Laparoscopic Suturing: A Survey of Surgical Residents. Education Surg. 2023;47(1):55-62.
7. Harper D, Lombardi A. Adapting Traditional Suturing Techniques for Laparoscopic Applications. Surg Techniques Rev. 2021;35(4):320-8.
8. Jain N (Ed). State of the Art, Atlas and Textbook of Laparoscopic Suturing. New Delhi: Jaypee Brothers Medical Publishers (P) Ltd.; 2006.
9. Kumar V, Saxena AK (Eds). Advanced Techniques in Laparoscopic Surgery. Berlin: Springer; 2020.
10. Lavelle JF, Sinclair MF. Automated Suturing Devices in Laparoscopic Surgery: A Comparative Analysis. Technol Surg. 2020;22(6):789-98.
11. Lee J, Kim S. Innovations in Laparoscopic Suturing Instruments. Int J Med Robot. 2022;18(1):e2210.
12. Lo I. (2008). Essential Principles of Tying Secure Arthroscopic Knots. [online] Available from https://www.vumedi.com/video/essential-principles-of-tying-secure-arthroscopic-knots/ [Last accessed May, 2024].
13. Mendez C, Gupta A. Laparoscopic Suturing: Mastery Through Technique and Practice. London: Elsevier Health Sciences; 2023.
14. Mishra RK (Ed). Textbook of Laparoscopy for Surgeons and Gynecologists, 4th edition. New Delhi: Jaypee Brothers Medical Publishers (P) Ltd.; 2021. pp. 900.
15. Mishra RK (Ed). Textbook of Practical Laparoscopic Surgery. New Delhi: Jaypee Brothers Medical Publishers (P) Ltd.; 2008.
16. Mishra RK. Textbook of Practical Laparoscopic Surgery. Jaypee Brothers Medical Publishers, New Delhi, 2007; pp. 104-23.
17. Morrison T, Jacobs LR. Teaching Laparoscopic Suturing: The Role of Simulation in Medical Schools. Med Teacher. 2021;43(7):778-84.
18. Nguyen L, Ho CP. Impact of Suture Materials on Laparoscopic Knot Reliability. Mat Surg. 2024;9(2): 200-10.
19. O'Reilly MP, Saunders BH. Virtual Reality Training for Laparoscopic Surgery. Cambridge: Cambridge University Press; 2022.
20. Patel R, Thompson J. The Role of Simulation in Learning Laparoscopic Suturing and Knotting. Med Education Online. 2021;26:1857289.
21. Rodriguez A, Davis SS. Robotic-Assisted Laparoscopic Knot Tying: Methods and Efficiency. Surg Innov. 2019;26(4):459-66.
22. Shimi SM, Lirici MM, Vander Velpen G, Cuschieri A. Comparative study of holding strength of slipknot using absorbable and nonabsorbable ligature materials. Surg Endosc. 1994;11:1285-91.
23. Smith JA, Patel VR (Eds). Principles of Laparoscopic Suturing and Knotting. New York: Springer; 2023.
24. Surgical Knots and Suturing Techniques. (2024). Available from https://en.wikipedia.org/wiki/Surgical_knot.
25. Wang Y, Thompson C. Innovations in Knot Tying Techniques for Minimally Invasive Surgery. Innov Surg. 2022;18(4):250-60.
26. Weston PV. A new clinch knot. Obstet Gynecol. 1991;78(1); 144-7.
27. Weston PV. A new clinch knot. Obstet Gynecol. 1991; 78:144-7.
28. Williams NE, Tan JL. Comparative Study of Knot Security in Laparoscopic Surgery. J Surg Res. 2020;245:217-23.
29. Zimmerman KA, Patel ND. Laparoscopic Knotting: A Visual Guide for Surgeons. Philadelphia: Lippincott Williams & Wilkins; 2022.

Square Knot

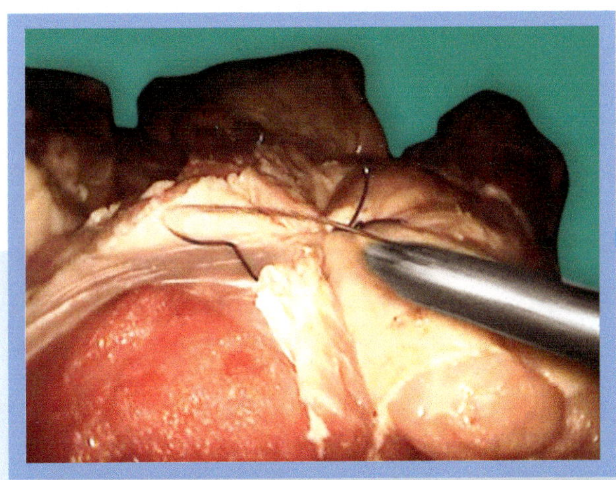

◼ INTRODUCTION

Tissue approximation in laparoscopic surgery encompasses a wide array of techniques, including extracorporeal knotting, loop ligatures, intracorporeal suturing and knotting, and the utilization of various suture assist devices. Proficiency in laparoscopic suturing and knotting instills a strong sense of confidence, enabling surgeons to reconstruct vital organs, repair inadvertent injuries, or control bleeding when other methods are either ineffective or unsuitable.

Among these techniques, intracorporeal suturing and knot tying are generally preferred in laparoscopic tissue approximation due to their versatility, flexibility, cost-effectiveness, and reliance on readily available equipment. However, in certain deep cavities and specific situations, extracorporeal knotting may be the preferred choice.

A skilled laparoscopic surgeon must possess the ability to perform laparoscopic suturing and knotting, as this skill is vital for enhancing the precision and safety of advanced and intricate procedures.

The square knot stands as a fundamental knot that every surgeon, whether engaged in open or laparoscopic surgery, must master. It is created by first tying a single half knot, followed by another half knot in the opposite direction. The sequence for a square knot is "right over left, left over right" or "left over right, right over left."

However, the square knot is susceptible to slippage when tissues are under tension. In case slippage occurs, it can be converted into a square slip knot and securely tied **(Figs. 1A to C)**.

Extracorporeal square knots are tied externally and then pushed down onto the tissue using a knot pusher. This method necessitates longer threads. Although extracorporeal knotting may seem simpler, it requires a systematic and careful approach to prevent tissue trauma and avoid contaminating or damaging the suture material.

◼ APPLICATION

- Laparoscopic tissue approximation, especially for tubular structures
- Ligation of the appendix during laparoscopic appendectomy
- Ligation of small blood vessels

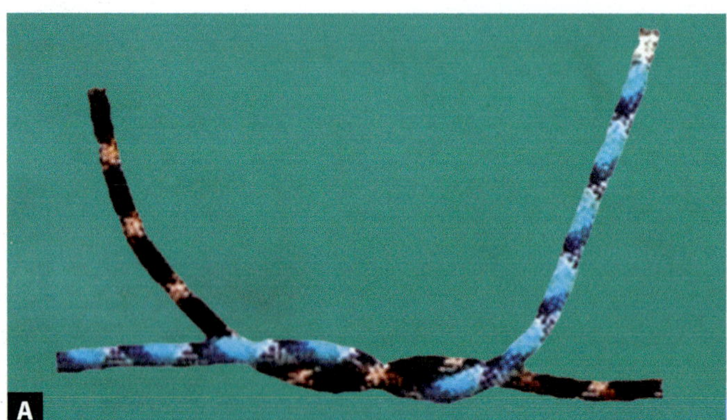

First part of square knot

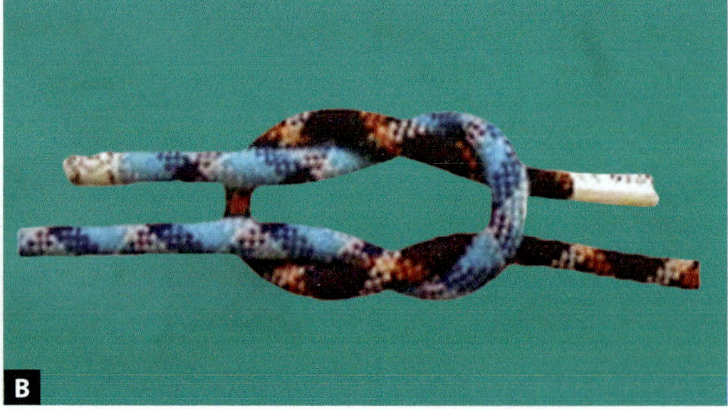

Left over right, under then through

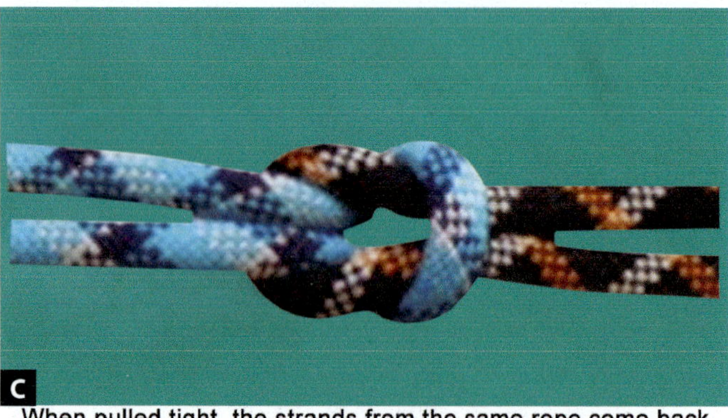

When pulled tight, the strands from the same rope come back out of the knot together in the same direction

Figs. 1A to C: Square knot.

- Various gynecological surgeries such as myomectomy and for vault closure during total laparoscopic hysterectomy.

ADVANTAGES

- Ability to secure the knot
- The use of standard tying method
- Only two half throws—thus, the knot size is small that the foreign body load is reduced.

DISADVANTAGES

- It cannot be used to tie large vessels.
- Not suitable for ligation of thick structures because it tends to loosen in such situations
- Cannot be used to approximate tissues requiring tension as in hernia repair
- Waste of thread since long thread is used for one tie; thus, the remaining thread thrown

STEPS OF EXTRACORPOREAL SQUARE KNOT

Step 1

A long suture (90 cm) with attached needle inserted into the abdominal cavity using Maryland forceps through 10 mm port with the aid of 5 mm reducer to avoid air leak and the needle dropped on the tissue to be sutured, but the tail of the thread remains outside the abdominal cavity.

Step 2

The needle is held by a needle holder at junction of the middle one third and proximal one third near the thread as shown in **Figures 2 and 3**.

Step 3

The needle passed in the tissue is to be approximated perpendicular and then the needle supinated to take the first bite as shown in **Figures 4 to 6**.

Step 4

The needle grasped and the second bite taken to approximate the two margins with help of Maryland forceps which support the tissue when the bite taken and needle removed from other side as shown in **Figures 7 and 8**.

Step 5

After the needle is passed from the other side of tissue, the thread is fed into the abdominal cavity, while the tail of

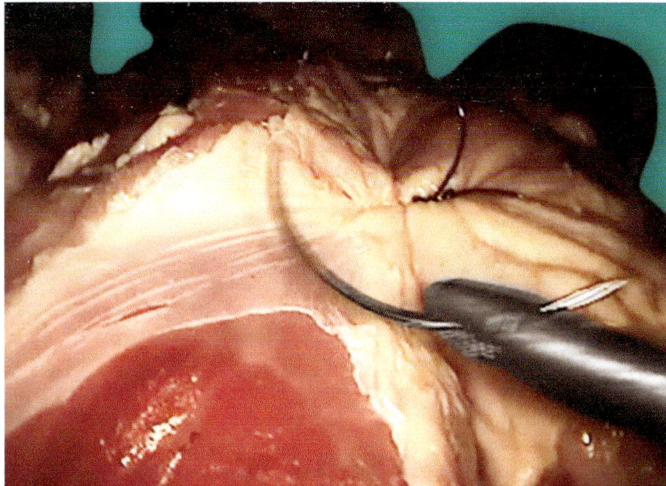

Fig. 2: The needle engaged into the needle holder.

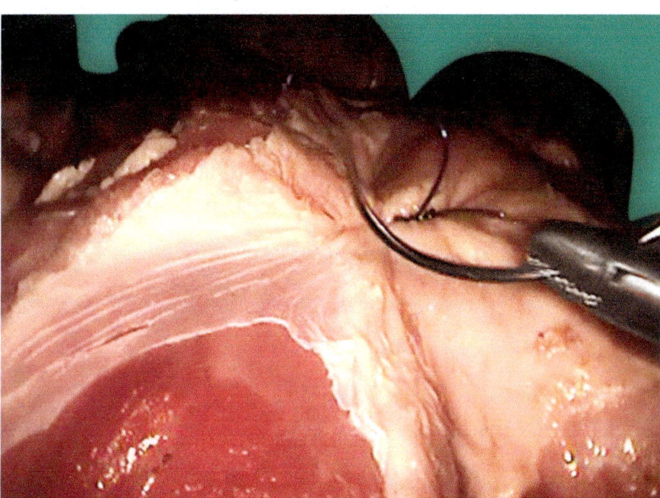

Fig. 3: The needle properly grasped by the needle holder.

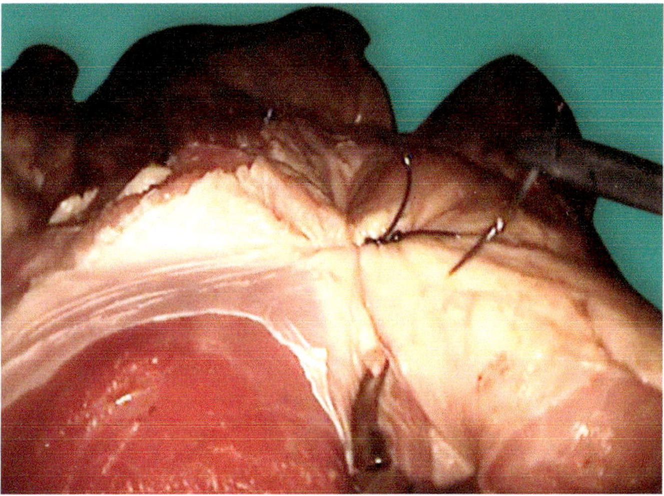

Fig. 4: The needle penetrates tissue perpendicularly, while the Maryland forceps supports the tissue for proper taking of bite.

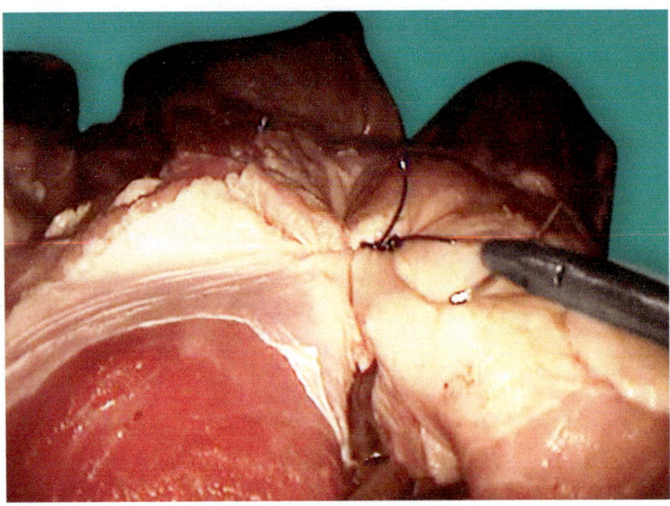

Fig. 5: How the bite is taken.

thread remains outside the abdominal cavity As shown in **Figures 9A to G**.

Step 6

The needle is brought out from the abdominal cavity using needle forceps through the port by grasping the thread close to the needle (**Figs. 10 and 11**).

Step 7

Extraperitoneal portion of the extracorporeal square knot: The first hitch extracorporeal square is formed by grasping the left limb, which should be shorter than the right limb, by artery forceps, and then passing it below the right limb, then over it and released, and the artery forceps passed

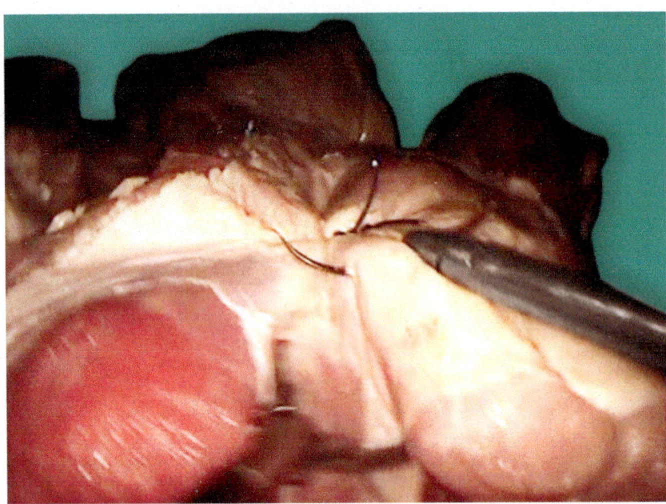

Fig. 6: First bite taken by supination of the needle.

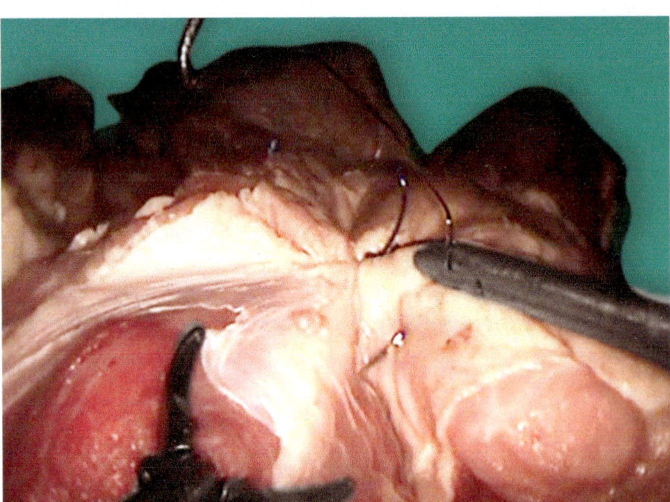

Fig. 7: Insertion of the needle into the second margin to be approximated.

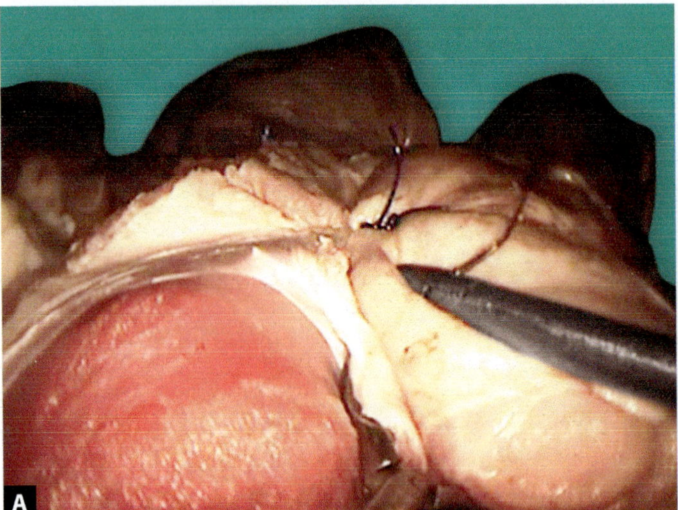

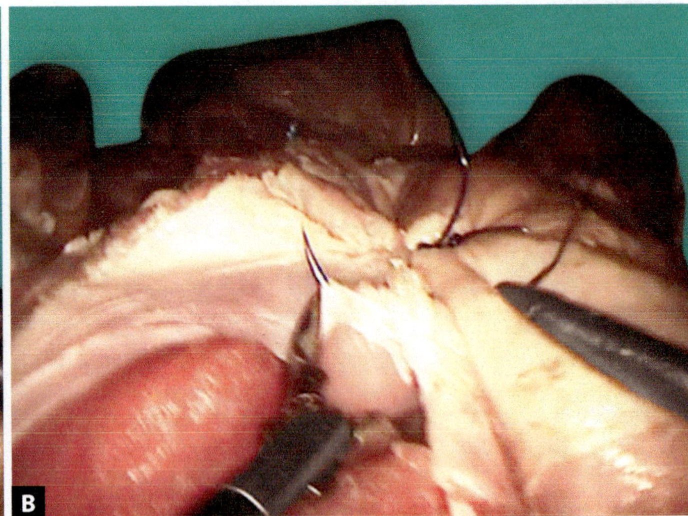

Figs. 8A and B: Maryland forceps aiding approximation of the tissue margins while the needle supinated to take proper bite.

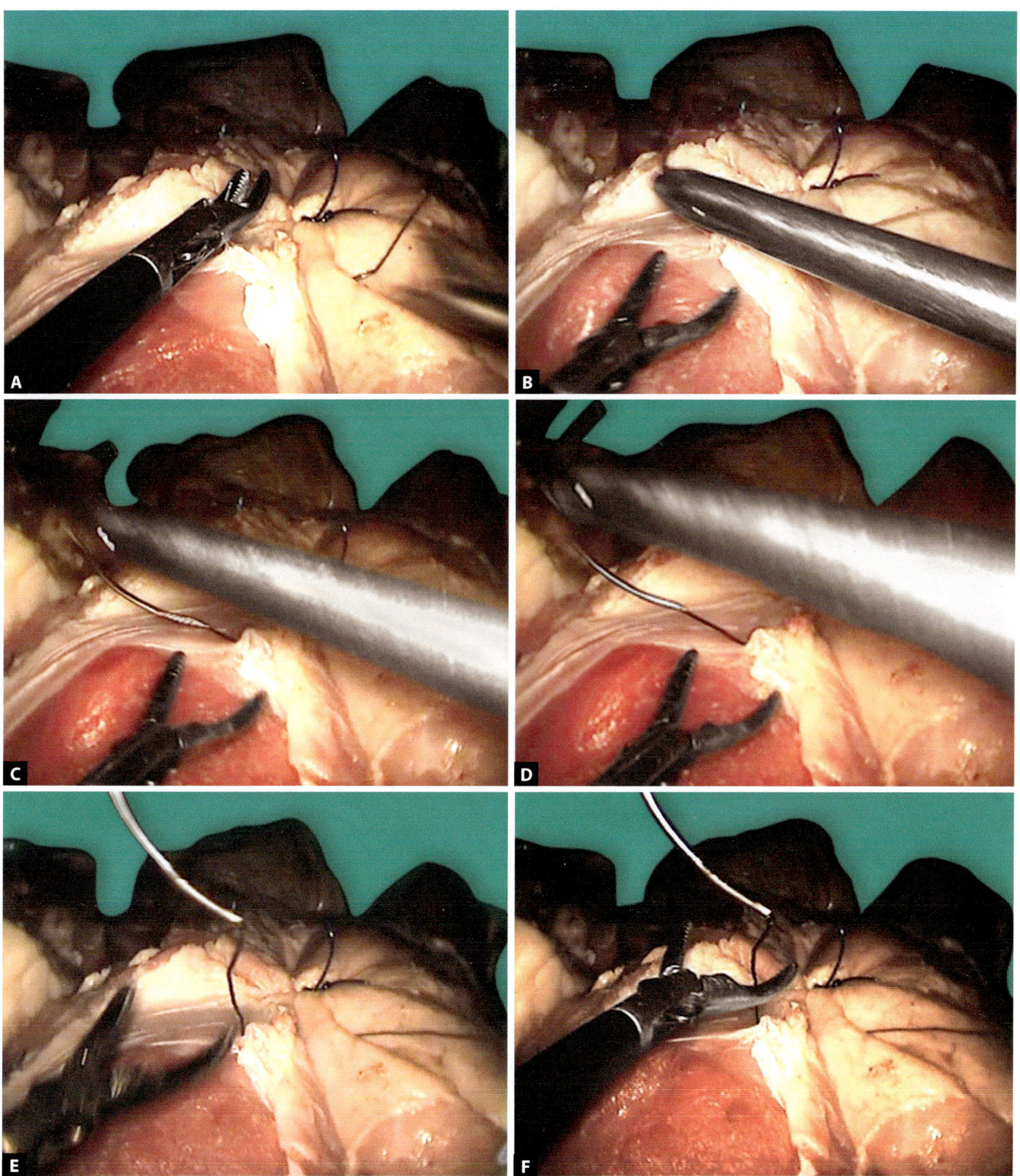

Figs. 9A to F

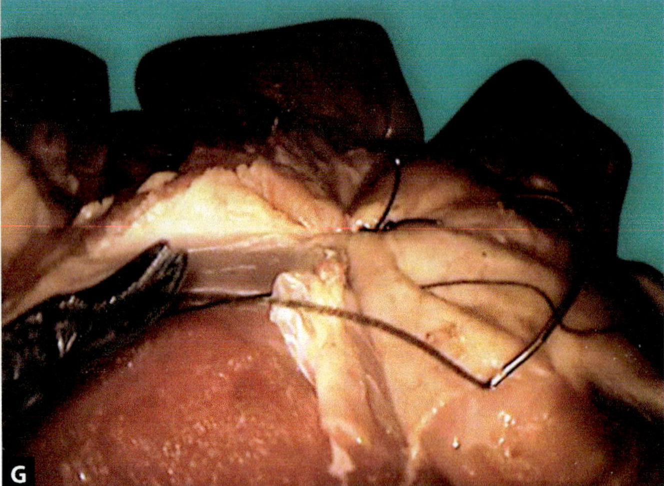

Figs. 9A to G: (A) Bite taken by the needle and (B) exit of the needle with the aid of the needle holder while the Maryland forceps stabilizing the tissue. Needle passage during bite and feeding in of the thread. (C to E) Delivery of the needle from suture margin with Maryland forceps supporting the tissue and (F and G) feeding in of the thread using Maryland forceps.

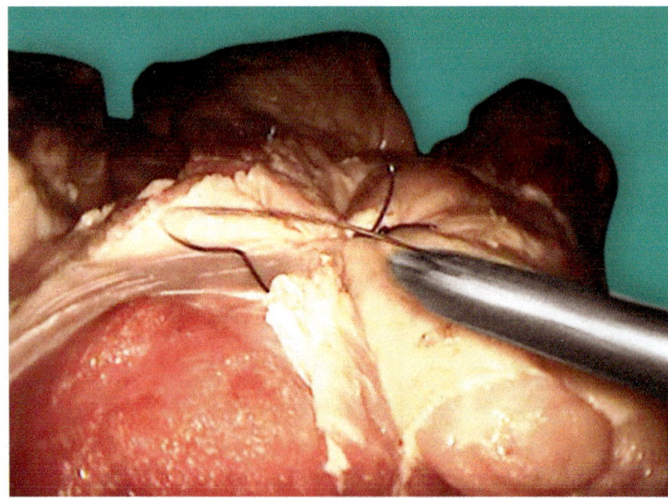

Fig. 10: Needle forceps grasping the thread close to the needle to take it out safely for external portion of the extracorporeal square knot.

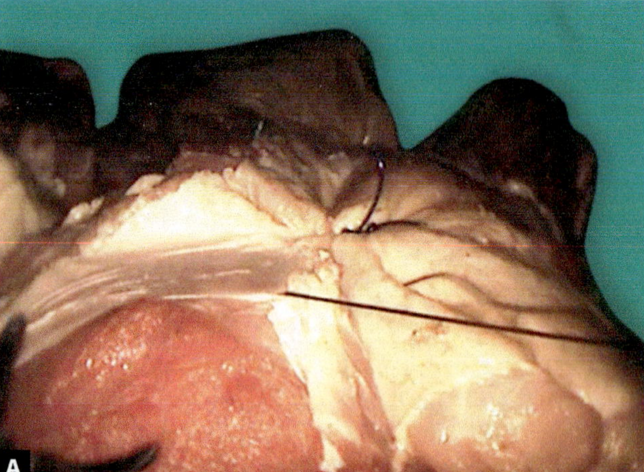

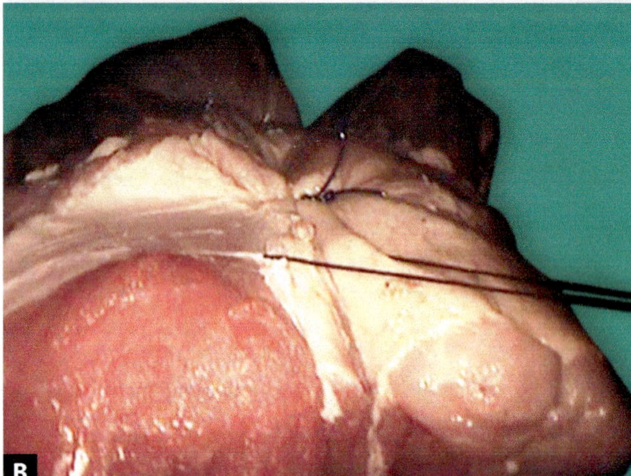

Figs. 11A and B: Two limbs of the thread whose ends are extracorporeal for the second stage of the knot.

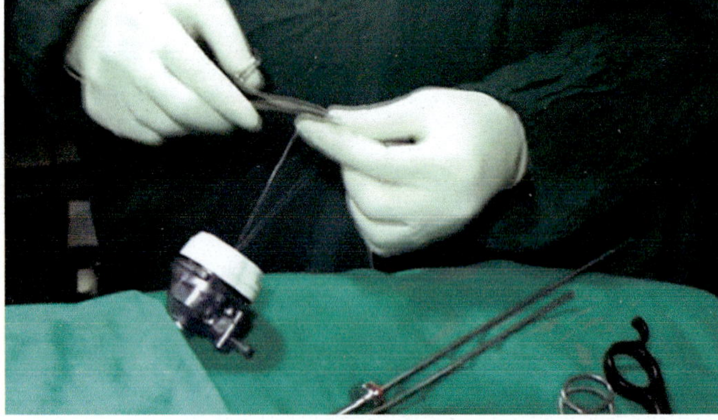

Fig. 12: Artery forceps grasping the left short limb and passing it below the long limb and back over it.

between the two limbs from below and it grasps the left short limb of the thread and then placed on the towel on the left side as shown in **Figures 12 and 13**.

Step 8

The tip of the long limb of the thread inserted into the eye on the tip of the knot pusher as shown in **Figures 14A to D**.

Step 9

The tip of the long limb of the thread held between the thumb and index finger of the right hand after it has passed through the eye of the needle holder and the knot

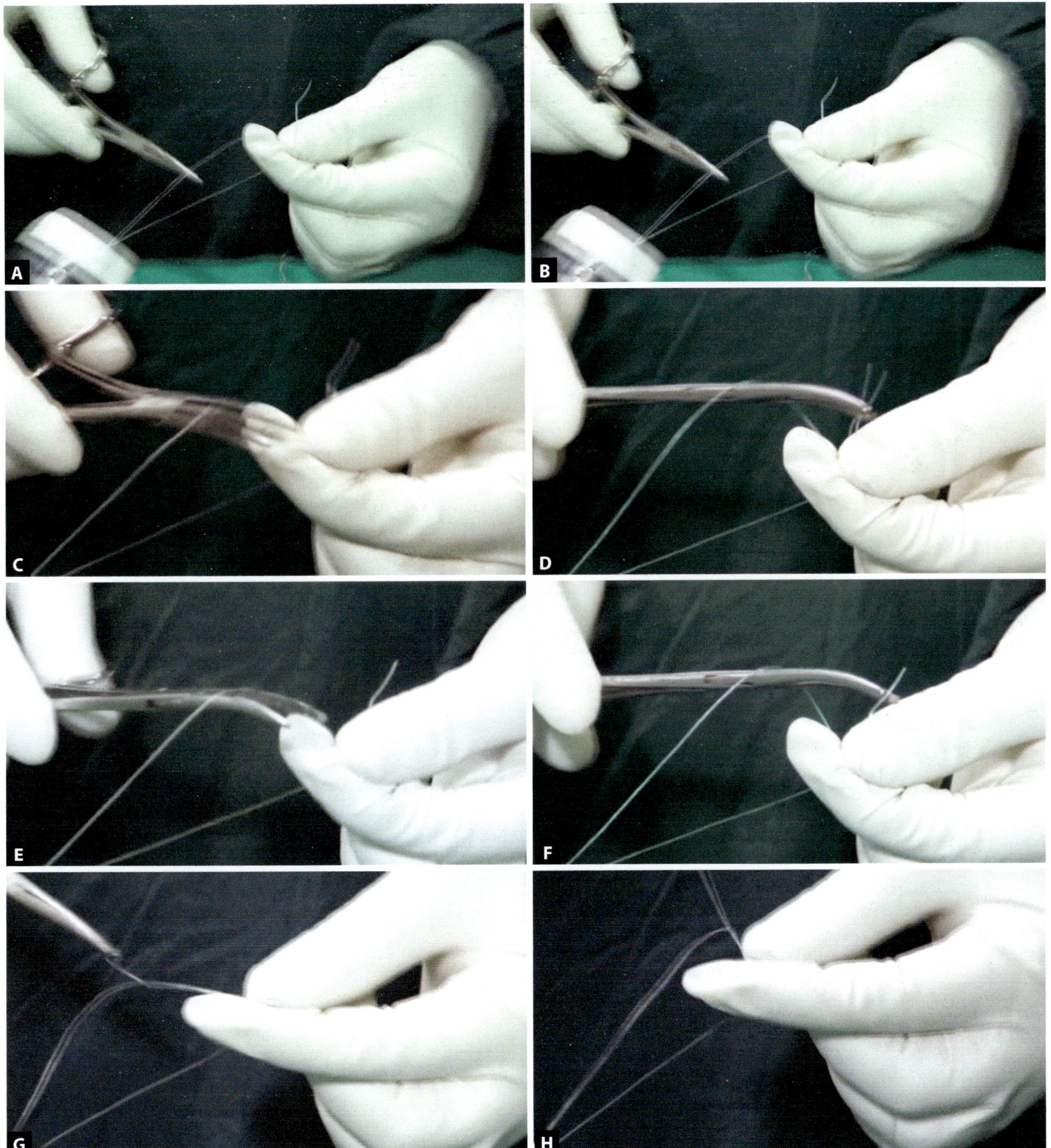

Figs. 13A to H

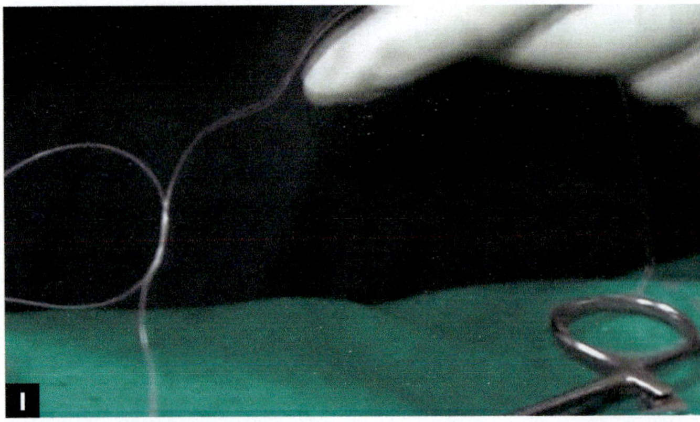

Figs. 13A to I: Artery forceps releases the short limb of the thread and passes in between the limbs of the thread from below and grasps again the tip of the short limb of the thread, thus forming the first hitch of the extracorporeal square knot.

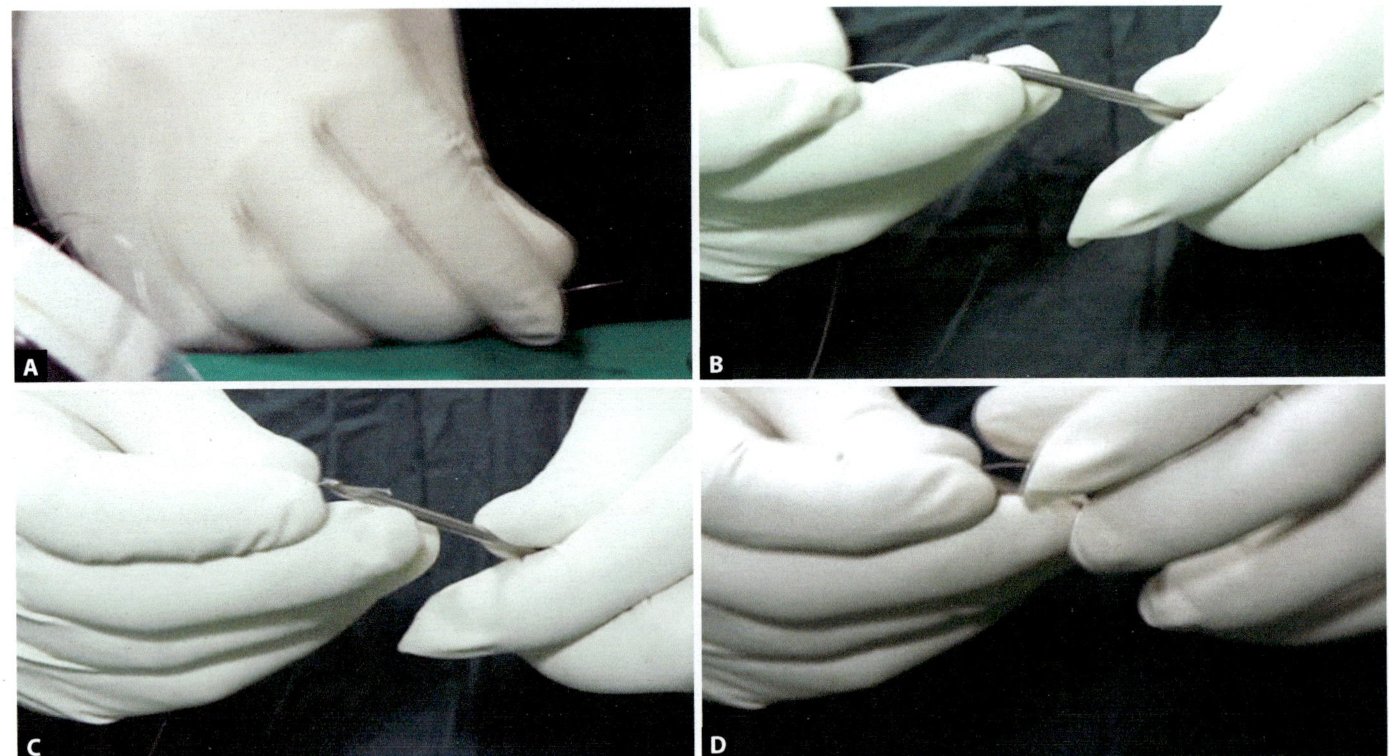

Figs. 14A to D: Insertion of the long limb of the thread into the knot pusher.

pusher advanced in front of the knot to enter the peritoneal cavity through the port to tie the knot as shown in **Figures 15A to H**.

Step 10

Intracorporeal portion of the extracorporeal square knot: The knot pusher inserted into the abdominal cavity through the port in front of the knot directed to the tissue sutured in steps 3 and 4 as shown in **Figures 16A to H**.

Step 11

The knot pusher pushed in front of the knot to beyond the tissue to be sutured to acquire the past point character. This is specific to extracorporeal square knot, the most important step to secure the knot as shown in **Figures 17A and B**.

Step 12

The knot is tied using the knot pusher by past point to secure the knot; this is the most important step in

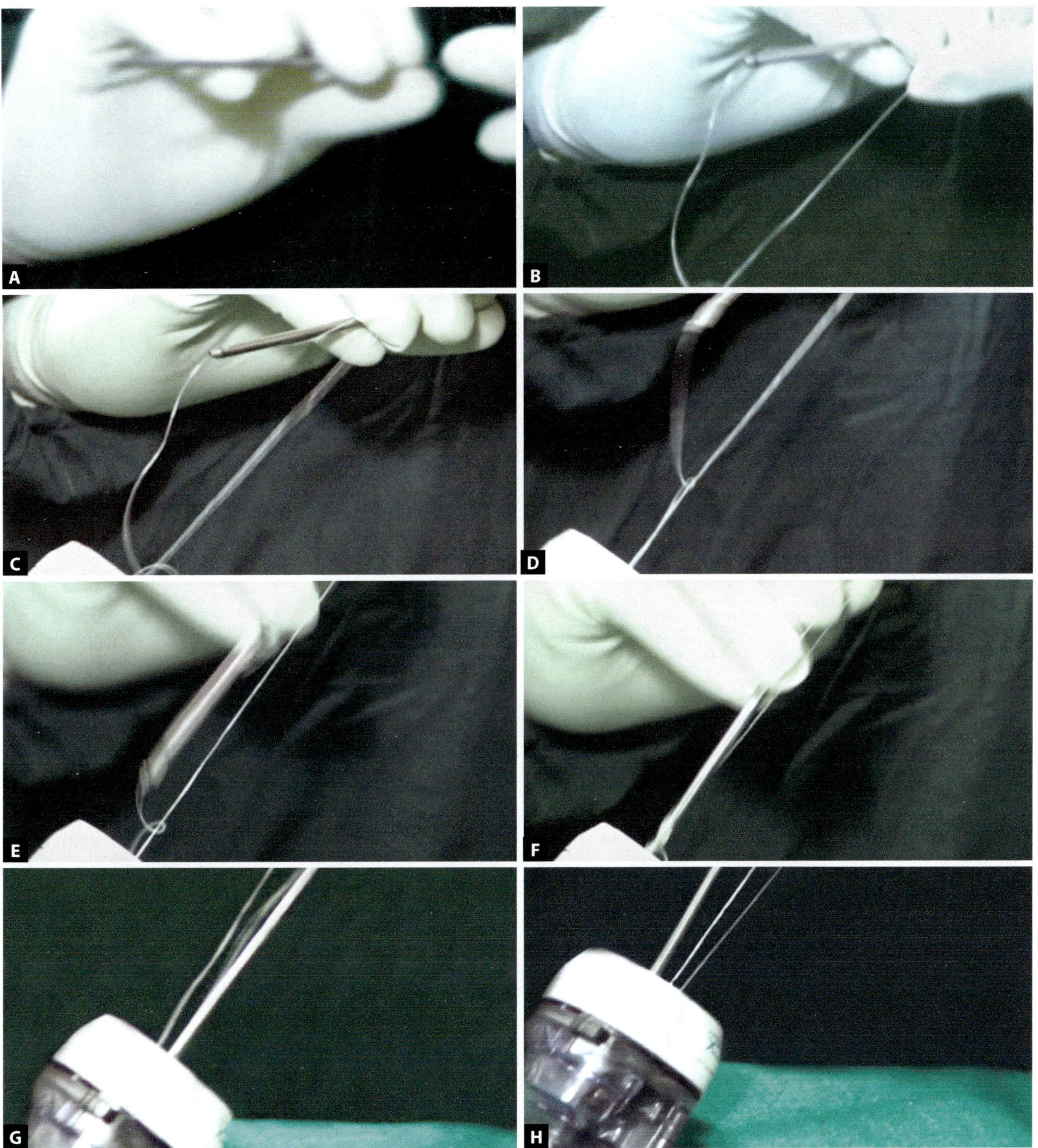

Figs. 15A to H: How the knot pusher pushes the knot into the port.

extracorporeal square knot and unique to it as in other extracorporeal knot the knot pusher is pushed behind the knot to tie it **(Fig. 18)**.

N.B.: The knot pusher must be pushed in front of the knot to get the past point character specific to extracorporeal square knot shown in the next step.

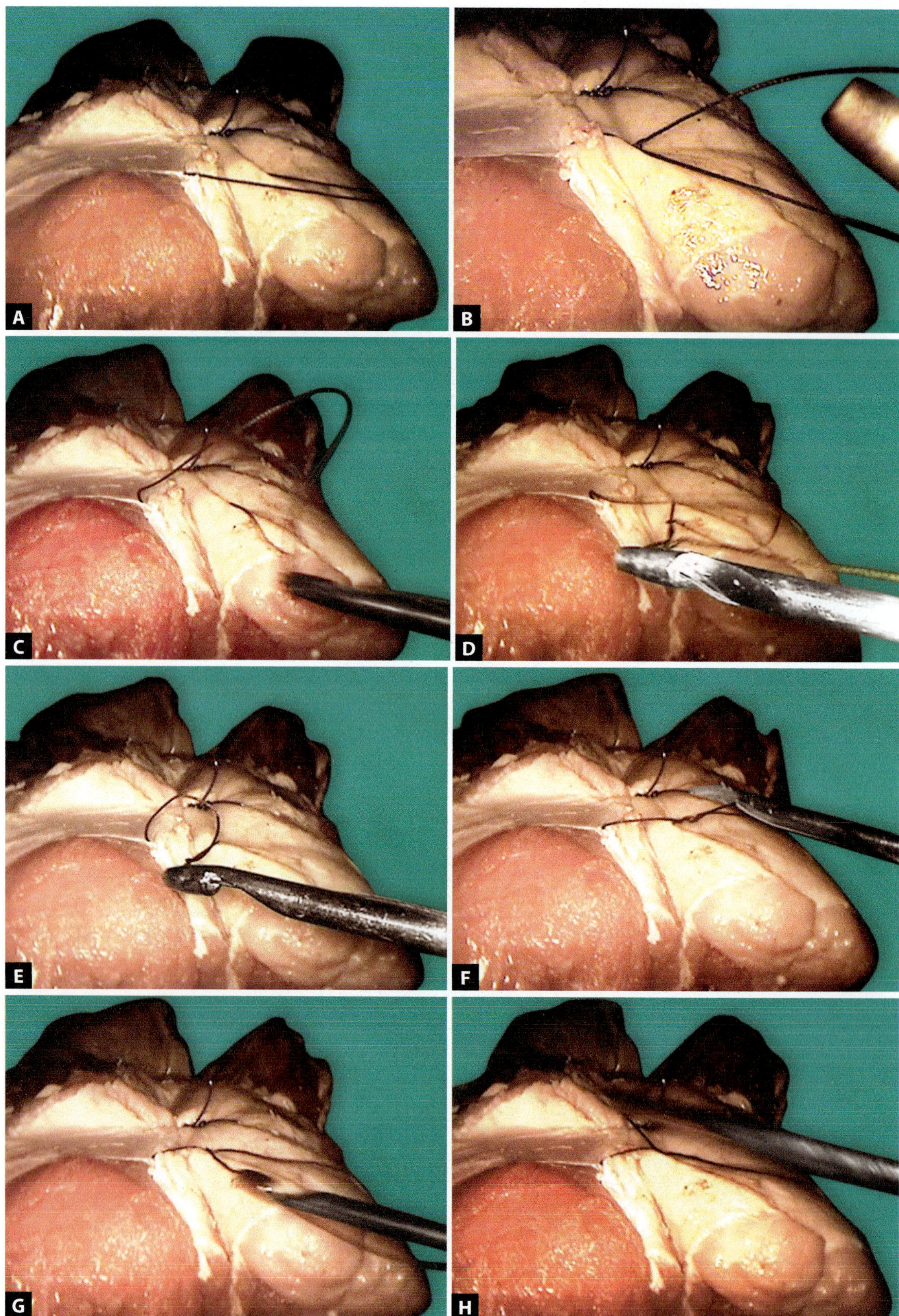

Figs. 16A to H: Introduce the knot pusher into the peritoneal cavity to tie the suture by passing the knot pusher in front of the knot.

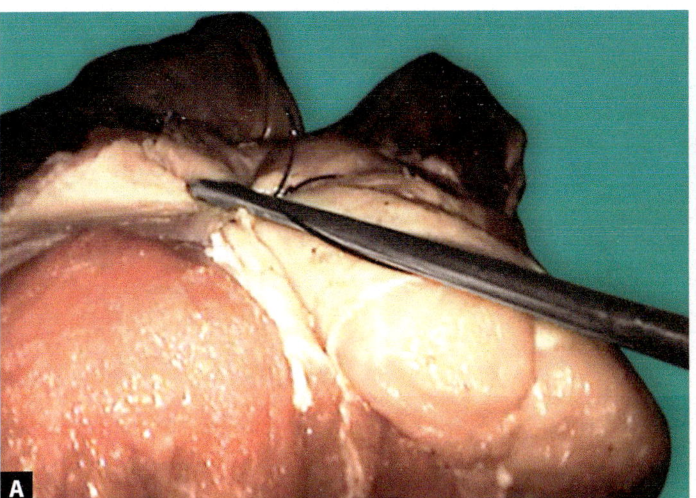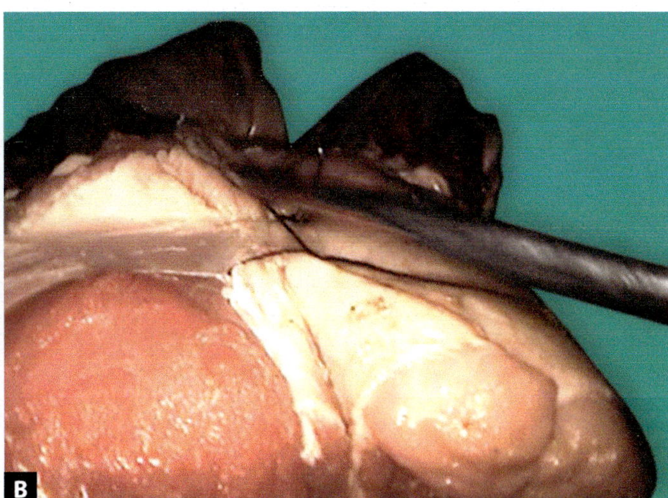

Figs. 17A and B: Knot pusher past point.

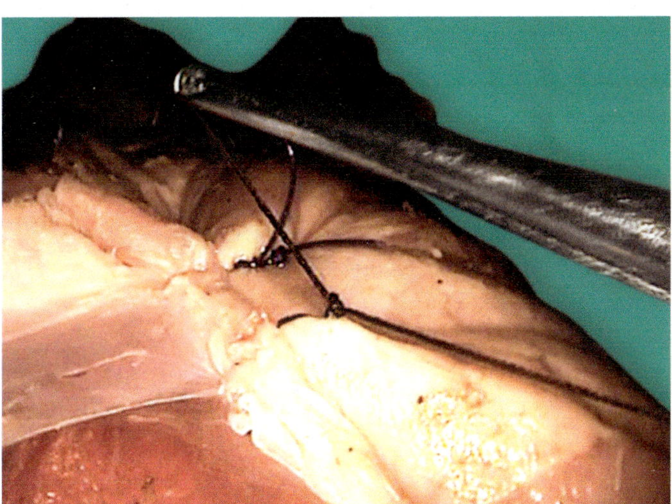

Fig. 18: Past point tying of the knot.

Step 13

The needle pusher is brought out of the abdominal cavity to prepare and push the knot; the thread is not removed from the knot pusher.

Step 14

The second hitch of the extracorporeal square knot is formed by passing the short limb of the thread above the long limb and then below and passed between the limbs from below and held by artery forceps, thus forming the first hitch of the extracorporeal square knot and then the knot pusher advanced in front of the knot and inserted into the port as shown in **Figures 19 and 20**.

Step 15

The knot pusher is advanced past point to tie the second hitch of the extracorporeal square knot as shown in **Figures 21A to G**.

Step 16

The suture is cut 5 mm from the knot as shown in **Figures 22 and 23**.

TASK ANALYSIS OF EXTRACORPOREAL SQUARE KNOT

- Take suture length 90 cm for extracorporeal square knot.
- The Endoski needles are generally preferred than the curved ones.
- For making an Endoski needle, the needle is held at one third from the tip by the needle holder and slightly away from that by the base of artery forceps.
- This will give you an Endoski needle in which two thirds of the needle is straight and one third is curved.
- Now, insert the Maryland in the reducer completely.
- Catch hold the tail of the suture and bring it out through the reducer.
- Reintroduce the Maryland in the reducer by the side of fed suture and catch the suture near the needle and hide the needle in the reducer.
- Now, introduce the Maryland and the reducer together in the abdomen with suture held near the needle.

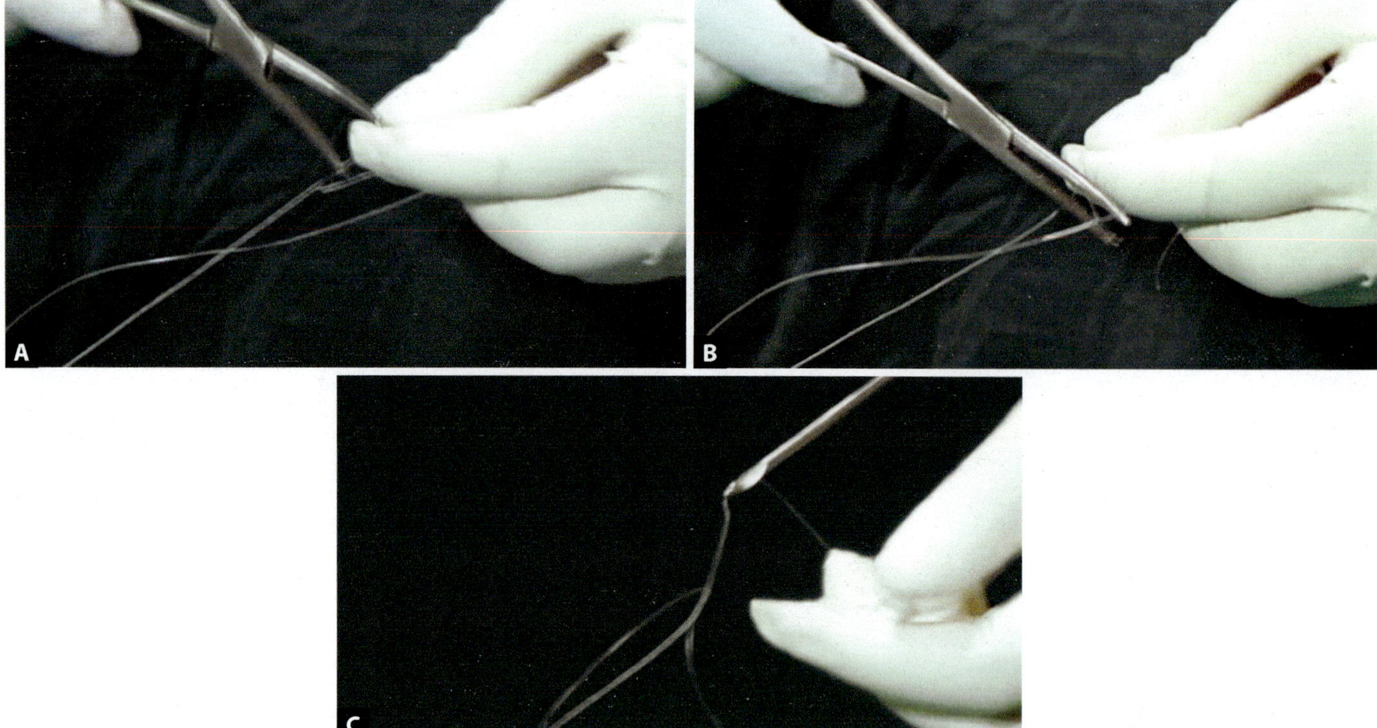

Figs. 19A to C: Formation of the second hitch of the extracorporeal square knot.

- Drop the needle over the tissue in a way that tip should be left and the tail should be right.
- Align the needle by pressing the needle by upper jaw of the needle holder at the junction of one third and two thirds.
- Stabilize the tissue by the left hand and prick the tissue by the needle and by rotating the tip of needle to keep it perpendicular to the tissue.
- Bringing the tip of the needle one third out, catch it with left hand instrument and keep the convex end of the instrument toward the tissue.
- Now, take another bite and hold the needle with the Maryland.
- The suture is now fed inside for a minimum of four times.
- At each feeding, minimum of 5 cm length of the suture should be inside.
- During the process of feeding, the camera person should focus the telescope toward the tip of cannula.
- With the help of the Maryland, the suture should be taken out.
- While taking out the suture, needle holder should support between the suture so that the tissue does not get cut through.

- Ask the assistant for the finger on the reducer and take a half knot, apply an artery forceps in the tail end and keep the needle end straight.
- Keep the Clark knot pusher near the knot and hook it forward.
- Slide the knot keeping the needle end of the suture straight and tail end of suture loose.
- Sliding process should be continuous; any stoppage or withdrawal of Clark knot pusher can make the knot pusher disengaged with the suture.
- Once Clark knot pusher reaches the tissue, do the past pointing to tighten the first half of square knot.
- Now, again bring the Clark knot pusher out and make another half knot and slide it.
- While sliding second time, take care that the same needle limb of suture should have to be straight and tail end is sliding.
- Past pointing is important to make the sliding knot to convert into square locked knot.
- Now, finally take a third time the half knot in similar fashion and each time do past pointing.
- Once the knot is tightened, bring out the knot pusher, take curve scissor, and cut the suture.

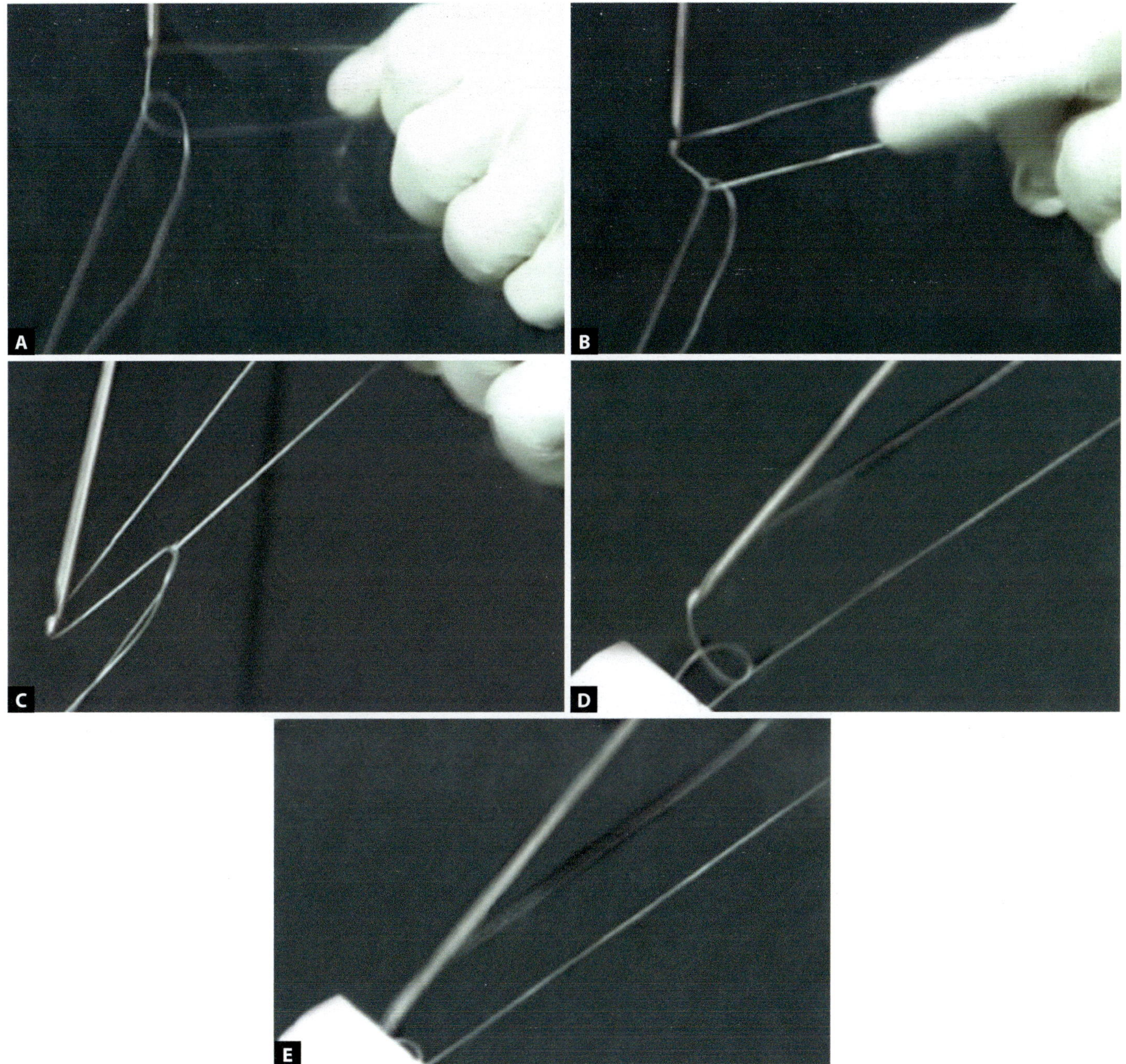

Figs. 20A to E: Knot pusher pushed in front of the knot into the abdomen

- It is basically used for the tissue which are under tension and strong enough to tolerate the past pointing.
- You should never use extracorporeal square knot for any tubular structure and blood vessels.
- This knot is useful for vault closure in total laparoscopic hysterectomy (TLH), myomectomy, fundoplication, and herniorrhaphy.

■ RECOMMENDATION

It is strongly advisable for surgeons to invest ample time in training to master the art of laparoscopic suturing and knotting. These skills are the differentiating factors between basic and advanced laparoscopic surgery. The square knot, being a versatile knot, finds utility in a wide

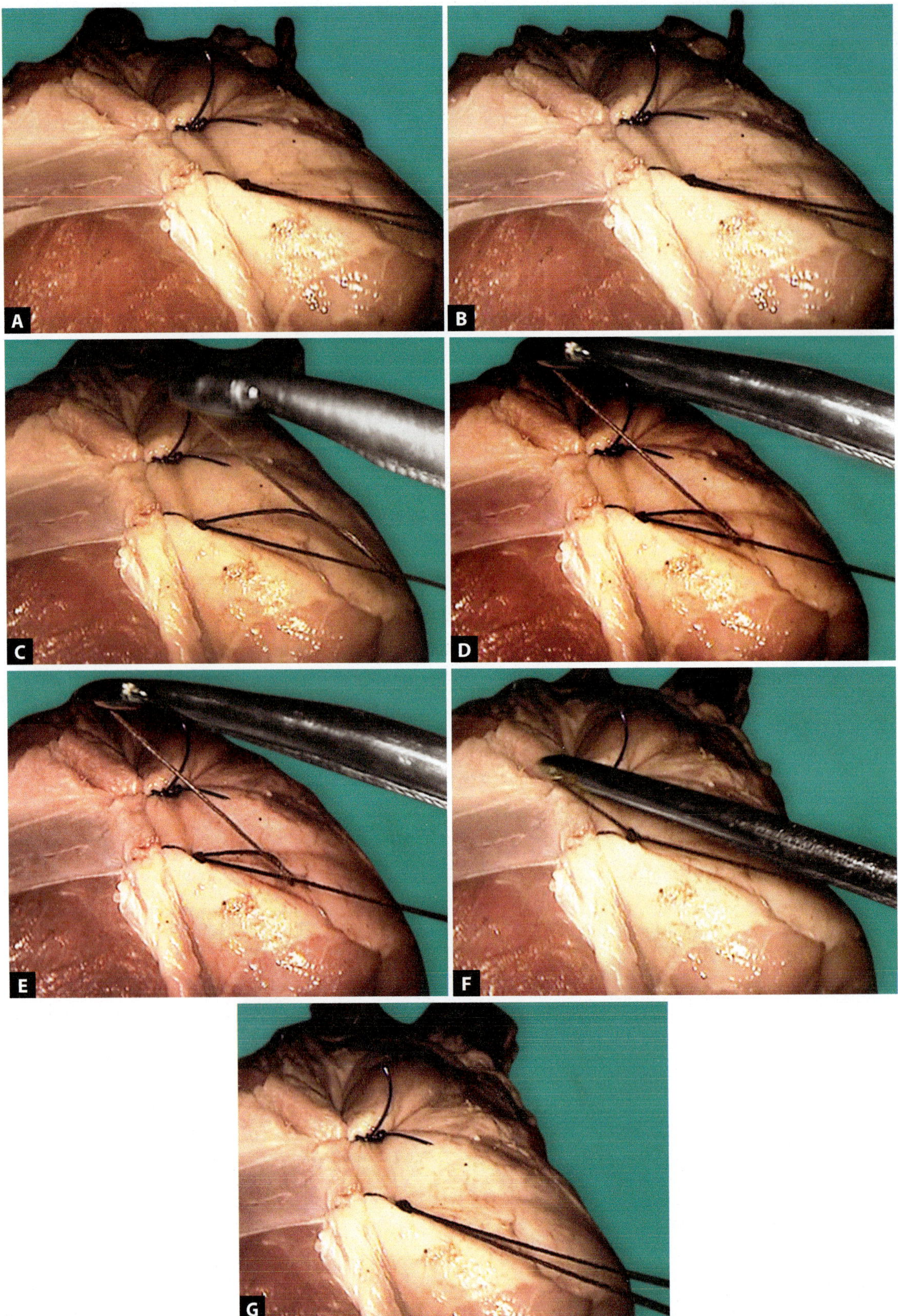

Figs. 21A to G: Knot tying using knot pusher by past point method.

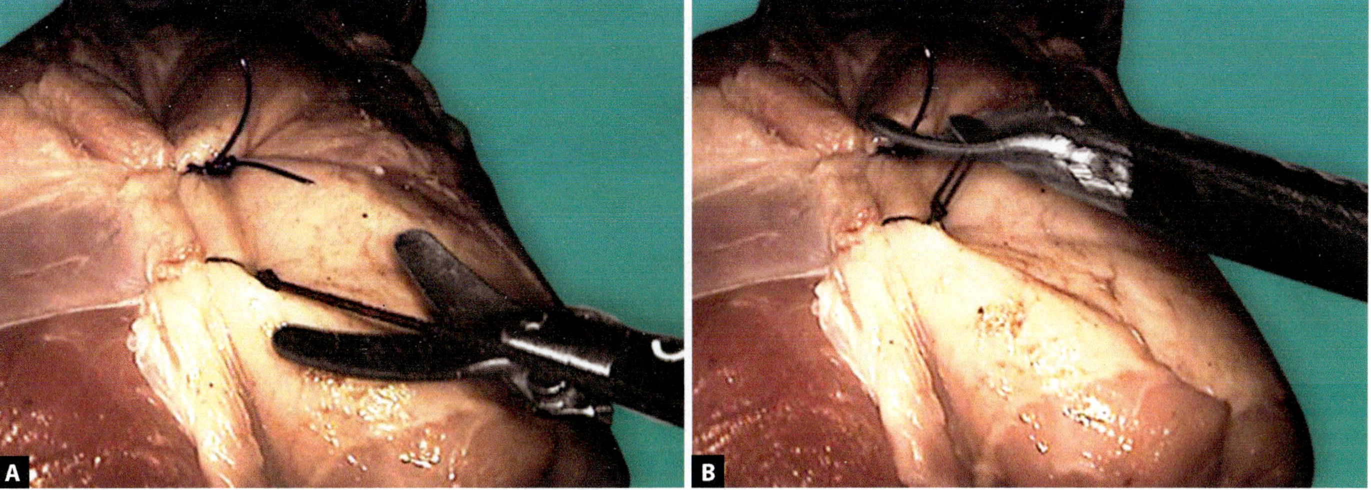

Figs. 22A and B: Cutting the suture after complete tying.

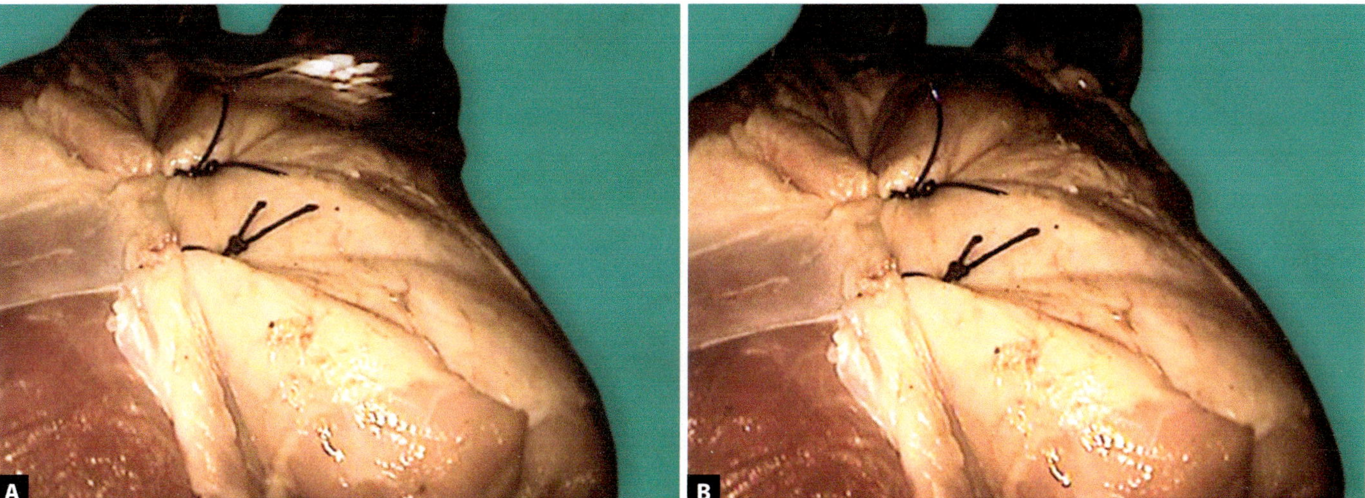

Figs. 23A and B: The final appearance of extracorporeal square knot.

spectrum of laparoscopic procedures, underscoring its significance in enhancing surgical proficiency.

CONCLUSION

The square knot remains a fundamental technique in laparoscopic surgery, essential for surgeons to master due to its versatility and reliability in various procedures. While intracorporeal suturing and knot tying are generally preferred for their flexibility and cost-effectiveness, extracorporeal knotting, such as the square knot, is invaluable in specific situations, particularly in deep cavities. Mastery of the square knot allows surgeons to perform precise tissue approximation, crucial for the success of advanced and intricate laparoscopic procedures.

Despite its susceptibility to slippage under tension, proper technique and careful execution can mitigate this issue, ensuring secure and effective tissue closure. Given its broad applications, from ligating small vessels to securing tubular structures, the square knot is an indispensable skill that enhances surgical proficiency and patient outcomes. It is recommended that surgeons invest significant time in training to perfect their suturing and knot-tying skills, solidifying their competence in both basic and advanced laparoscopic surgery.

BIBLIOGRAPHY

1. Chen MH, Khalil H (Eds). Laparoscopic Suturing Techniques for Surgeons. Oxford: Oxford University Press; 2022.

2. Choi E, Kim DY. The Use of Biodegradable Sutures in Laparoscopic Surgery. J Biomed Mat. 2024;15(3):438-45.

3. Fernandez R, Martin CJ. Ergonomics in Laparoscopic Suturing: Minimizing Surgeon Fatigue. J Ergonomics Surg. 2023;17(3):145-54.

4. Gomez R, Lee T. Evolution of Suturing Techniques in Laparoscopic Surgery. J Minim Invasive Sur. 2021;28(2):123-32.

5. Gupta S, Mehra R. Barriers to Learning Laparoscopic Suturing: A Survey of Surgical Residents. Education Surg. 2023;47(1):55-62.

6. Harper D, Lombardi A. Adapting Traditional Suturing Techniques for Laparoscopic Applications. Surg Techniques Rev. 2021;35(4):320-8.

7. Kumar V, Saxena AK (Eds). Advanced Techniques in Laparoscopic Surgery. Berlin: Springer; 2020.

8. Lavelle JF, Sinclair MF. Automated Suturing Devices in Laparoscopic Surgery: A Comparative Analysis. Technol Surg. 2020;22(6):789-98.

9. Lee J, Kim S. Innovations in Laparoscopic Suturing Instruments. Int J Med Robot. 2022;18(1):e2210.

10. Mendez C, Gupta A. Laparoscopic Suturing: Mastery Through Technique and Practice. London: Elsevier Health Sciences; 2023.

11. Mishra RK (Ed). Textbook of Laparoscopy for Surgeons and Gynecologists, 4th edition. New Delhi: Jaypee Brothers Medical Publishers (P) Ltd.; 2021. pp. 900.

12. Mishra RK. Textbook of Practical Laparoscopic Surgery. Jaypee Brothers Medical Publishers, New Delhi, 2007; pp. 104-23.

13. Morrison T, Jacobs LR. Teaching Laparoscopic Suturing: The Role of Simulation in Medical Schools. Med Teacher. 2021;43(7):778-84.

14. Nguyen L, Ho CP. Impact of Suture Materials on Laparoscopic Knot Reliability. Mat Surg. 2024;9(2):200-10.

15. O'Reilly MP, Saunders BH. Virtual Reality Training for Laparoscopic Surgery. Cambridge: Cambridge University Press; 2022.

16. Patel R, Thompson J. The Role of Simulation in Learning Laparoscopic Suturing and Knotting. Med Education Online. 2021;26:1857289.

17. Rodriguez A, Davis SS. Robotic-Assisted Laparoscopic Knot Tying: Methods and Efficiency. Surg Innov. 2019;26(4):459-66.

18. Shimi SM, Lirici MM, Vander Velpen G, Cuschieri A. Comparative study of holding strength of slipknot using absorbable and nonabsorbable ligature materials. Surg Endosc. 1994;11:1285-91.

19. Smith JA, Patel VR (Eds). Principles of Laparoscopic Suturing and Knotting. New York: Springer; 2023.

20. Surgical Knots and Suturing Techniques. (2024). Available from https://en.wikipedia.org/wiki/Surgical_knot.

21. Wang Y, Thompson C. Innovations in Knot Tying Techniques for Minimally Invasive Surgery. Innov Surg. 2022;18(4):250-60.

22. Williams NE, Tan JL. Comparative Study of Knot Security in Laparoscopic Surgery. J Surg Res. 2020;245:217-23.

23. Zimmerman KA, Patel ND. Laparoscopic Knotting: A Visual Guide for Surgeons. Philadelphia: Lippincott Williams & Wilkins; 2022.

7

CHAPTER

Surgeon's Knot

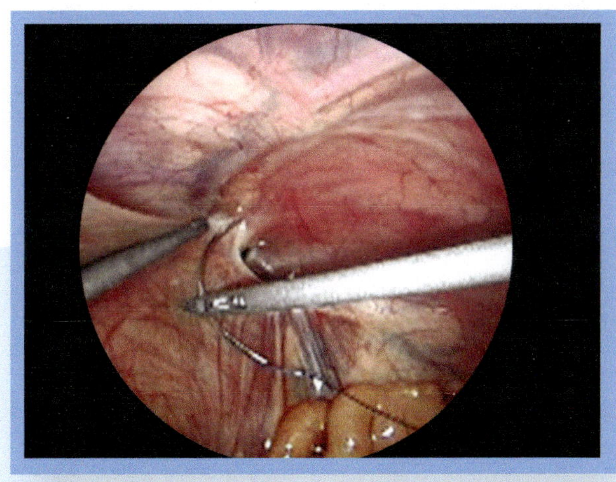

◼ INTRODUCTION

Intracorporeal suturing and knot tying pose some of the most formidable challenges in laparoscopic surgery. The inherent loss of depth perception, diminished tactile feedback, and visual impediments make the precise placement of well-tied knots a demanding and time-consuming endeavor. The suturing technique must be adapted based on the specific instruments being employed. While ongoing research is focused on the development of new needle holders and automated suturing systems, we introduce a straightforward technique that can be effectively utilized with basic surgical instruments.

The realm of laparoscopic surgery, with its minimally invasive techniques, has transformed the surgical field, offering numerous benefits over traditional open surgery, including reduced pain, quicker recovery times, and minimized scarring. A pivotal skill in this domain is the ability to perform a laparoscopic surgeon's knot, which is both an art and a science, requiring precision, dexterity, and an in-depth understanding of the anatomy and surgical principles.

The laparoscopic surgeon's knot, also known as the intracorporeal surgeons knot, is a technique used to securely tie sutures within the body during laparoscopic procedures. This knotting technique is crucial in situations where manual knot tying is impractical due to the limited access and visibility inherent in minimally invasive surgeries.

The execution of a laparoscopic surgeon's knot requires a set of specialized instruments, including needle drivers, scissors, and graspers, all of which are designed to operate through small incisions. The choice of suture material also plays a critical role, with preferences varying based on the tissue type, the need for absorbability, and the required strength of the suture.

One of the primary challenges in laparoscopic knot tying is the lack of tactile feedback, which surgeons typically rely on in open surgeries. To overcome this, laparoscopic surgeons develop a heightened sense of spatial awareness and learn to rely heavily on visual cues from the laparoscopic camera. Additionally, mastering the coordination between hand movements and the instruments' actions is crucial for executing precise and secure knots.

Achieving proficiency in tying laparoscopic surgeon's knots requires extensive practice and training.

Simulation-based training models, including virtual reality simulators and physical models, provide valuable platforms for surgeons to hone their skills in a risk-free environment. Moreover, mentorship and observation of experienced laparoscopic surgeons play a significant role in the learning process.

The laparoscopic surgeon's knot is a testament to the sophistication and advancement of minimally invasive surgery. Its successful execution demands not only technical skill and precision but also an in-depth understanding of the principles of laparoscopy. As the field continues to evolve, so will the techniques and technologies too that enhance the efficacy and safety of laparoscopic surgeries, benefiting both surgeons and patients alike. The journey of mastering the laparoscopic surgeon's knot is both challenging and rewarding, representing a blend of art and science that is at the heart of modern surgery.

◼ INSTRUMENTATION

Needle (Fig. 1)

While conventional open surgical needles with a half-circle design can indeed be utilized endoscopically, the Endoski needle, developed in Dundee, represents a needle specifically engineered for endoscopic applications. It stands as a hybrid, combining features of both straight and half-circle needles. The Endoski needle is equipped with atraumatic suture and features a straight shaft with a terminal tapering curve that corresponds to a quarter of a circle, essentially resembling a miniature ski in shape.

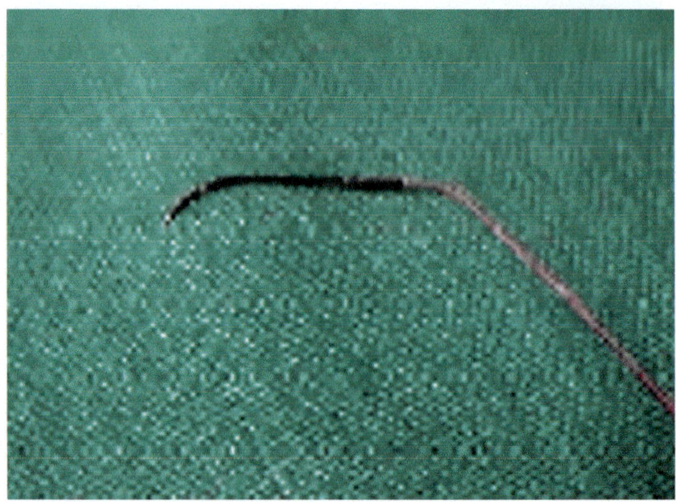

Fig. 1: Endoski needle.

The shaft itself is a modified rectangle, gradually transitioning to a rounded shape toward the tip, ensuring that the curved section of the needle maintains a rounded profile. This unique design facilitates easier handling of the shaft by the jaws of the needle holder and ensures a smooth passage of the curved portion of the needle through tissues during endoscopic procedures.

Needle Holders

The most commonly used is 5 mm Cuschieri needle holders. These have single-action, tapered jaws. The handles are spring loaded and the most recent versions have diamond coating for gripping the suture material without damage. A relaxed "open hand" grip is strongly recommended for these instruments. Please note that there are a wide variety of needle holders (or drivers). In practice, it is vital for each surgeon to become accustomed to a particular type and use that pair all the time. This is crucial for efficient and safe suturing **(Figs. 2 to 4)**.

Needle holder should grasp the needle rock solid hard to prevent rotation. Hence, until now, reusable needle holders are available. Needle holders have different types of jaws. Flat grasping surface makes it possible to turn needle in all direction as in conventional surgery. Dome-shaped indentation at the tip automatically orients the needle in a particular direction, although this function is not always useful; it can sometimes make it easier to grasp the needle. If a surgeon or gynecologist wants to perform any advanced laparoscopic procedure, one should develop the art of laparoscopic suturing and knotting. Laparoscopic knotting and suturing should be learnt on a good quality endotrainer **(Figs. 5 and 6)**. The art and science of laparoscopic suturing and knotting is explained later in tissue approximation technique. Surgeon should slowly expertise these techniques. They will develop their confidence once capable of suture inside abdominal cavity and as a result, conversion rate will also decrease.

Numerous automatic laparoscopic suturing devices have been developed to assist with intracorporeal suturing. However, it is essential to note that none of these devices can completely replace manual laparoscopic suturing. This is because these devices are limited to functioning within specific tissue planes that are suitable for their particular applications.

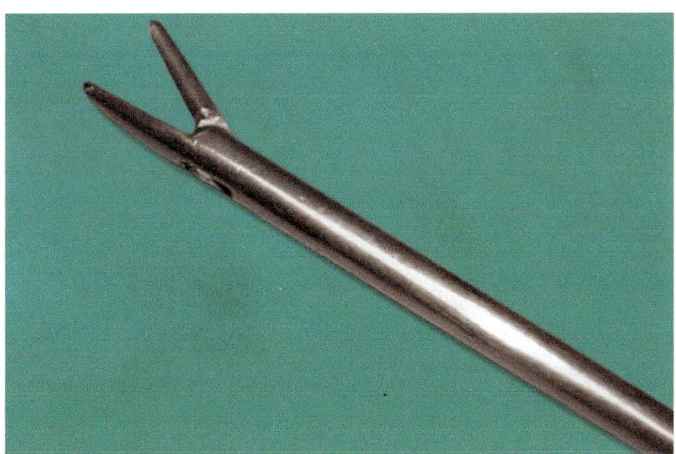

Fig. 2: Jaw of needle holder.

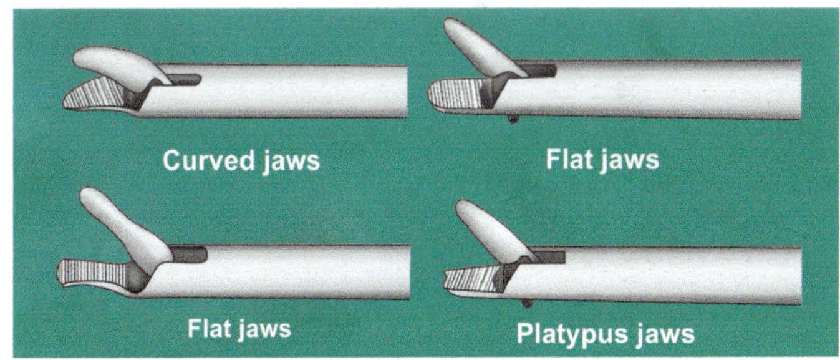

Fig. 4: Different types of jaws of needle holders.

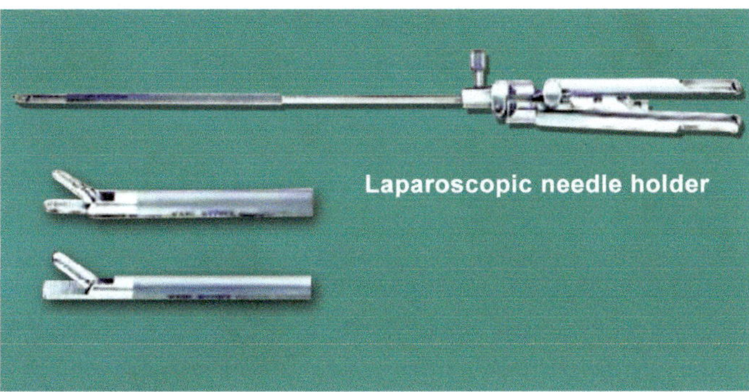

Fig. 3: Laparoscopic straight-handle needle holder.

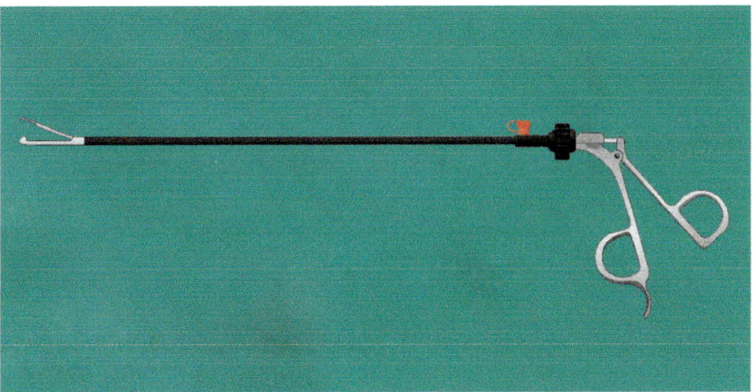

Fig. 5: Laparoscopic autosuturing instrument.

Needle Control

Introduction into the Body Cavity

We recommend the use of the introducer tube to protect all ligatures and sutures from the cannula valve mechanisms.

The suture material on the Endoski needle is trimmed to a suitable length. For a continuous suture, this will be approximately 15–20 cm.

The *suture length must never exceed 20 cm* as this will result in very difficult intracorporeal suturing since the length is magnified (2.5 times) by the imaging system and long suture can result in trapping in the suture (**Fig. 7**).

To begin, the needle holder is introduced through an introducer tube. The tail end of the suture is positioned alongside the tip of the needle and the needle holder grasps the suture at its midpoint. Subsequently, the needle and the tail are carefully withdrawn into the introducer tube

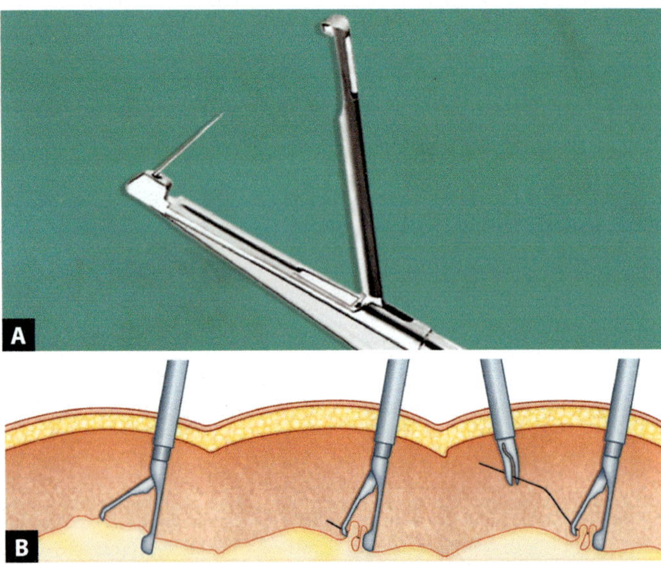

Figs. 6A and B: (A) Autosuturing devices; (B) Laparoscopic autosuturing device.

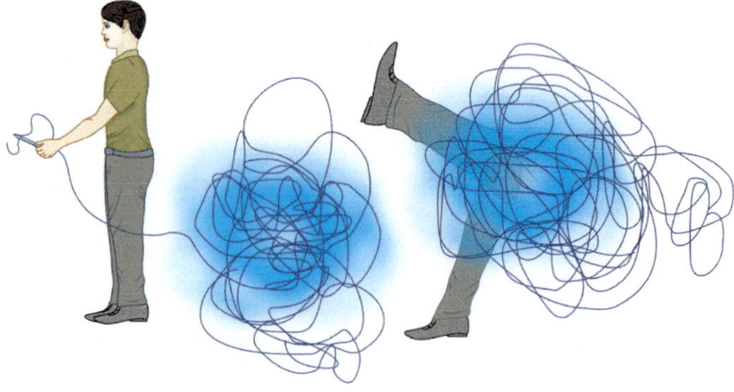

Fig. 7: Laparoscopic surgeon trapped with too big suture length.

until neither is visible. At this point, the introducer tube can be maneuvered through a port, allowing the needle to be extricated from the tube. The suture is then guided into the abdominal cavity and positioned on a convenient surface, such as the flat, smooth anterior surface of the stomach.

■ TO INSERT THE NEEDLE

- Begin by passing the needle holder through the reducing tube.
- Using the needle holder, grasp the suture material at a midpoint between the needle's tip and the tail of the thread.
- Carefully pull the suture and needle completely inside the tube until they are no longer visible.
- Insert the tube through an appropriate port.
- Extrude the needle and suture from the tube by advancing the needle holder and place them on a secure surface, such as the anterior surface of the stomach.

Manipulation

- A trailing needle is a needle in a secure position.
- Always maintain visual contact with a held needle.
- Keep the tips of both needle holders within your field of view.
- Ensure that two needle holders do not cross each other by moving parallelly from one side to the other.

The ability to precisely position the needle within the jaw of the needle holder is one of the foundational skills that should be mastered. It is highly beneficial to practice this skill as it greatly simplifies subsequent tasks. Initially, this task can be frustrating until you become proficient at it.

To begin, arrange the needle into the desired orientation on the tissues, ideally on a serosal surface rather than fatty tissue. Recommended techniques to achieve the correct needle positioning on the tissues include the "nudge," "push," and "twist" techniques. Demonstrations of these maneuvers can be particularly valuable for learning purposes.

Position

The needle should be positioned correctly in the jaws of the needle holder. The ideal way to do this is to grasp the needle with the tips of the jaws, perpendicular to the shaft of the needle. Grasping the needle by the back of the jaws can impair precision and reduce the grasping force, which can make the needle more likely to swivel.

For a right-handed surgeon, the needle should be held in the right-hand needle holder with the tip pointing to the left. The tip of the needle should also point upward and the shaft of the needle should make an obtuse angle with the shaft of the holder.

The following are the key elements in achieving this correct positioning:
- The position of the needle on the tissue
- The angle of approach of the needle holder
- The way in which the needle is picked up.

Adjustments to the angle can be made using the following:
- The other needle holder
- The surrounding tissue
- The tensioned suture material

Here are some additional tips for positioning the needle correctly in the needle holder:
- Hold the needle holder in your dominant hand with the thumb and ring finger in the rings.
- Place the middle finger on top of the finger ring for support.
- Use your index finger to stabilize the tips of the needle holder.
- Approach the needle from the side, with the tips of the needle holder perpendicular to the shaft of the needle.
- Gently close the jaws of the needle holder around the needle, making sure to grasp it in the correct orientation.
- Once the needle is secure, you can adjust the angle of the needle holder as needed.

With a little practice, you will be able to position the needle correctly in the needle holder every time. This will help you to sew more precisely and avoid needle swivel, which can cause complications.

Passage Through the Tissues

- Begin by positioning the needle appropriately within the needle holder and identify the location of the initial entry point. Place the sharp tip of the needle precisely at this point to ensure it enters the tissue at a right angle.
- As approximately half of the needle's curve (around 2.0 mm) has penetrated the tissue, supinate the wrist and lift it slightly. This motion helps in smoothly passing the curved section of the needle through the tissue.

- Once the needle's point is observed to emerge at the exit point, maintain your grasp on it. Then, the assisting needle holder should securely grip the end of the needle (not the tip) before it is released by the dominant needle holder.
- For the second bite, in another edge of the tissue, the dominant needle holder can retrieve the needle directly from the assisting needle holder, provided the needle is positioned favorably for direct transfer. Otherwise, it may be more ergonomic to release the needle and then pick it up again using the dominant holder.
- After both edges of the tissue have been passed, release the needle, and use an instrument-to-instrument technique to pull the suture to the desired point through the tissues.
- It is important to note that a trailing needle, one that follows naturally, causes less harm than a needle held rigidly in the holder. Always ensure that a grasped needle remains within your field of view.

Tensioning

To initially apply tension to a continuous suture, gently pull it through the suture material. Further tightening can be achieved using the dominant needle holder, but caution is essential to prevent fraying or damaging the suture. The open jaws of the needle holder are positioned alongside the suture as it exits from the tissues. These open jaws can then be employed to apply counterpressure on the tissues while the suture is pulled taut by the assisting needle driver.

To maintain tension in a suture line, occasional locking sutures are utilized and the assistance of an assistant is appropriately coordinated. In clinical practice, an assistant maintains tension on the suture line using a specialized suture holder designed to avoid damaging the suture. These holders feature rounded jaws for this purpose.

■ MICROSURGICAL TYING

This sequence of actions is meticulously choreographed to ensure a precise and streamlined process with an emphasis on efficiency, minimal wasted movement, and structured coordination. These key points are worth noting:
- The distinct roles of the passive and active holders in the process.
- The formation of the initial "C" shape and its relationship to the suture's tail.

- The deliberate evaluation of positioning during the procedure.
- The utilization of the natural bias of the thread.
- The execution of appropriate rotations involving both the active and passive needle holders, which must be synchronized.
- The significance of keeping the ends of both needle holders within the surgical field for continuous monitoring.
- The importance of employing two-handed techniques for efficient suturing.

■ TASK ANALYSIS OF SURGEON'S KNOT

- Cutting the suture 20 cm
- Inserting the Maryland in the reducer
- Holding the suture in the middle
- Hiding in the reducer
- Inserting in the abdomen with the reducer
- Dropping over the tissue in a way that tip should be left and the tail should be right
- Aligning the needle with the following three techniques:
  - Pressing the needle by upper jaw of the needle holder at the junction of one third and two thirds.
  - Holding the needle by left hand at the curvature and pulling the suture up near the needle by the right hand.
  - Hang the needle by left hand like a pendulum and go with the open jaw of the needle holder keeping the moving jaw to the left and dragging it to the right.
- Stabilize the tissue with the left hand and prick the tissue by the needle and by rotating the tip of needle to keep it perpendicular to the tissue.
- Bringing the tip of the needle one third out and catch it with left hand instrument and keeping the convex end of the instrument toward the tissue.
- Guard the tissue by the needle holder, keeping concave part toward the tissue and pulling the needle by left hand instrument.
- Hold the suture by the needle holder as soon as needle is out.
- Guard the suture by the Maryland and pull the suture by needle holder to make a tail of 2 cm.
- A "C" shape will form and keep the left-hand instrument above and in the center of the "C."
- Bring the tip of the needle holder near the tip of the Maryland and rotate the needle holder to make a loop.
- Keep the Maryland static and take two loose wrap by the needle holder.

- Move the instrument together to catch the tail by the Maryland.
- After catching the tail, do not pull the tail, but move the needle holder toward the tip of the Maryland.
- Drop the suture away from the Maryland and come again to catch the needle end of the suture near the knot and tie the first knot.
- Catch the suture now with your left hand to make a reverse "C."
- Now, keep the needle holder static in the center and above of the reverse "C."
- Hold the suture with Maryland and bring the tip of the Maryland near the tip of needle holder.
- Rotate the Maryland to make a loop.
- Needle holder will be static and Maryland will take a single wrap.
- Needle holder will catch the tail, but the tail should not be pulled.
- Maryland will slide the loop in the direction of the tip of the needle holder.
- Maryland will drop the suture away from the knot and will come again to hold the suture near the knot.
- Needle holder and Maryland will move away from each other in tissue plane to tie the second knot.
- Suture will be held again by the needle holder to make a "C."
- Maryland will be static in the center and above of the "C."
- Needle holder will come near the tip of the Maryland with the suture and will be rotated to make a loop.
- Needle holders will move around the tip of Maryland to take a single wrap.
- Maryland will hold the tail and needle holder will slide the wrap in the direction of the tip of the Maryland.
- Needle holder will leave the suture away from the knot and come again to catch the suture near the knot.
- Needle holder and Maryland by holding the suture will move in the opposite direction to tighten the last knot in the tissue plane.
- Hold the needle at the end of the suture with the Maryland and remove the needle holder.
- Introduce the scissor in the right port and cut the suture.
- Hide the suture in the reducer by pulling the Maryland and pull Maryland and the reducer together out.
- Push the Maryland to eject the needle out.

■ STEPS OF SURGEON'S KNOT

Surgeon's knot contains a double wrap on the first throw, followed by two opposing, alternating single throws. In other words, it is a double knot followed by a square knot (Reef knot) **(Figs. 8A to H)**.

Figures 9 to 32 depict the various steps of tying a surgeon's knot.

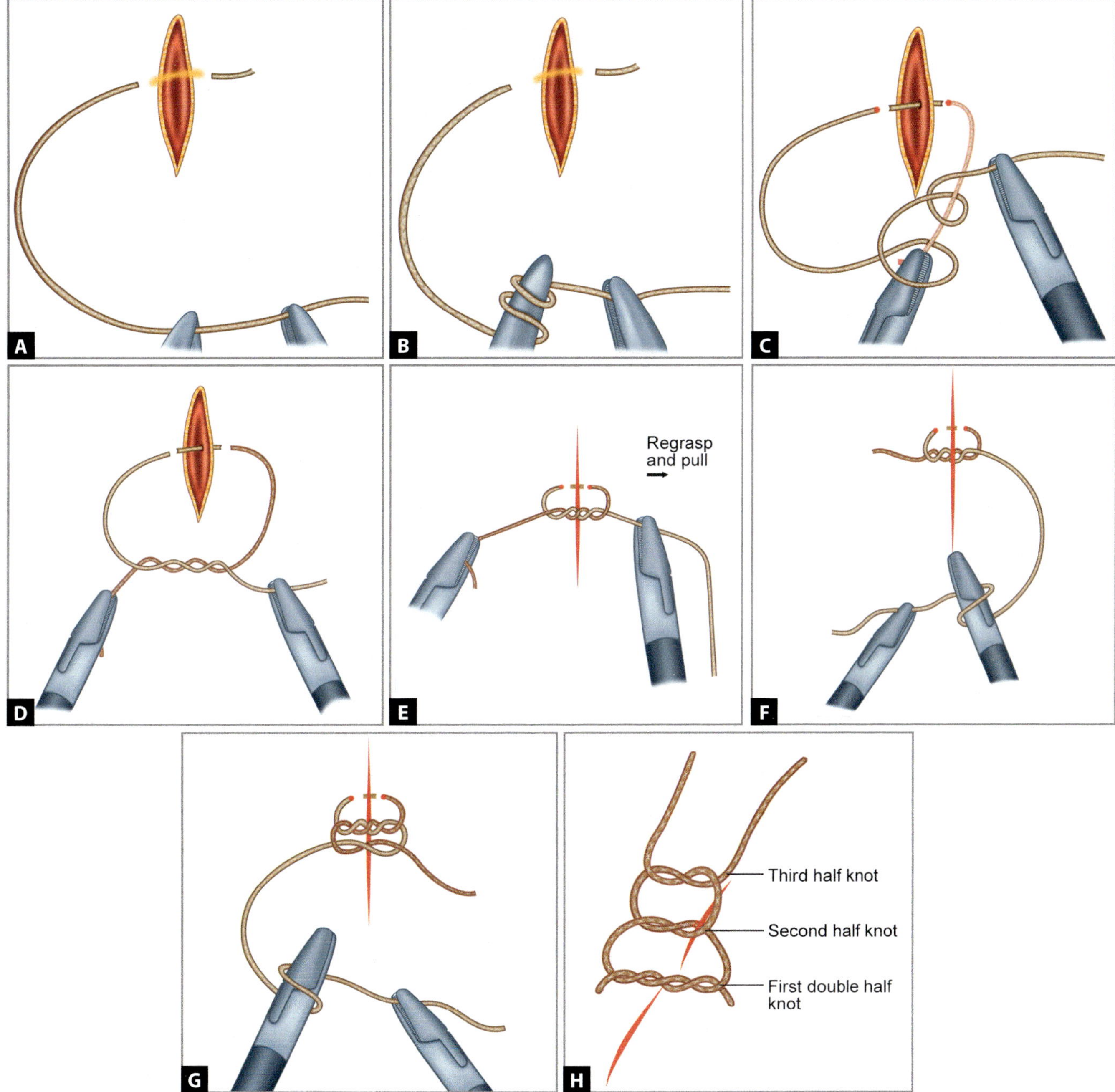

Figs. 8A to H: (A) "C" loop is made; (B) The instrument of the side of "C" should be kept above the "C" and two winds are taken with the help of right instrument; (C) Winds are slipped in the line of left instrument; (D) Knot is tightened with the help of both the instruments; (E) First knot of surgeon's knot is complete; (F) A reverse "C" is made and single wind is taken over the right instrument with the help of left instrument; (G) Again "C" loop is made and single winds are taken to complete surgeons knot; (H) Surgeon's knot contains double wrap on the first throw, followed by two opposing, alternating single throws.

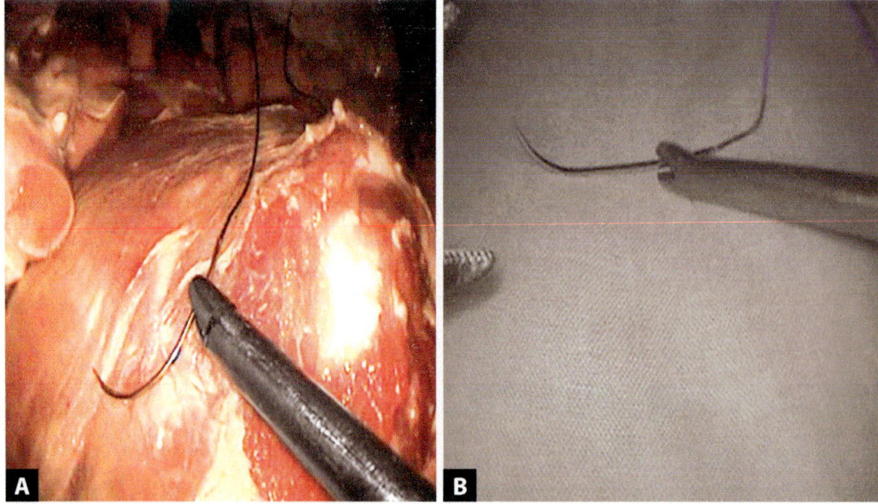

Figs. 9A and B: *Step 1:* The needle is held at right angles to its body at the junction of two thirds and one third.

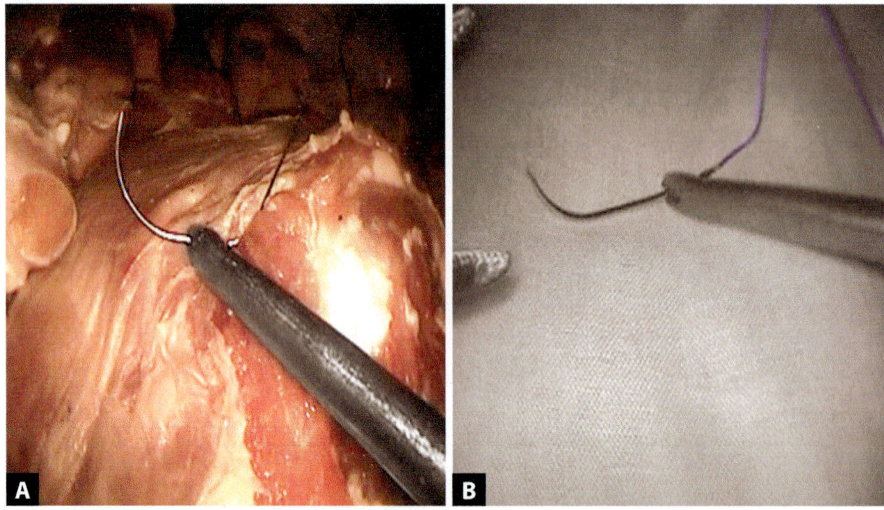

Figs. 10A and B: *Step 2:* With pressure over the needle with the upper jaw, it can be made horizontal and held firmly with the needle holder.

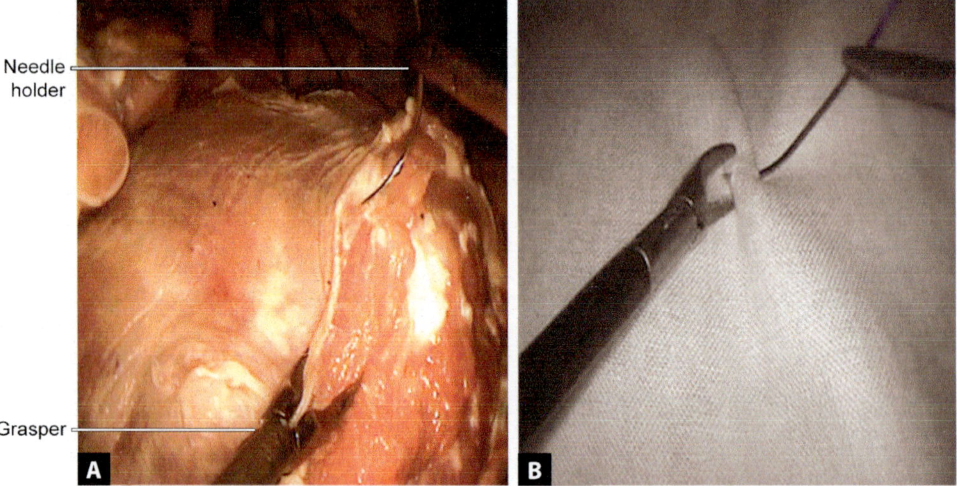

Figs. 11A and B: *Step 3:* The needle held firmly in the needle holder is pushed through the tissue at right angles with the other grasper supporting the tissue.

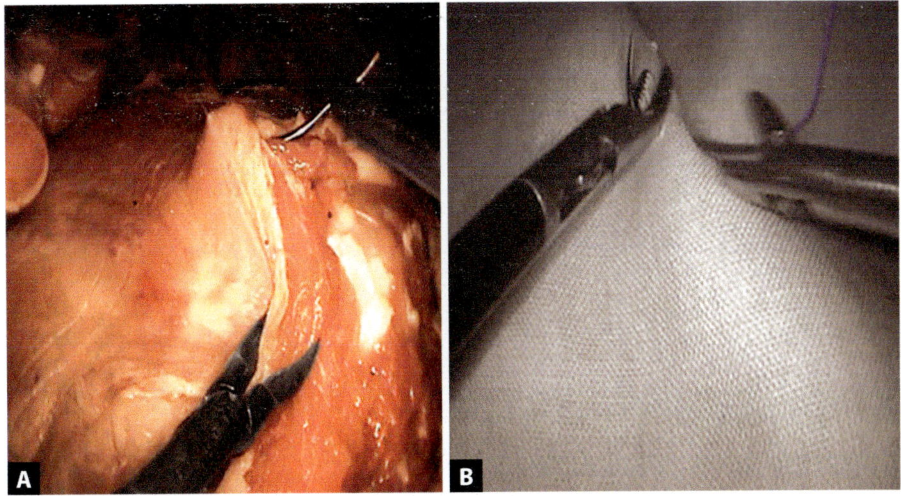

Figs. 12A and B: *Step 4:* With the needle held firmly in the needle holder, it is pushed through the tissue with support given by the grasper in the other hand.

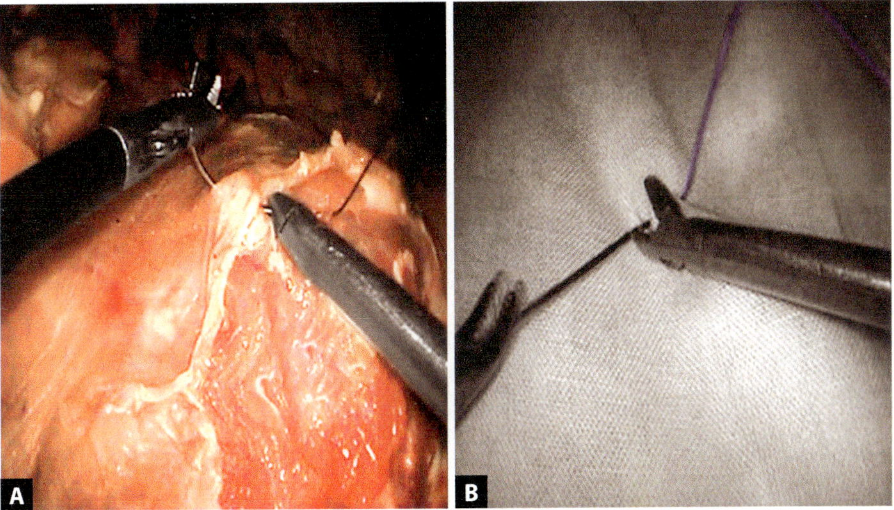

Figs. 13A and B: *Step 5:* Before the needle has gone through completely, it is held by the grasper in the other hand.

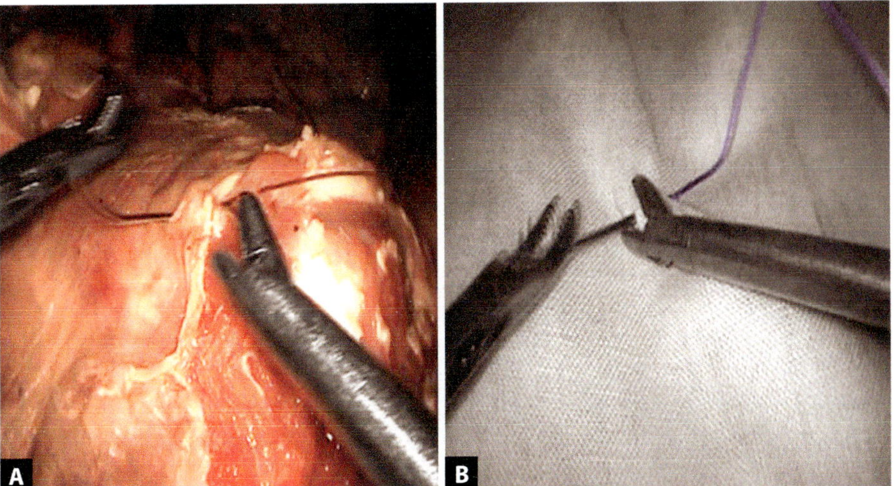

Figs. 14A and B: *Step 6:* The needle is released by the needle holder and left hand instrument is ready to hold the proximal portion of the needle.

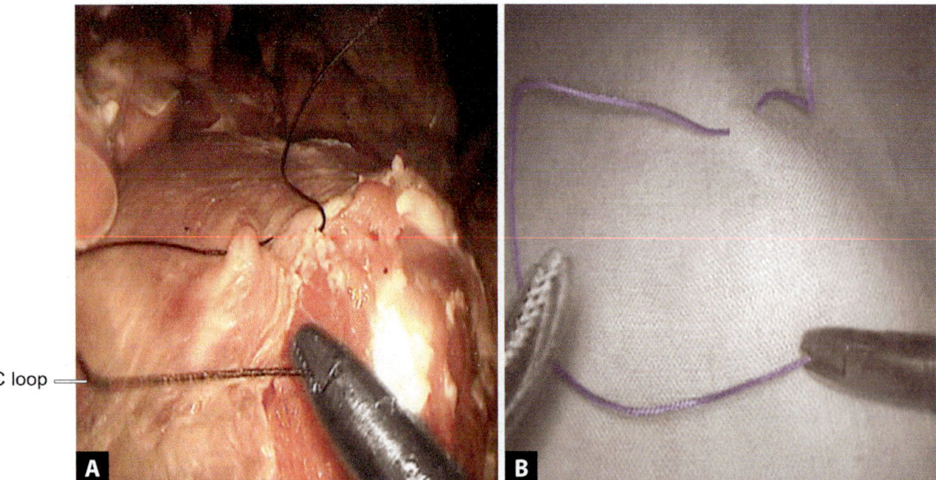

Figs. 15A and B: *Step 7:* Suture behind the needle is held by the needle holder in such a way as to form a "C" loop in front of the suture passed through the tissue.

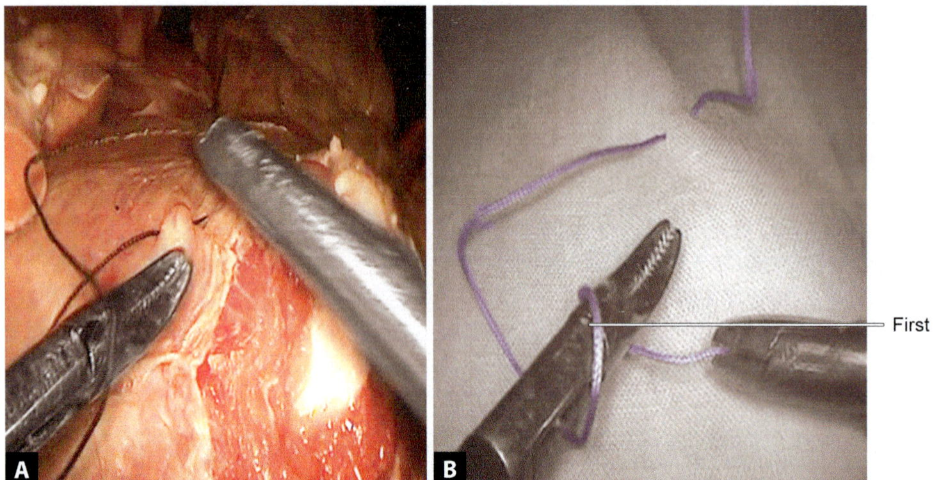

Figs. 16A and B: *Step 8:* With the needle holder holding the suture, a loop is thrown around the grasper from above, keeping the grasper stationary in front of the future knot.

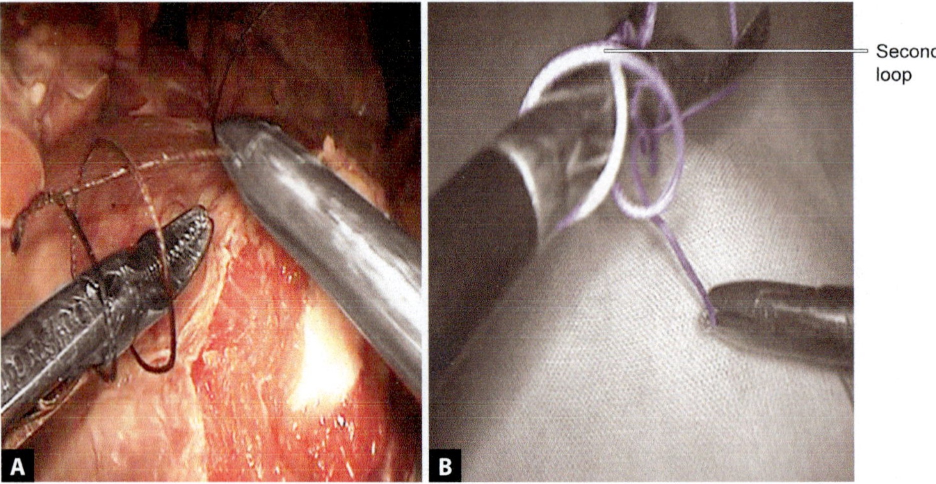

Figs. 17A and B: *Step 9:* One more loop is thrown around the stationary grasper with the suture held by the needle holder by advancing it through the loops.

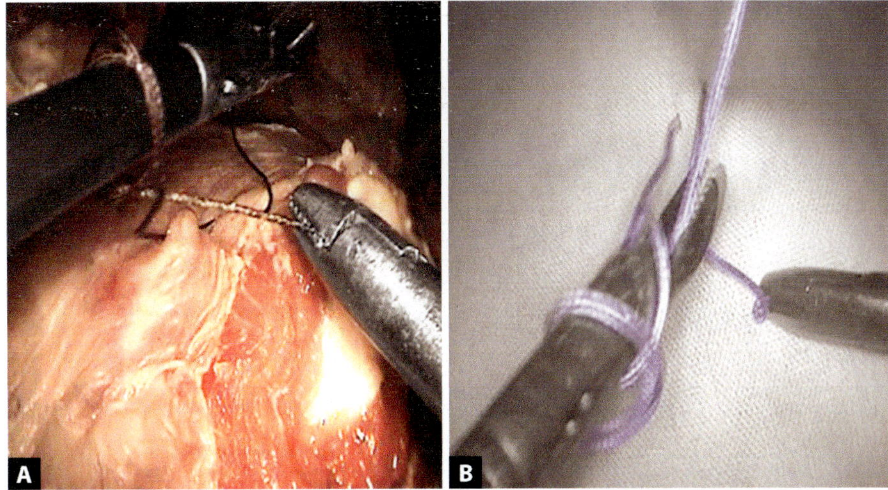

Figs. 18A and B: *Step 10:* The original end of the suture is grasped by the grasper.

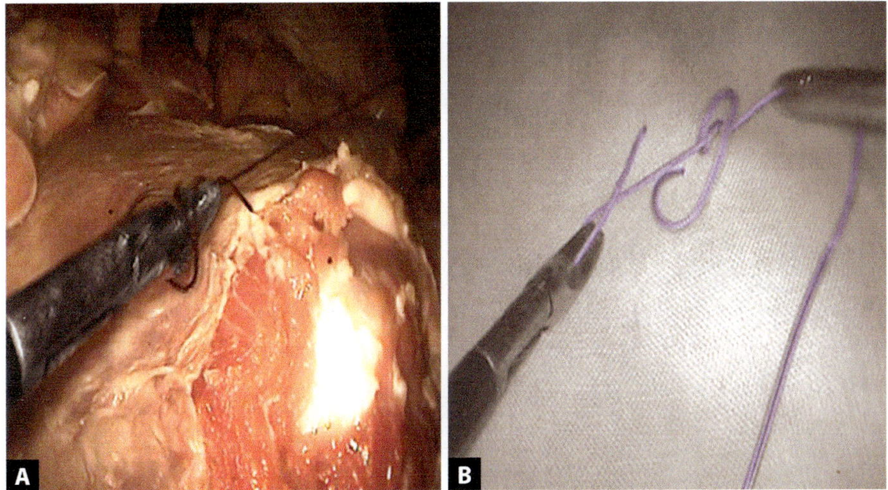

Figs. 19A and B: *Step 11:* Both the ends of the suture are pulled in the opposite directions by the needle holder and the grasper.

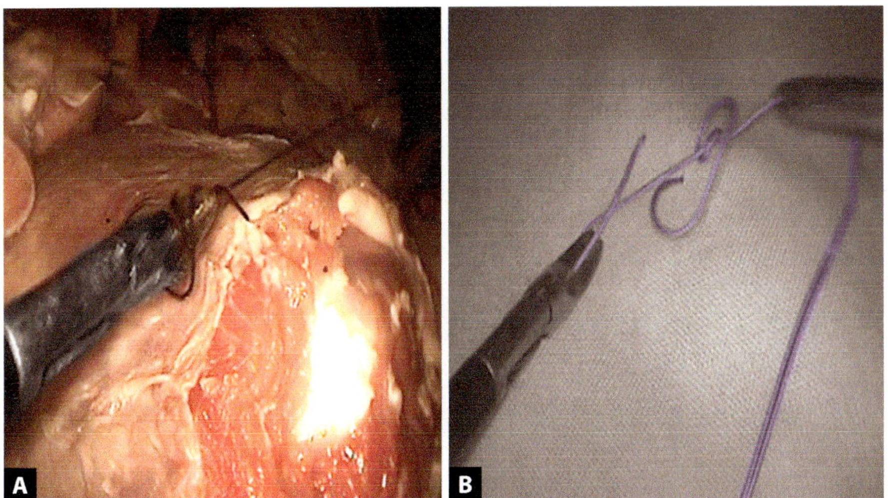

Figs. 20A and B: *Step 12:* Applying even pull from both the ends, knot is tied well, changing the grasp of the needle holder nearer.

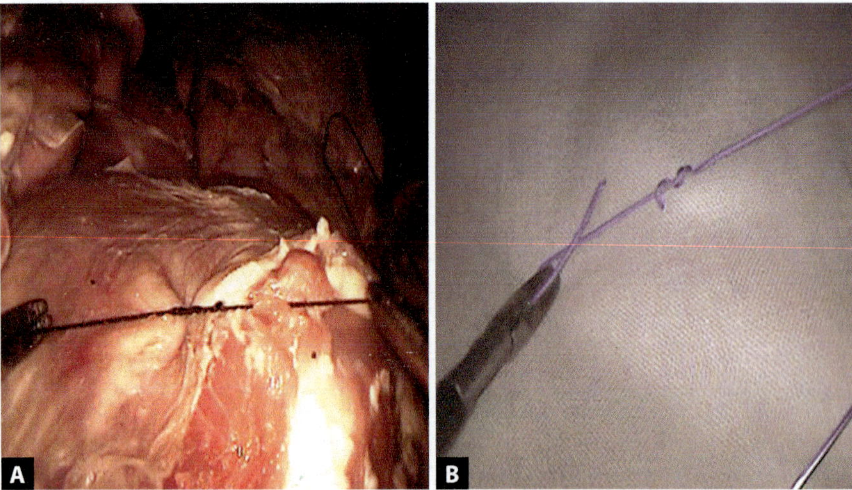

Figs. 21A and B: *Step 13:* First double knot is tied.

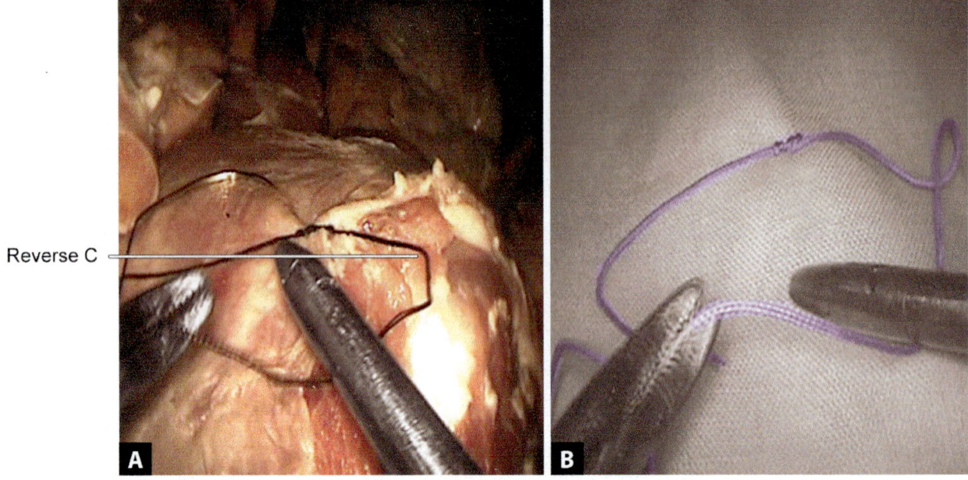

Reverse C

Figs. 22A and B: *Step 14:* Holding the suture in the grasper a reverse C loop is formed in front of the knot, keeping the needle holder in the center.

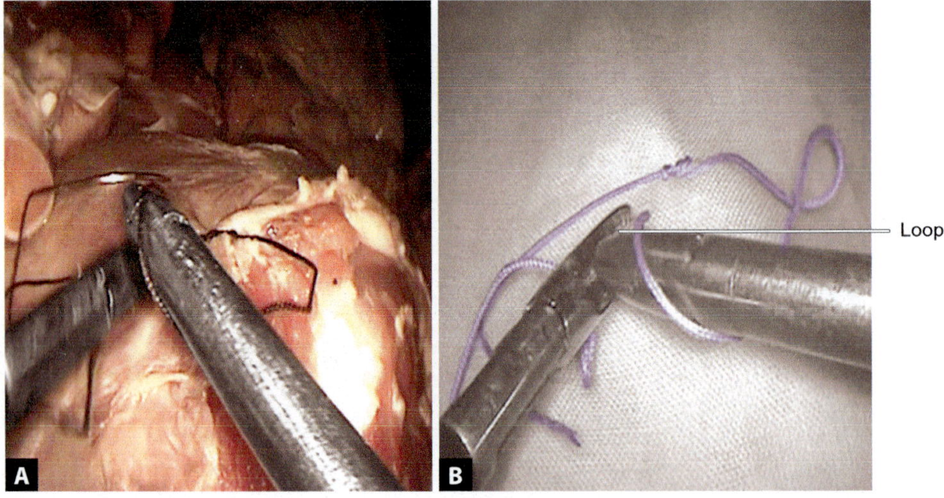

Loop

Figs. 23A and B: *Step 15:* Keeping the needle holder stationary in front of the knot, a loop is thron by the grasper with the suture sliding it above the needle holder.

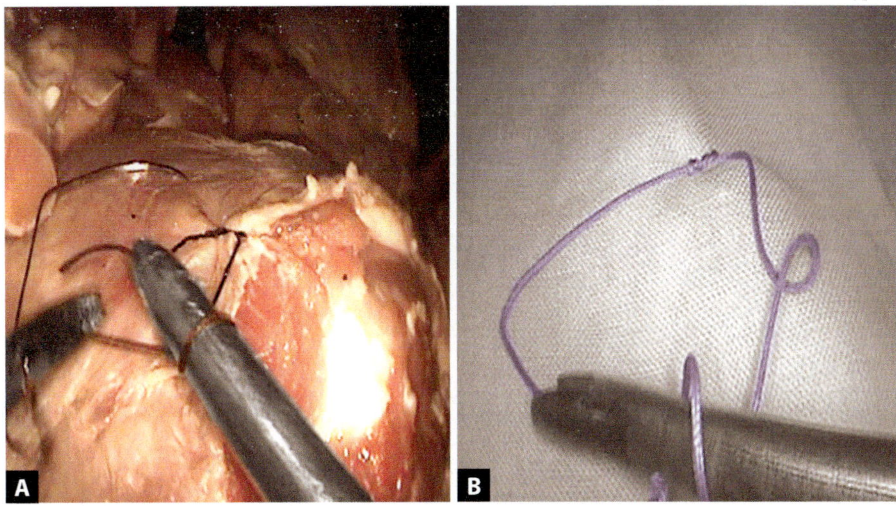

Figs. 24A and B: *Step 16:* By pushing through the loop, needle holder picks up the end of the suture.

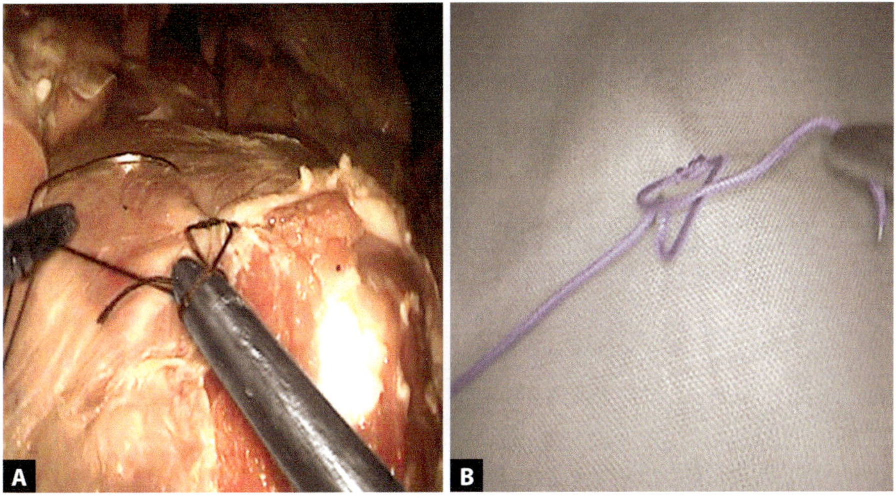

Figs. 25A and B: *Step 17:* Both the ends of the suture are pulled in opposite directions to complete the second knot.

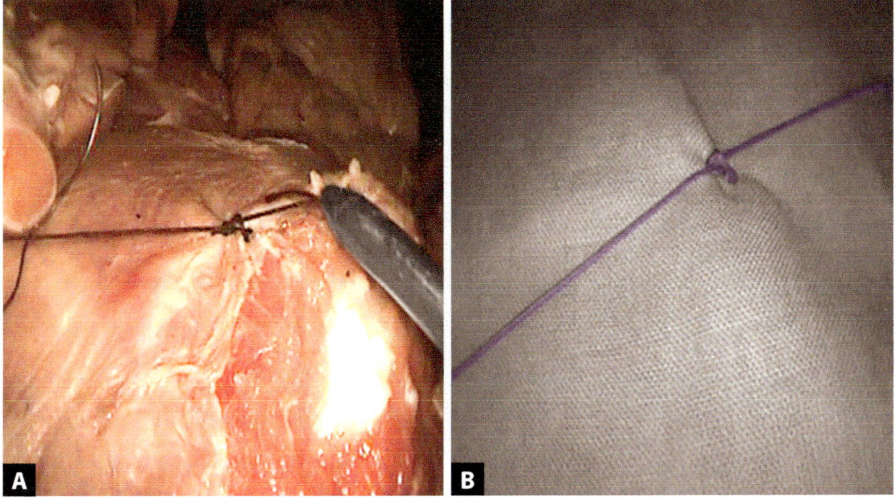

Figs. 26A and B: *Step 18:* Second knot is firmly placed over the first with even pull used from both ends of the suture.

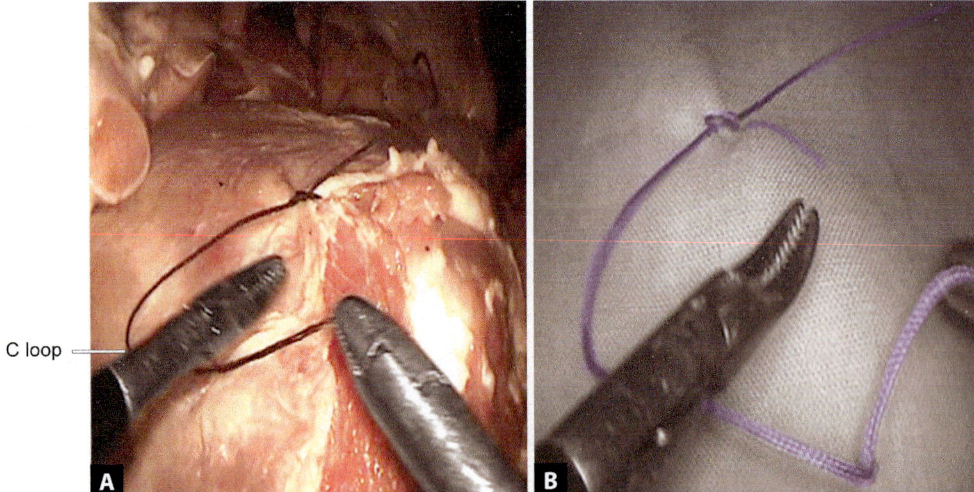

Figs. 27A and B: *Step 19:* Again a C loop is formed by the suture held by the needle holder with grasper kept stationary above the suture in front of the knot at the center of the C.

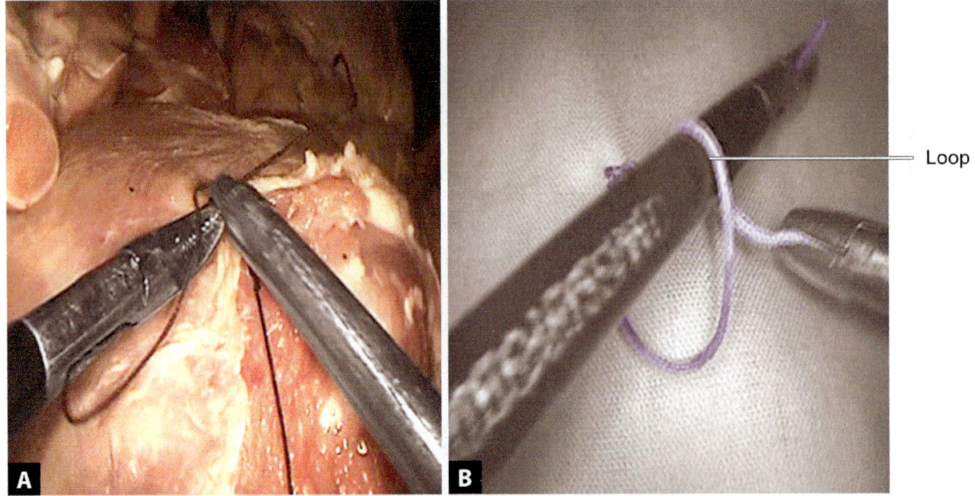

Figs. 28A and B: *Step 20:* The needle holder holding the suture at the end of the C loop throws a loop around the grasper in front of the knot.

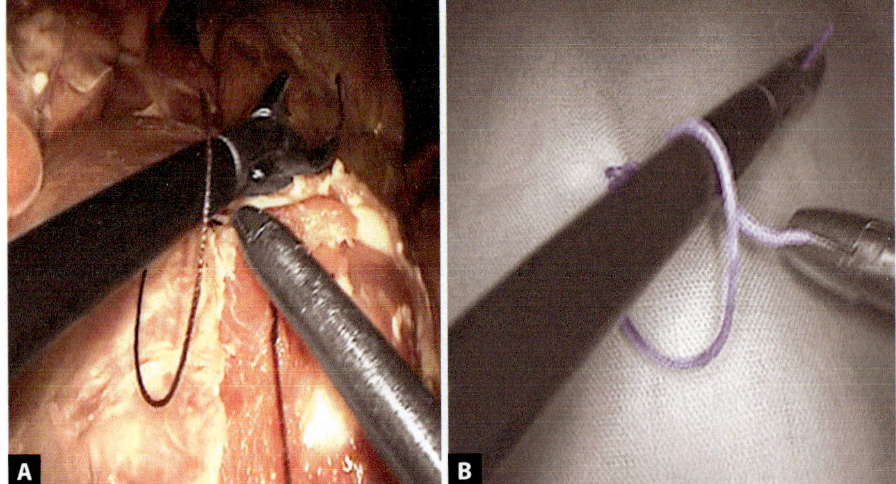

Figs. 29A and B: *Step 21:* By pushing through the loop, grasper picks up the end of the suture.

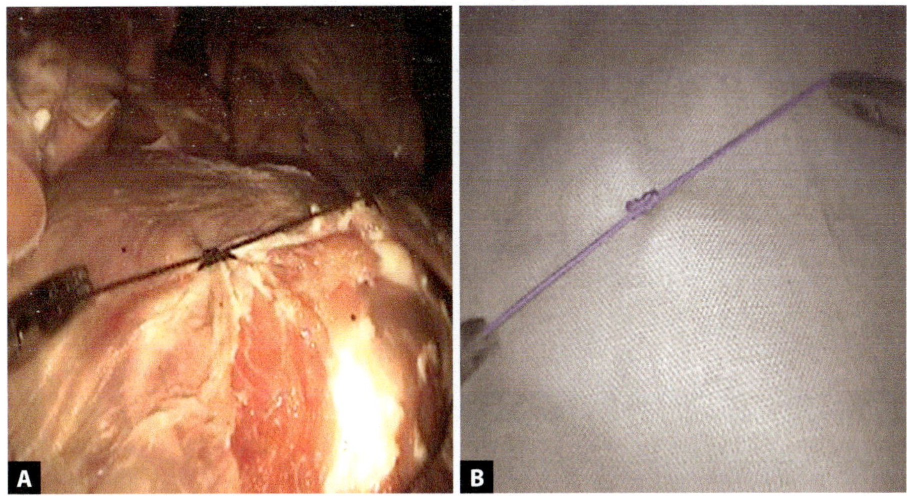

Figs. 30A and B: *Step 22:* By applying even tension, ends of the suture are pulled in the opposite directions to complete the third knot.

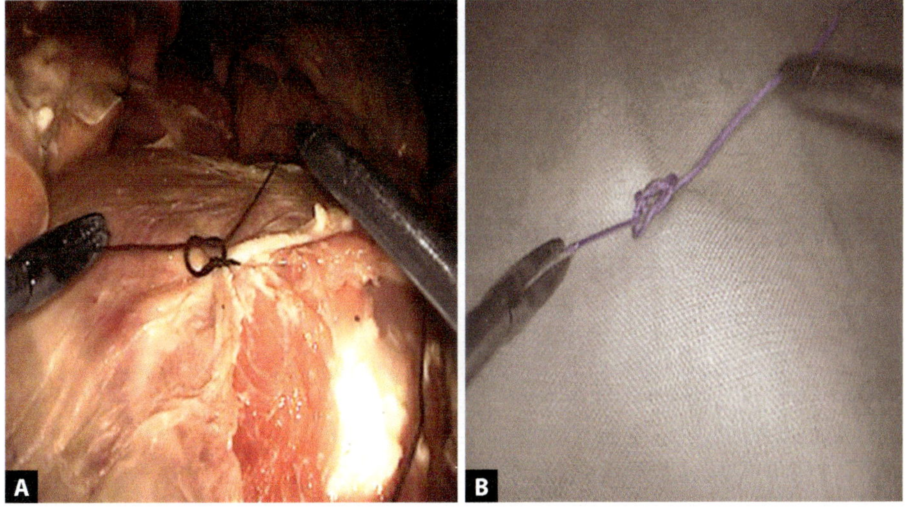

Figs. 31A and B: *Step 23:* Third knot is second half of the Reef knot (Square knot).

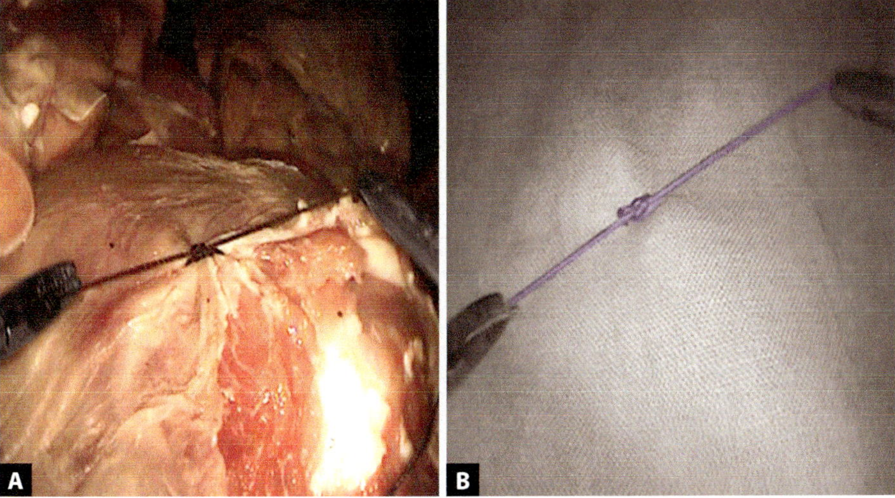

Figs. 32A and B: Surgeon's knot is firmly holding the tissue together under tension.

ADVANTAGES

The surgeon's knot is a strong knot and hence, it can be used wherever a robust ligature is needed, such as for tying blood vessels or for intracorporeal interrupted suturing where tissue approximation is required, as in cases of enterotomy or bladder injury. Adding the extra double knot before tying a Reef knot increases its friction, thereby enhancing its strength. This knot can also be used to secure two dissimilar strands of suture, as in the surgeon's loop. It is also referred to as a double surgeon knot and is used to connect monofilaments of similar or dissimilar sizes.

DISADVANTAGES

Due to its nonsliding nature, it is unsuitable for extracorporeal knotting. Additionally, it proves challenging to use in situations deep within the pelvic cavity or at the end of a suture line, where the working space is limited, such as in the repair of inguinal or femoral hernias for peritoneal closure.

It is also very time-consuming as compared to other knots due to its composite nature with three knots.

Extra throws do not increase the strength of a properly tied knot, but they do add to its bulk and therefore to any potential tissue reaction, especially when buried.

CLINICAL APPLICATIONS

The surgeon's knot is a versatile knot and can be used in any bowel or visceral injury. This is also used in end-to-end anastomosis of bowel or fallopian tube **(Figs. 33 to 36)**.

The surgeon's knot, a modification of the square knot, is a versatile and secure knot that holds great importance in laparoscopic surgery. It is renowned for its strength, stability, and adaptability in various surgical scenarios. Its application extends across a wide range of procedures, including tissue approximation, ligation of blood vessels, and the closure of cavities, among others.

- *Tissue approximation:* In laparoscopic surgery, precise tissue approximation is crucial. Surgeons often use the surgeon's knot to securely bring together tissue edges, ensuring they remain in place during the healing process. This is particularly vital in procedures such as intestinal anastomosis or gastric bypass surgeries.
- *Hemostasis:* The knot's reliability is instrumental in controlling bleeding during laparoscopic surgery. Surgeons can confidently use the surgeon's knot to ligate blood vessels, ensuring that the sutures hold firm and minimize the risk of postoperative bleeding.
- *Closure of cavities:* In laparoscopy, surgeons may need to close cavities, such as the peritoneum or abdominal wall securely. The surgeon's knot excels in this regard, providing a robust closure that helps prevent complications such as herniation.

ADVANTAGES OF THE SURGEON'S KNOT IN LAPAROSCOPY

- *Security:* The surgeon's knot is celebrated for its robust and secure hold. This is of utmost importance in laparoscopic surgery, where precision and reliability are paramount.
- *Adaptability:* Laparoscopic procedures often require quick adjustments and meticulous control. The surgeon's knot's adaptability allows for easy manipulation and fine-tuning as needed during surgery.
- *Strength:* The knot's strength ensures that tissues remain in their intended positions, reducing the risk of complications like leaks or bleeding.
- *Ease of learning:* While mastering laparoscopic surgery is a complex process, learning to tie a surgeon's knot is a foundational skill. Its relative simplicity makes it accessible to surgeons at various stages of their careers.

CHALLENGES AND CONSIDERATIONS

While the surgeon's knot is a valuable tool in laparoscopic surgery, it is essential to acknowledge its limitations. For instance, in certain deep cavities or challenging anatomical locations, manipulating the knot may be cumbersome. Surgeons must also consider the materials used for sutures, as the knot's effectiveness can vary depending on the type of suture material employed.

CONCLUSION

The surgeon's knot is an indispensable component of the laparoscopic surgeon's toolkit. Its adaptability, strength, and reliability make it a go-to choice for securing tissues, ligating blood vessels, and closing cavities during minimally invasive surgeries. While it has its challenges, mastering the surgeon's knot is a fundamental skill for laparoscopic surgeons, ensuring the success and safety of these groundbreaking procedures. As laparoscopic techniques continue to evolve, the surgeon's knot remains a steadfast ally in the pursuit of better patient outcomes and enhanced surgical precision.

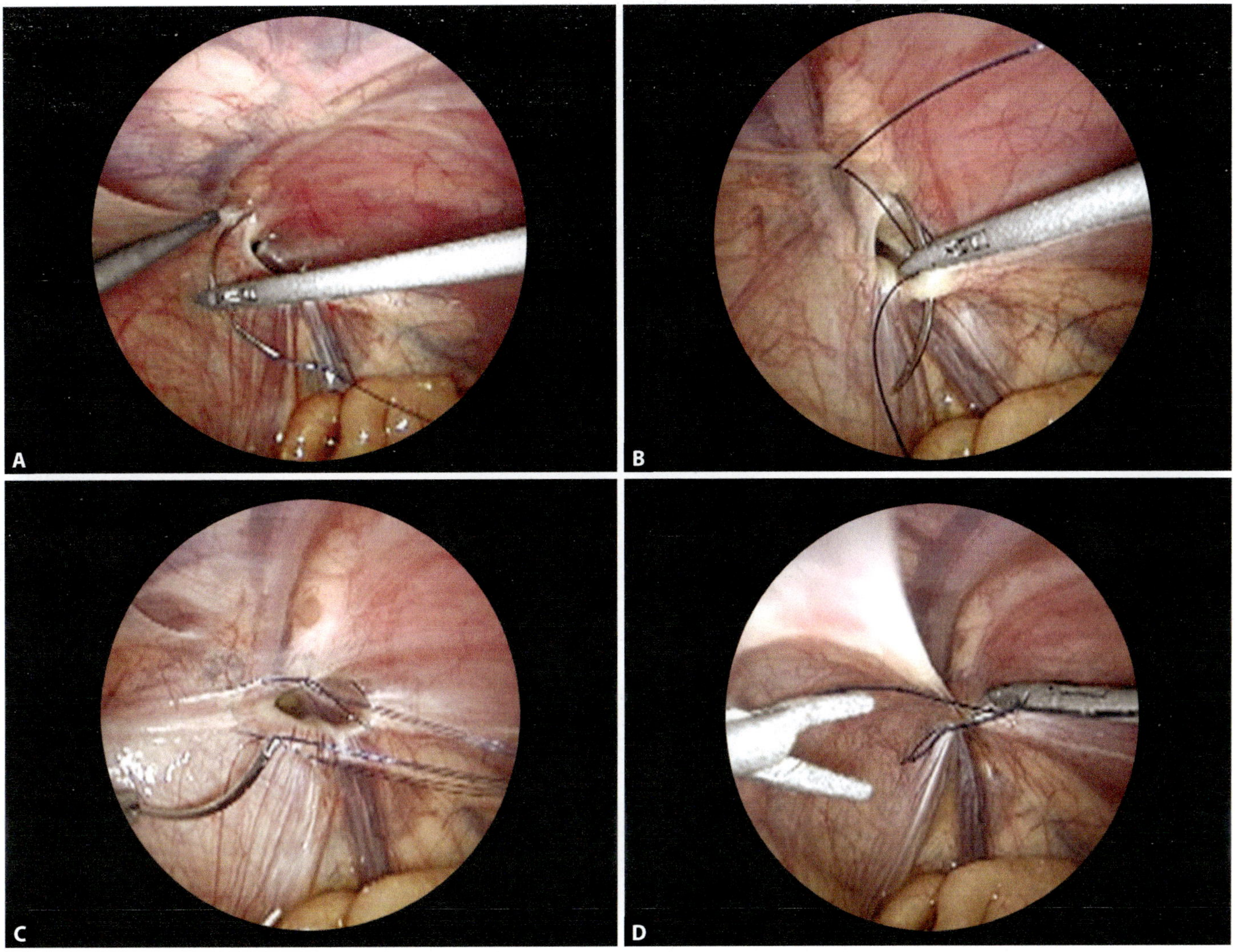

Figs. 33A to D: Purse string suture with surgeon's knot for pediatric inguinal hernia repair.

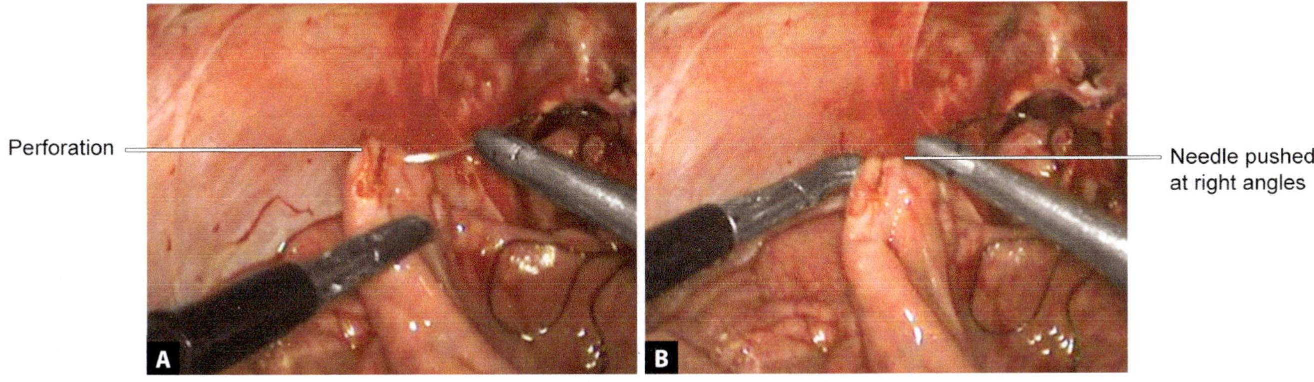

Figs. 34A and B

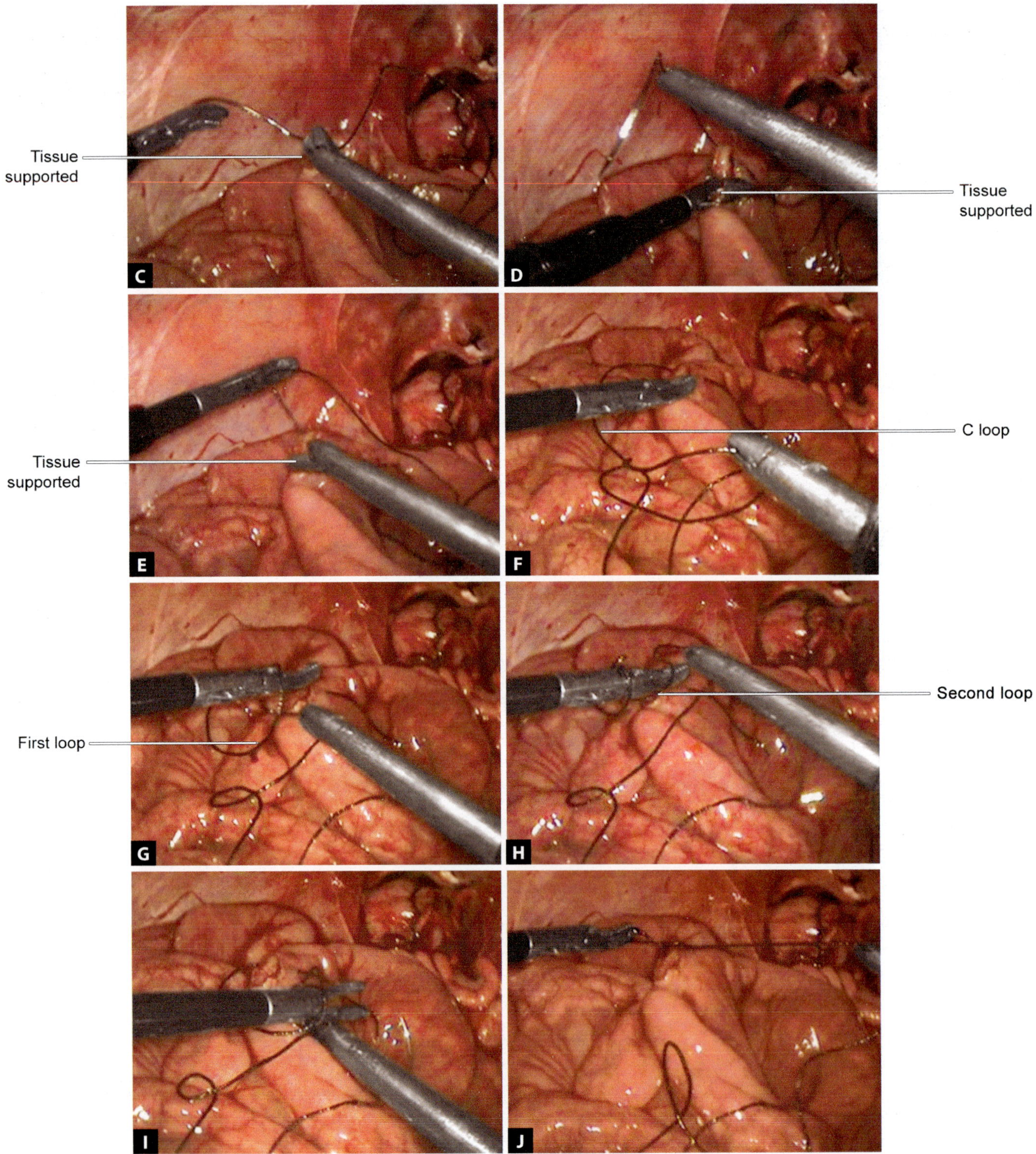

Tissue supported
C
Tissue supported
D
Tissue supported
E
C loop
F
First loop
G
Second loop
H
I
J

Figs. 34C to J

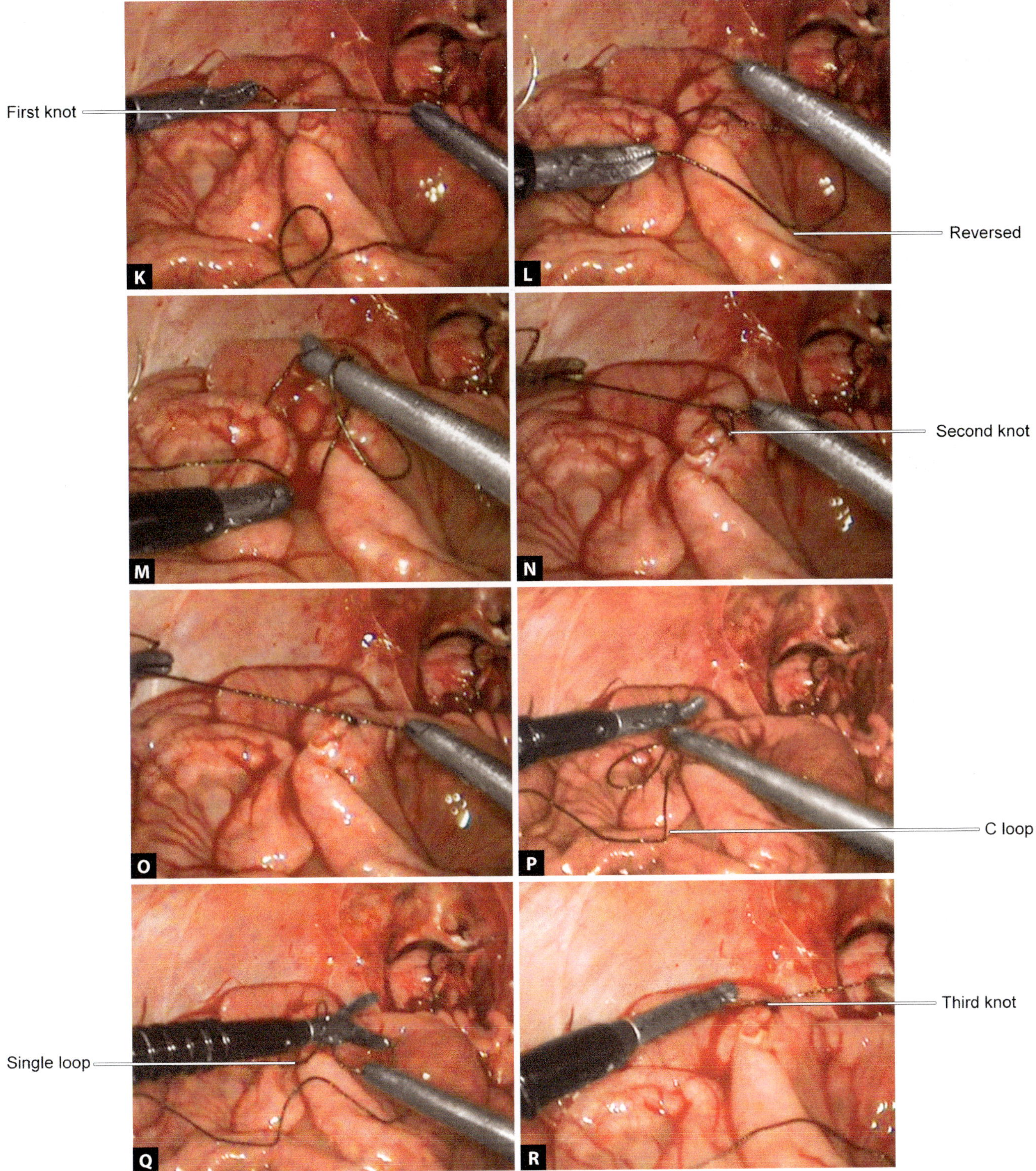

Figs. 34A to R: Closure of Ileal perforation using a surgeon's knot.

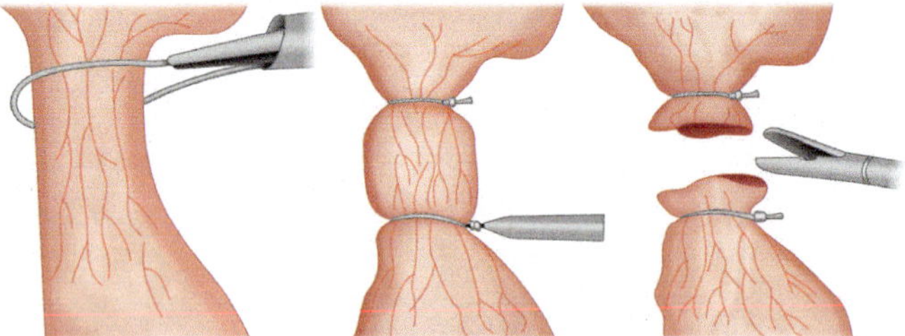

Fig. 35: Extracorporeal knot can be used in case of adhesion with omentum.

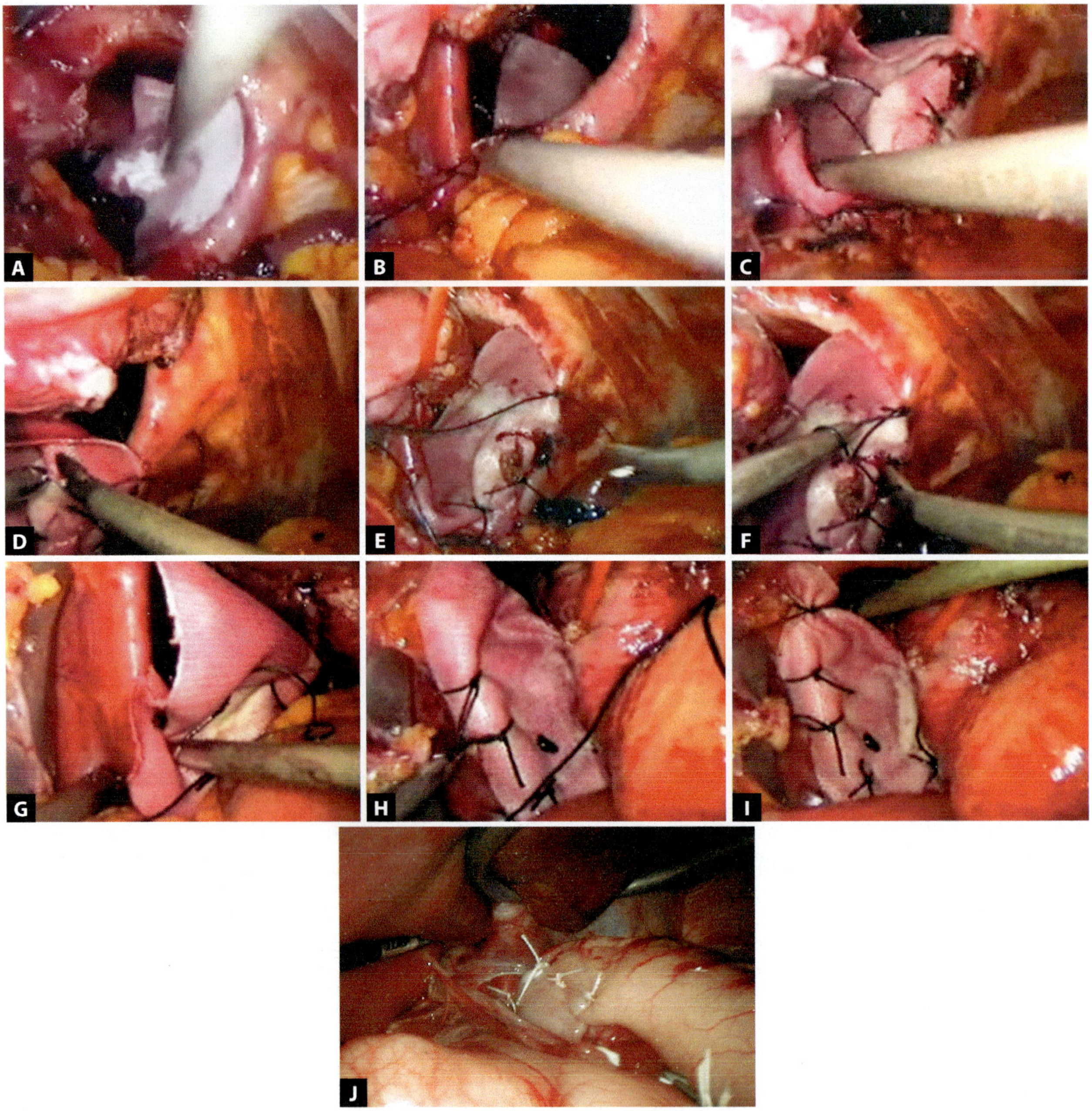

Figs. 36A to J: (A to I) Mesh is fixed with diaphragm with the help of intracorporeal sutures using surgeon's knot; (J) Fixation of wrap in fundoplication by intracorporeal sutures using surgeon's knot.

◼ BIBLIOGRAPHY

1. Berci G, Cuschieri A, Sackier JM, Nyhus LM, Judge C. (Eds.). Problems in General Surgery—Laparoscopic Surgery. Philadelphia: Lippincott Company; 1991.
2. Brunicardi FC, Anderson D, Billiar TR, Dunn DL, Hunter JG, Pollock RE (Eds.). Schwartz's Manual of Surgery. New York: McGraw Hill LLC; 2006.
3. Chen MH, Khalil H (Eds). Laparoscopic Suturing Techniques for Surgeons. Oxford: Oxford University Press; 2022.
4. Choi E, Kim DY. The Use of Biodegradable Sutures in Laparoscopic Surgery. J Biomed Mat. 2024;15(3):438-45.
5. DeMott, K. (2002). Knots: Stop at three throws deep in the Pelvis (Surgical Tips and Tricks). [online] Available from [https://www.thefreelibrary.com/Knots%3A+ Stop+at+three+throws+deep+in+the+Pelvis. +(Surgical+ Tips+and...-a083759858](https://www.thefreelibrary. com/Knots%3A+Stop+at+three+throws+deep+in+ the +Pelvis.+(Surgical+Tips+and...-a083759858) [Last accessed May, 2024].
6. Fernandez R, Martin CJ. Ergonomics in Laparoscopic Suturing: Minimizing Surgeon Fatigue. J Ergonomics Surg. 2023;17(3):145-54.
7. Gomez R, Lee T. Evolution of Suturing Techniques in Laparoscopic Surgery. J Minim Invasive Sur. 2021;28(2):123-32.
8. Gupta S, Mehra R. Barriers to Learning Laparoscopic Suturing: A Survey of Surgical Residents. Education Surg. 2023;47(1):55-62.
9. Harper D, Lombardi A. Adapting Traditional Suturing Techniques for Laparoscopic Applications. Surg Techniques Rev. 2021;35(4):320-8.
10. Kumar V, Saxena AK (Eds). Advanced Techniques in Laparoscopic Surgery. Berlin: Springer; 2020.
11. Kyle Leming J, Dorman K, Brydges R, Carnahan H, Dubrowski A. Tensiometry as a measure of improvement in knot quality in undergraduate medical students. Adv Health Sci Educ Theory Pract. 2007;12(3):331-44.
12. Lavelle JF, Sinclair MF. Automated Suturing Devices in Laparoscopic Surgery: A Comparative Analysis. Technol Surg. 2020;22(6):789-98.
13. Lee J, Kim S. Innovations in Laparoscopic Suturing Instruments. Int J Med Robot. 2022;18(1):e2210.
14. Mendez C, Gupta A. Laparoscopic Suturing: Mastery Through Technique and Practice. London: Elsevier Health Sciences; 2023.
15. Mishra RK (Ed). Textbook of Laparoscopy for Surgeons and Gynecologists, 4th edition. New Delhi: Jaypee Brothers Medical Publishers (P) Ltd.; 2021. pp. 900.
16. Mishra RK. Textbook of Practical Laparoscopic Surgery. Jaypee Brothers Medical Publishers, New Delhi, 2007; pp. 104-23.
17. Morrison T, Jacobs LR. Teaching Laparoscopic Suturing: The Role of Simulation in Medical Schools. Med Teacher. 2021;43(7):778-84.
18. Nguyen L, Ho CP. Impact of Suture Materials on Laparoscopic Knot Reliability. Mat Surg. 2024;9(2): 200-10.
19. O'Reilly MP, Saunders BH. Virtual Reality Training for Laparoscopic Surgery. Cambridge: Cambridge University Press; 2022.
20. Patel R, Thompson J. The Role of Simulation in Learning Laparoscopic Suturing and Knotting. Med Education Online. 2021;26:1857289.
21. Rodriguez A, Davis SS. Robotic-Assisted Laparoscopic Knot Tying: Methods and Efficiency. Surg Innov. 2019;26(4):459-66.
22. Schubert DC, Unger JB, Mukherjee D, Perrone JF. Mechanical performance of knots using braided and monofilament absorbable sutures. Am J Obstet Gynecol. 2002;187(6):1438-40; discussion 1441-2.
23. Shimi SM, Lirici MM, Vander Velpen G, Cuschieri A. Comparative study of holding strength of slipknot using absorbable and nonabsorbable ligature materials. Surg Endosc. 1994;11:1285-91.
24. Smith JA, Patel VR (Eds). Principles of Laparoscopic Suturing and Knotting. New York: Springer; 2023.
25. Surgical Knots and Suturing Techniques. (2024). Available from https://en.wikipedia.org/wiki/Surgical_knot.
26. Shimi SM, Lirici M, Vander Velpen G, Cushieri A. Comparative study of holding strength of slipknot using absorbable and nonabsorbable ligature materials. Surg Endosc. 1994;8(2)93-6.
27. Wang Y, Thompson C. Innovations in Knot Tying Techniques for Minimally Invasive Surgery. Innov Surg. 2022;18(4):250-60.
28. Williams NE, Tan JL. Comparative Study of Knot Security in Laparoscopic Surgery. J Surg Res. 2020;245:217-23.
29. Zimmerman KA, Patel ND. Laparoscopic Knotting: A Visual Guide for Surgeons. Philadelphia: Lippincott Williams & Wilkins; 2022.

Tumble Square Knot

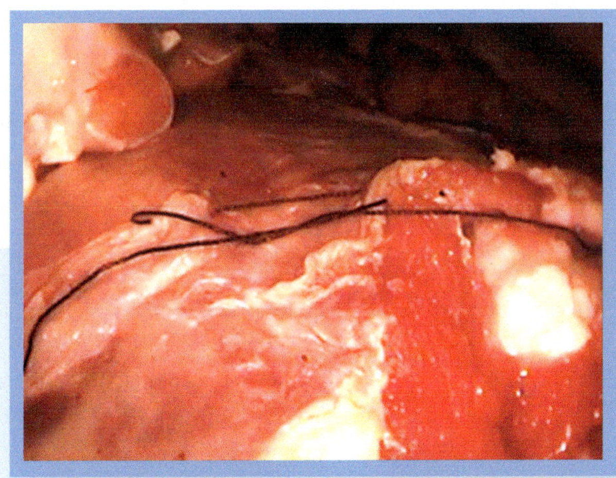

◾ INTRODUCTION

The laparoscopic tumble square knot is an epitome of surgical innovation, embodying the advances in minimally invasive surgery that have dramatically transformed patient care. This specialized knotting technique, designed for the precise and constrained environment of laparoscopic surgery, has gained prominence due to its reliability, efficiency, and adaptability. This chapter delves into the origins, methodology, applications, advantages, and future implications of the laparoscopic tumble square knot, underscoring its significance in the modern surgical landscape.

◾ ORIGINS AND METHODOLOGY

The laparoscopic tumble square knot was developed in response to the unique challenges posed by minimally invasive surgery. Traditional suturing and knotting techniques, while effective in open surgery, often proved cumbersome and less reliable when translated to the laparoscopic context, where surgeons operate through small incisions using specialized instruments and cameras. The tumble square knot emerged as a solution, leveraging the principles of friction and leverage to create a secure and tight knot that can be executed in the limited space of laparoscopic surgery.

The technique involves creating a loop with the suture material, then "tumbling" the free end through this loop in a specific manner that allows for the formation of a square knot when tension is applied. This method can be repeated to stack multiple knots for added security, ensuring that the suture holds the tissue edges together effectively throughout the healing process.

◾ APPLICATIONS IN SURGERY

The laparoscopic tumble square knot is versatile, finding applications across a broad range of surgical procedures. It is particularly valuable in gastrointestinal surgery, gynecology, and urology, where secure tissue approximation is crucial for successful outcomes. Its reliability and the speed with which it can be executed make it an essential technique in surgeries where time is of the essence, such as in emergency repairs of internal organs.

◾ ADVANTAGES OVER TRADITIONAL TECHNIQUES

The primary advantage of the laparoscopic tumble square knot is its adaptability to the laparoscopic environment. Other benefits include:

- *Security:* The knot's design ensures it remains tight and secure, reducing the risk of postoperative complications such as leaks or wound dehiscence.
- *Efficiency:* Surgeons can execute the knot quickly, reducing operative time and potentially minimizing patient exposure to anesthesia.
- *Minimized tissue trauma:* The technique allows for precise tension control, avoiding excessive pressure on the tissues and promoting better healing.
- *Learnability:* Despite its effectiveness, the technique can be mastered with practice, making it accessible to surgeons at various skill levels.

◾ FUTURE IMPLICATIONS AND INNOVATIONS

As surgical techniques continue to evolve, the principles underlying the laparoscopic tumble square knot are likely to inspire further innovations. The integration of robotic surgery platforms, for instance, could enhance the precision and consistency of this knotting technique. Advanced imaging and augmented reality could also provide real-time guidance to surgeons, making the execution of such knots even more accurate and reliable.

Moreover, the continued refinement of suture materials, combined with innovative knotting techniques, promises to further reduce surgical complications and improve patient outcomes. Research into biomechanics and tissue healing could lead to customized knotting strategies tailored to specific surgical procedures or patient needs.

The laparoscopic tumble square knot represents a significant advancement in the field of minimally invasive surgery. Its development not only addresses the specific challenges of laparoscopic procedures but also exemplifies the ongoing pursuit of surgical excellence. As technology advances, the integration of new tools and techniques will likely expand the applications and effectiveness of this knotting method. Ultimately, the laparoscopic tumble square knot stands as a testament to the innovation and adaptability at the heart of modern surgery, promising better care and outcomes for patients worldwide.

One noteworthy intracorporeal knot in this context is the tumble square knot. Essentially, it begins as a standard square knot and then transforms into a slip knot, allowing for a sliding configuration. This knot is particularly useful in laparoscopic procedures.

For this type of knot, surgeons typically use suture materials like polyglactin 710 and polydioxanone (PDS). The suture length employed should generally be less than 24 centimeters to ensure optimal performance and maneuverability during laparoscopic tissue approximation.

This knot is particularly useful for approximating tissues that are under tension. For instance:

- *Posthysterectomy vaginal vault closure:* It is employed to suture the vault of the vagina after a total laparoscopic hysterectomy.
- *Burch suspension:* It is employed in procedures like the Burch suspension, where tissue tension needs to be managed.
- *Fundoplication:* It is used during fundoplication surgeries for gastroesophageal reflux disease (GERD); it can aid in securing tissues.
- *Myomectomy:* Surgeons use it to suture the seromuscular layer after performing a myomectomy.
- *Duodenal perforation closure:* It can be utilized to close ruptures in cases of duodenal perforation, ensuring a secure and stable closure.

The tumble square knot's ability to handle tension makes it a valuable tool in various laparoscopic procedures where tissue approximation is critical.

ADVANTAGES

The advantages of tumble square knot are as follows:

- It is a very secure knot.
- Easy to apply
- Faster to apply
- Requires less suture

DISADVANTAGES

Disadvantages of tumble square knot are as follows:

- It can cut through tissues.
- Slippery suture materials like Prolene cannot be used since the knots will tend to become loose.
- Braided suture material may also cause problems since there will be difficulty in sliding the knot.

TASK ANALYSIS OF TUMBLE SQUARE KNOT

- Cutting the suture = 24 cm
- Inserting the Maryland in the reducer
- Holding the suture in the middle
- Hiding in the reducer
- Inserting the needle in the abdomen with the reducer
- Dropping over the tissue in a way that the tip should be on the left and the tail should be on the right
- Align the needle by the following three techniques:

1. Pressing the needle by the upper jaw of the needle holder at the junction of one-third proximal and two-third distal of the needle.
2. Holding the needle by the left hand at the curvature and pulling the suture up near the needle by the right hand
3. Hang the needle by left hand like a pendulum and go with the open jaw of the needle holder keeping the moving jaw to the left and dragging it to the right.

- Stabilize the tissue with the left hand and prick the tissue by the needle and by rotating the tip of needle to keep it perpendicular to the tissue.
- Bringing the tip of the needle 1/3rd out and catch it with left-hand instrument, keeping the convex end of the instrument toward the tissue.
- Guard the tissue by the needle holder keeping the concave part toward the tissue and pulling the needle by left-hand instrument
- Hold the needle by the needle holder as soon as the needle is out and take bite at the other side of the tissue to be approximated and then pull the needle with Maryland while supporting the tissue with the needle holder and once the needle is out, hold the suture with the needle holder.
- Guard the suture by the Maryland and pull the suture by the needle holder to make a tail. The length of the tail should be defect plus 2 cm.
- A "C" shape will form and keep the left-hand instrument above and in the center of the "C".
- Bring the tip of the needle holder near the tip of the Maryland and rotate the needle holder clockwise to make a loop.
- Keep the Maryland static and take one loose wrap by the needle holder.
- Move both the instruments together to catch the tail by the Maryland.
- After catching the tail do not pull the tail but move the needle holder toward the tip of the Maryland. The knot should be placed toward the left side with the tail facing upward. The knot should not be placed in the middle or on the right side.
- Drop the suture away from the Maryland and keeping the loop loose, hold the suture with the Maryland and make a reverse "C"
- Now, keep the needle holder static at the center and above the reverse "C"
- Hold the suture with Maryland and bring the tip of Maryland near the tip of the needle holder.

- Rotate the Maryland anticlockwise to make a loop.
- Keeping the needle holder static, take a single wrap with Maryland.
- The needle holder will catch the tail but the tail should not be pulled.
- Maryland will slide the loop in the direction of the tip of the needle holder.
- Maryland will drop the suture and then tighten the knot. It will be a square knot.
- Now, pull the needle end and the limb on the same side as the needle end in the opposite direction to convert the square knot into a slip knot. i.e., tumbling.
- Now, slip the knot with the help of Maryland to tighten the tissue and bring them together till the buttock sign is formed. The knot should be held with 3rd or 4th serrated jaw of the Maryland. It should not be held with the tip or with the base.
- Now, hold the long end with Maryland and the tail with needle holder and pull the tail to untumble the slip knot to square knot and lock the knot.
- Keep the Maryland steady and hold the needle end with the needle holder and pull it to make "C".
- Now, hold the suture with the needle holder and keep Maryland steady and at the center of "C".
- Rotate the needle holder clockwise to make a loop and take one wrap over the Maryland with the needle holder.
- Both the instruments move together to hold the tail with the Maryland and the needle holder will slide the wrap in the direction of the tip of the Maryland
- The needle holder will leave the suture away from the knot and come again to catch the suture near the knot
- The needle holder and Maryland by holding the suture will move in the opposite direction to tighten the last knot in the tissue plane.

- Hold the needle at the end of the suture with the Maryland and remove the needle holder.
- Introduce the scissor in the right port and cut the suture.
- Hide the suture in the reducer by pulling Maryland and the reducer together out.
- Push the Maryland to eject the needle.

Steps

The steps to tie a tumble square knot are given as follows (**Figs. 1 to 11**):

1. Take a bite of the tissue to be approximated. Similarly, the other edge of tissue is also taken. Pull the needle end of the thread in, keeping at least 4 cm of tail end free (**Figs. 1A to C**).
2. A "C" loop is made with the thread keeping the left-hand instrument above the "C". One wind is taken around the tip of instrument with the needle holder (**Figs. 2A to C**).
3. A half knot is then made, which must be away from the suture line (**Figs. 3A and B**).
4. A reverse "C" is then made keeping the tip of the needle holder above and middle of the "C". A wind is made with left-hand instrument (**Figs. 4A and B**).
5. The tail end of the thread is pulled by the needle holder. An opposite half knot is, thus, made (**Figs. 5A and B**).
6. The needle end of the thread and the thread of the same side beyond the knots are pulled in opposite directions to help the knots tumble (**Figs. 6A and B**).
7. When the knots have tumbled and the closed jaw of Maryland is used to slide the tumbled knots toward the tissue of approximation (**Figs. 7A and B**).
8. Knots are tightened to approximate the edge of tissues (**Figs. 8A and B**).

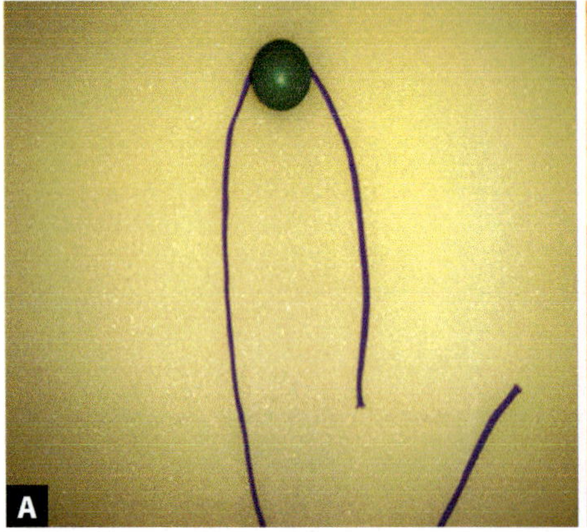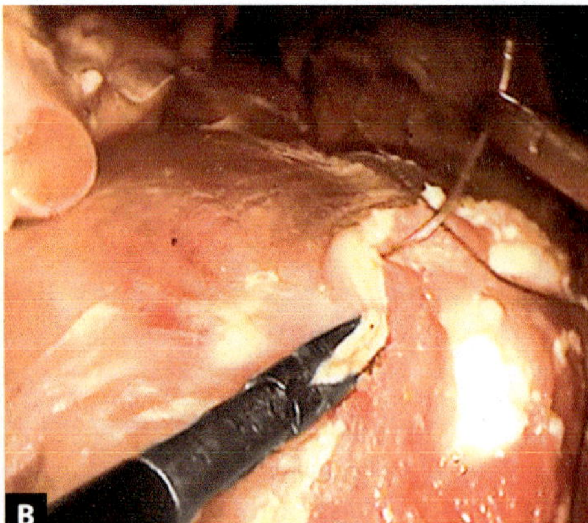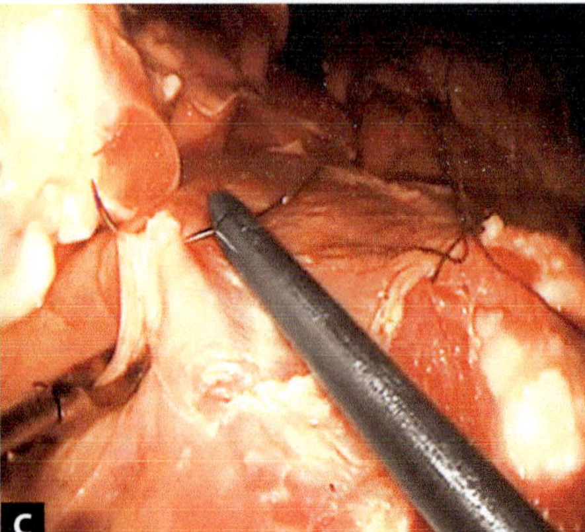

Figs. 1A to C: Step 1.

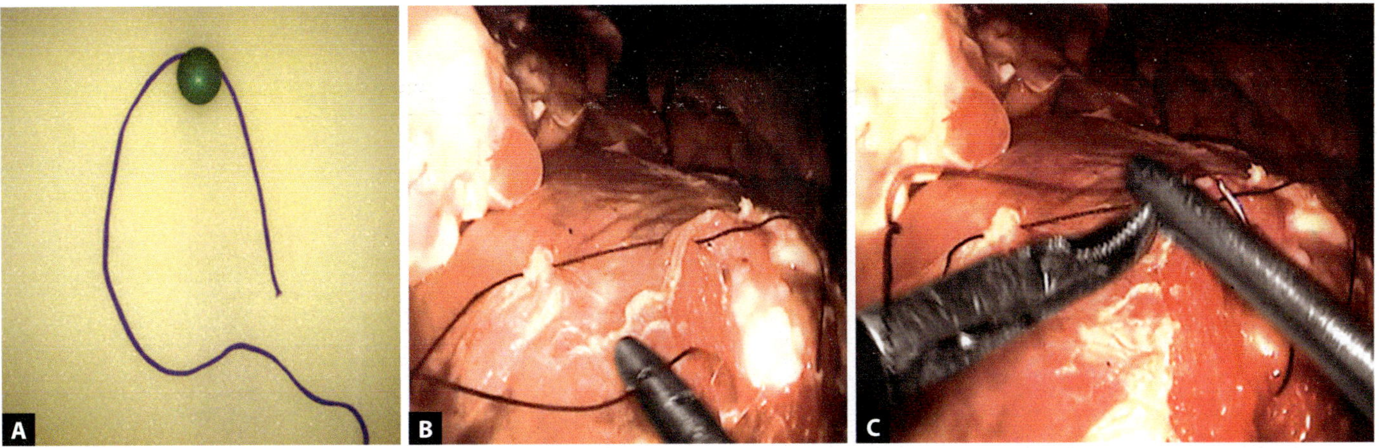

Figs. 2A to C: Step 2.

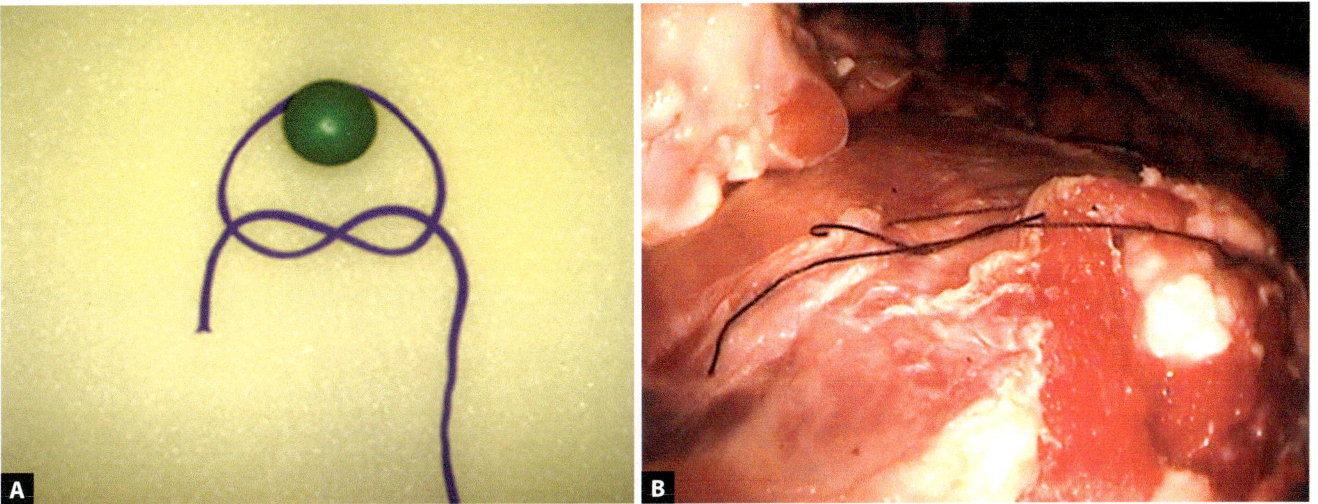

Figs. 3A and B: Step 3.

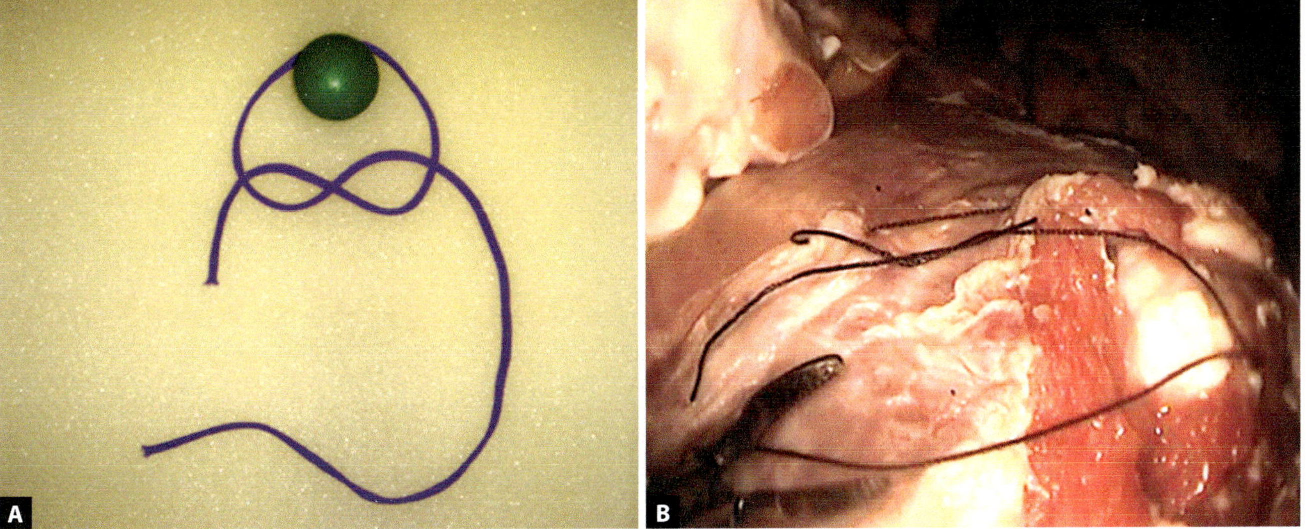

Figs. 4A and B: Step 4.

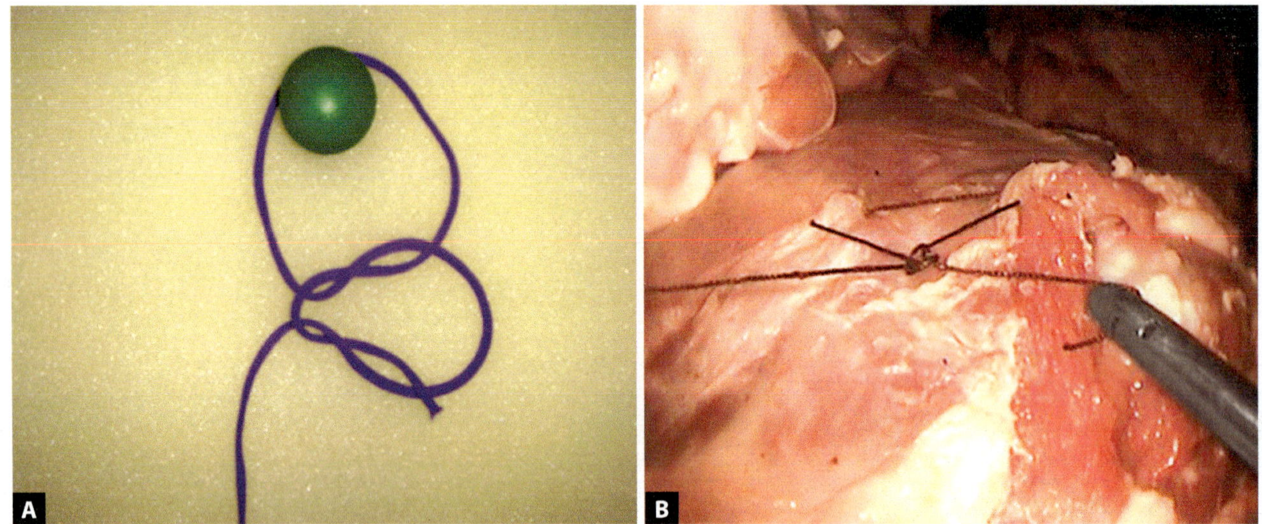

Figs. 5A and B: Step 5.

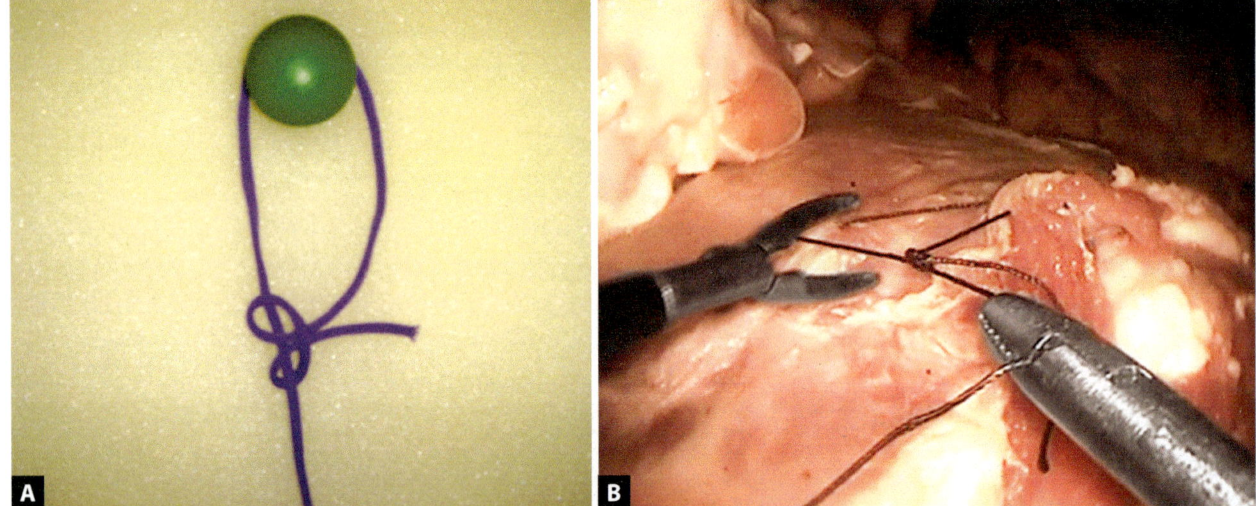

Figs. 6A and B: Step 6.

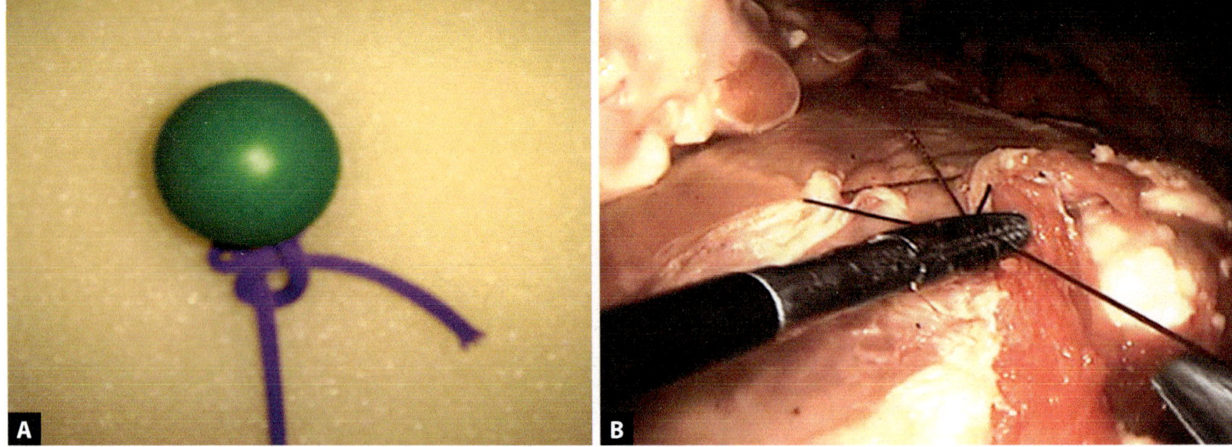

Figs. 7A and B: Step 7.

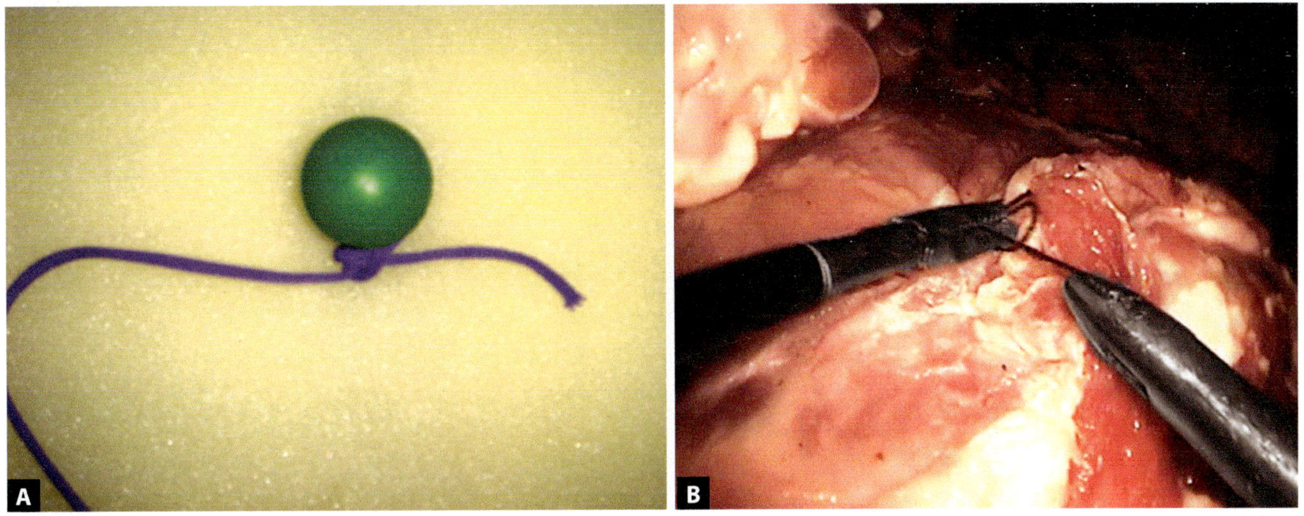

Figs. 8A and B: Step 8.

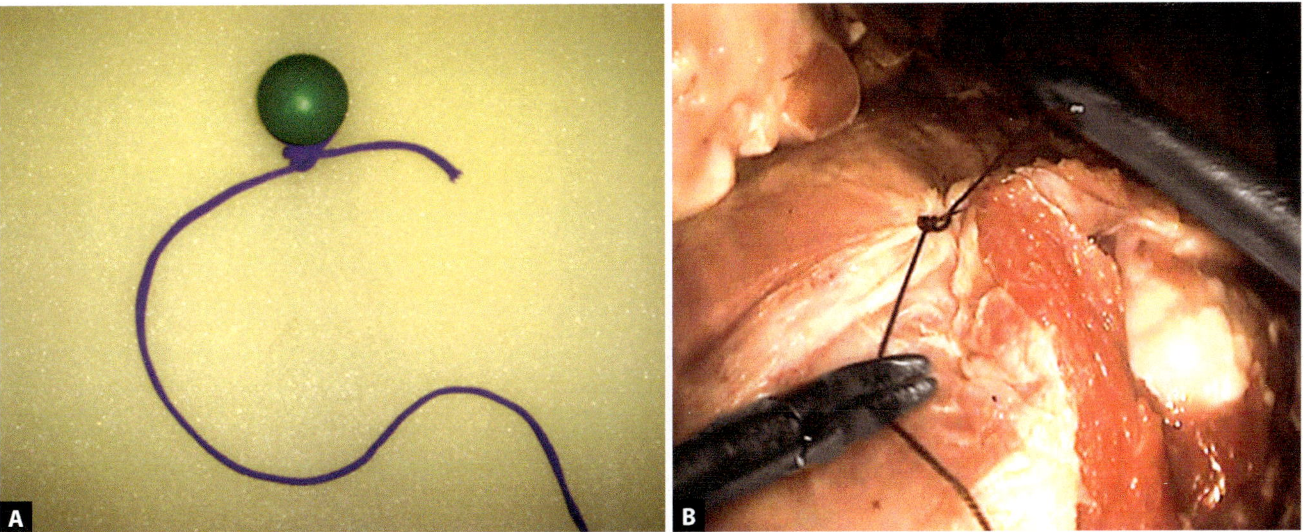

Figs. 9A and B: Step 9.

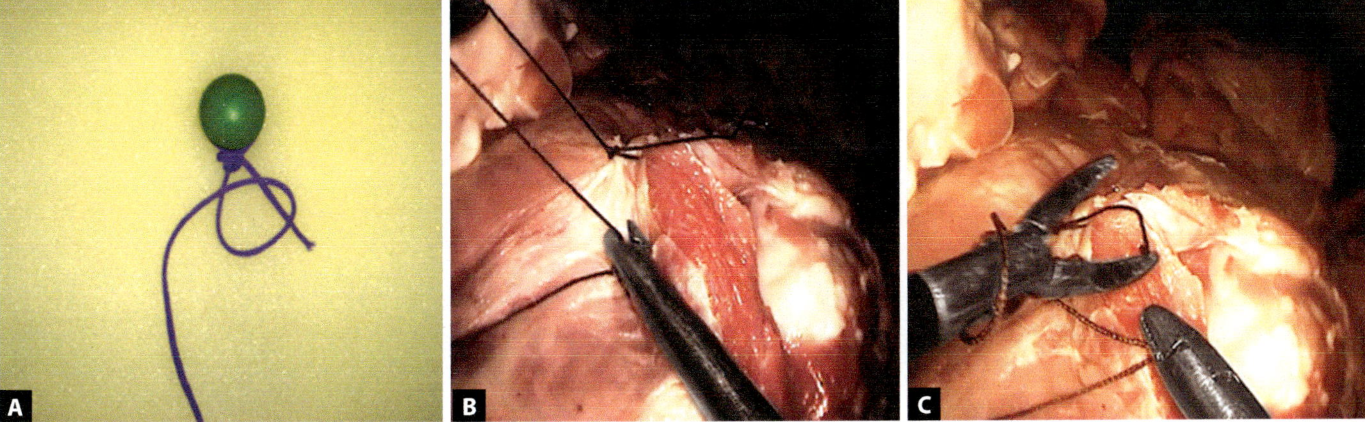

Figs. 10A to C: Step 10.

9. Now, both ends of the thread are pulled to untumble the knot **(Figs. 9A and B)**.
10. A "C" loop is then made and as in step 2 and a wind is taken over left-hand instrument **(Figs. 10A to C)**.
11. A half knot is then completed and the ends of the suture are tightened **(Figs. 11A and B)**.

■ CLINICAL APPLICATIONS

Figures 12 and 13 show tumble square knot being applied during fundoplication. This knot can be applied over any structure which is under tension.

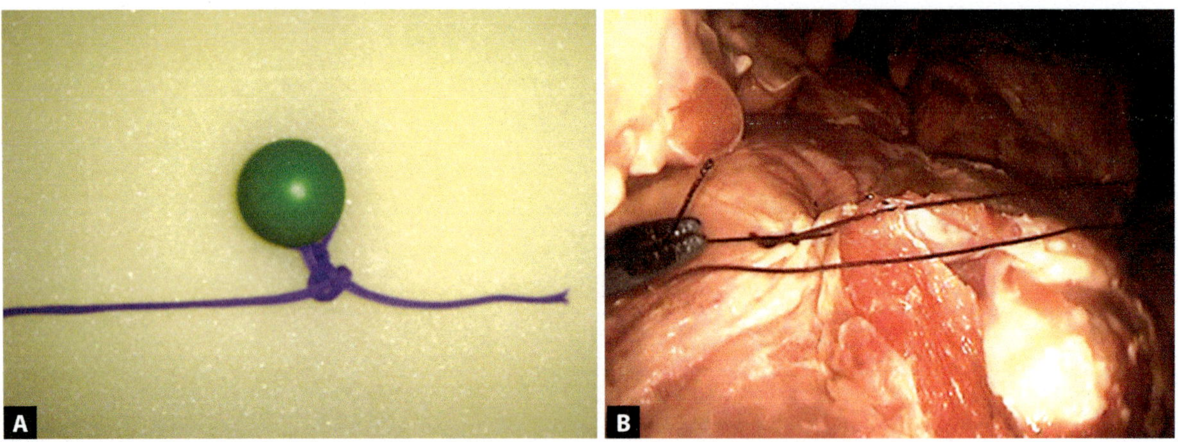

Figs. 11A and B: Step 11.

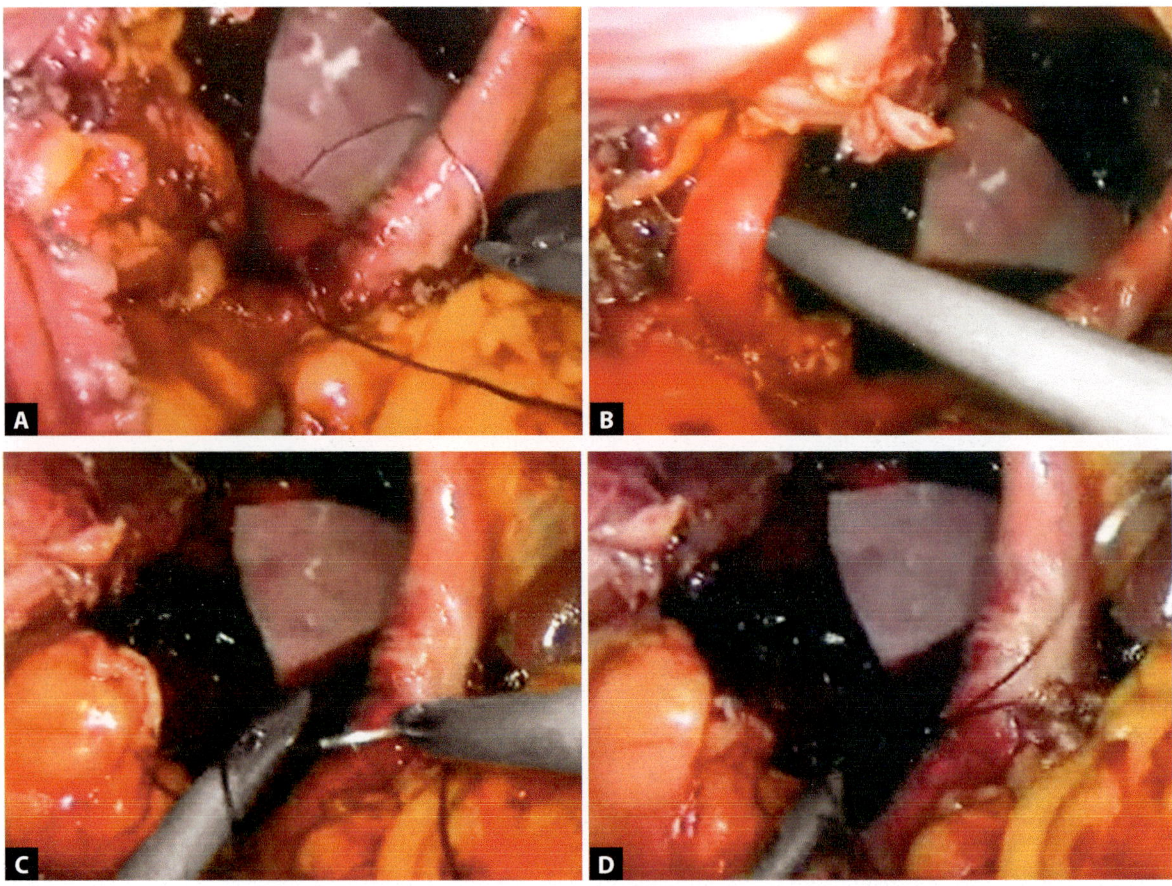

Figs. 12A to D:

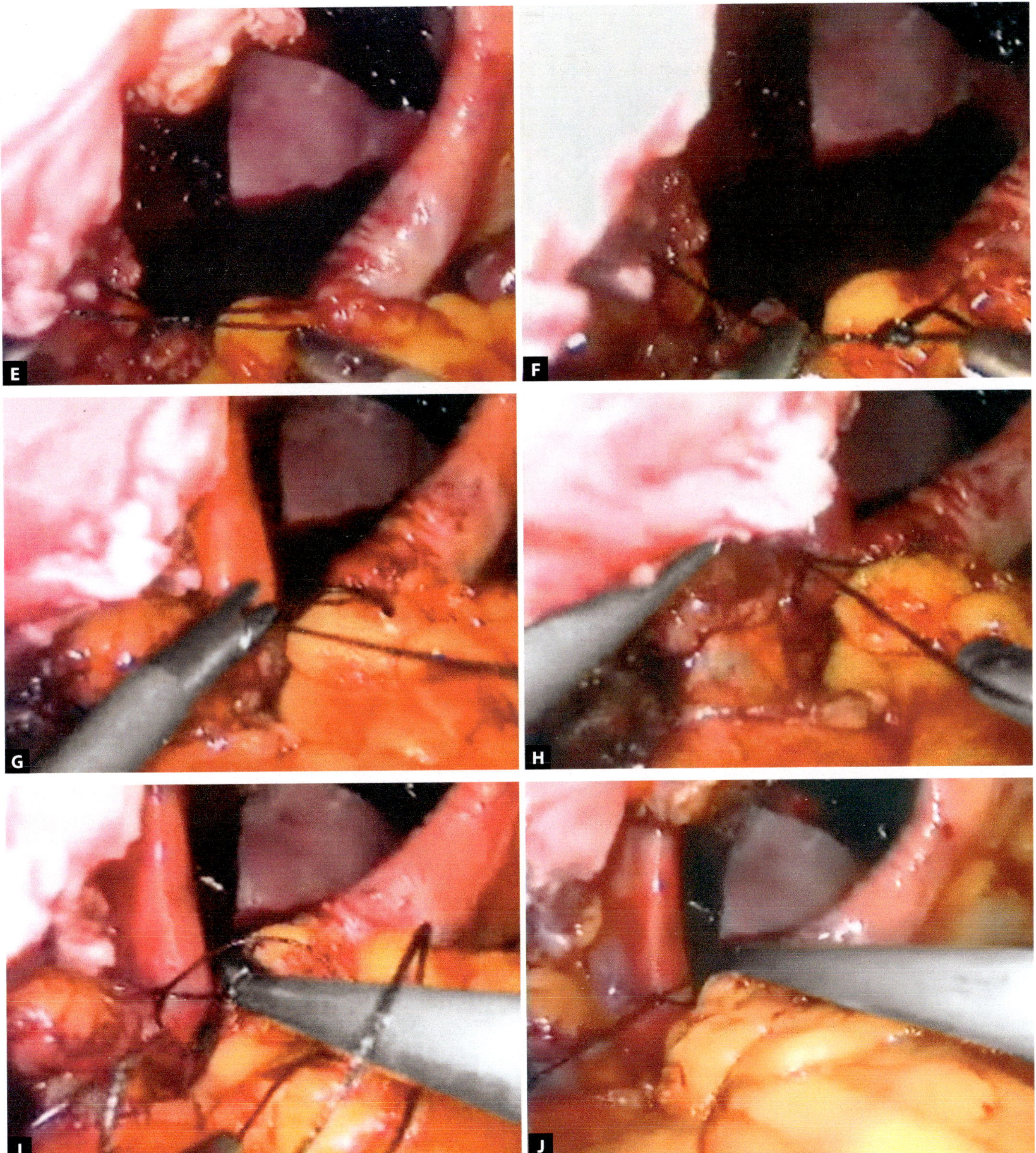

Figs. 12A to J: (A) Needle is being passed through the left crus of the diaphragm; (B) The right crus is taken next; (C) A half knot is being made; (D) A half knot is made in one direction to tumble the knot; (E) Knot is approximated; (F) Same side of the suture is pulled in opposite directions to tumble the knot; (G) Needle holder is used to slide the knot down to approximate both crura. (H) Opposite ends of the suture are pulled to untumble the knot. (I) Another half knot is made to secure the tumble square knot; (J) Finally, the knots are tightened.

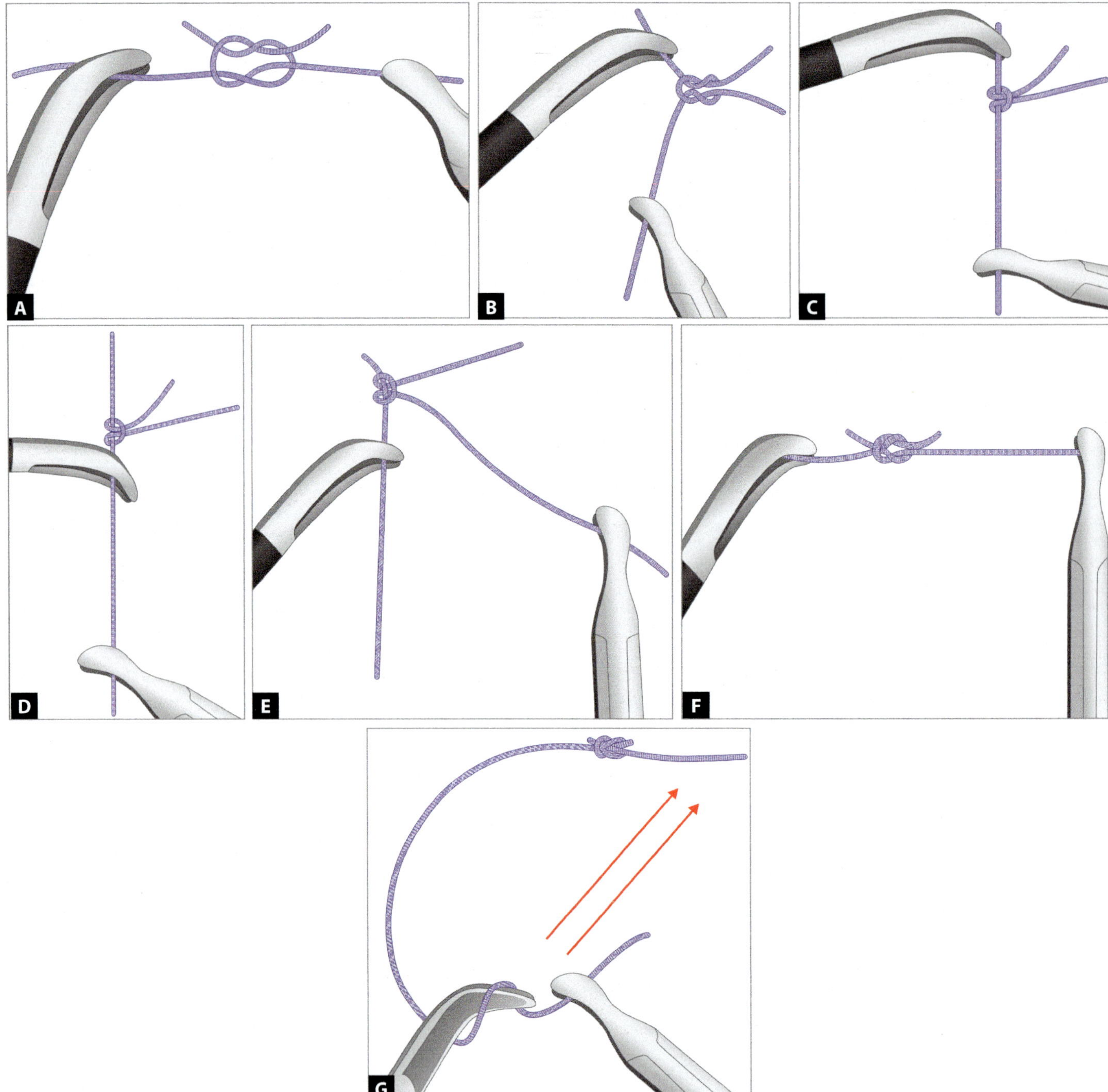

Figs. 13A to G: (A) A square knot is tied; (B) Same side of thread should be straightened with the help of two Marylands or needle holders; (C) After straightening the same side of thread, it is ready to slide; (D) Closed jaw of Maryland forceps will slide the knot; (E and F) After tightening, the knot is locked again by pulling both the thread; (G) This is a simple square knot which can be changed to slipping configuration by tightening of a same side of thread.

■ CONCLUSION

Laparoscopic knots must meet specific criteria: they should be safe, straightforward to execute, provide secure closure, and be replicable. Although intracorporeal suturing and knot tying initially demand manual dexterity, regular practice can transform them into routine tasks.

When operating within the abdominal cavity, utilizing the tumble square knot offers advantages over extracorporeal knot tying. This includes avoiding the seesaw effect and minimizing tissue tugging. Extracorporeal knot tying can involve the challenging task of passing lengthy suture material through tissues and the same port, which the tumble square knot circumvents.

◼ BIBLIOGRAPHY

1. Chen MH, Khalil H. Laparoscopic Suturing Techniques for Surgeons. Oxford: Oxford University Press; 2022.
2. Choi E, Kim DY. The Use of Biodegradable Sutures in Laparoscopic Surgery. Journal of Biomedical Materials. 2024;15(3):438-45.
3. Fernandez R, Martin CJ. Ergonomics in Laparoscopic Suturing: Minimizing Surgeon Fatigue. Journal of Ergonomics in Surgery. 2023;17(3):145-54.
4. Gomez R, Lee T. Evolution of Suturing Techniques in Laparoscopic Surgery. J Minim Invasive Surg. 2021;28(2):123-32.
5. Gupta S, Mehra R. Barriers to Learning Laparoscopic Suturing: A Survey of Surgical Residents. Education in Surgery. 2023;47(1):55-62.
6. Harper D, Lombardi A. Adapting Traditional Suturing Techniques for Laparoscopic Applications. Surgical Techniques Review. 2021;35(4):320-8.
7. Kumar V, Saxena AK. Advanced Techniques in Laparoscopic Surgery. Berlin: Springer; 2020.
8. Lavelle JF, Sinclair MF. Automated Suturing Devices in Laparoscopic Surgery: A Comparative Analysis. Technology in Surgery. 2020;22(6):789-98.
9. Lee J, Kim S. Innovations in Laparoscopic Suturing Instruments. Int J Med Robot. 2022;18(1):e2210.
10. Mendez C, Gupta A. Laparoscopic Suturing: Mastery Through Technique and Practice. London: Elsevier Health Sciences; 2023.
11. Mishra RK. Textbook of Laparoscopy for Surgeons and Gynecologists, 4th edition. New Delhi: Jaypee Brothers Medical Publishers (P) Ltd; 2021.
12. Morrison T, Jacobs LR. Teaching Laparoscopic Suturing: The Role of Simulation in Medical Schools. Medical Teacher. 2021;43(7):778-84.
13. Nguyen L, Ho CP. Impact of Suture Materials on Laparoscopic Knot Reliability. Materials in Surgery. 2024;9(2):200-10.
14. O'Reilly MP, Saunders BH. Virtual Reality Training for Laparoscopic Surgery. Cambridge: Cambridge University Press; 2022.
15. Patel R, Thompson J. The Role of Simulation in Learning Laparoscopic Suturing and Knotting. Medical Education Online. 2021;26:1857289.
16. Rodriguez A, Davis SS. Robotic-Assisted Laparoscopic Knot Tying: Methods and Efficiency. Surgical Innovation. 2019;26(4):459-66.
17. Shimi SM, Lirig M, Vander-Velpen G, Cusehieri A. Comparative study of holding strength of slipknot using absorbable and nonabsorbable ligature materials. Surg Endosc. 1994;11:1285-91.
18. Smith JA, Patel VR (Eds). Principles of Laparoscopic Suturing and Knotting. New York: Springer; 2023.
19. Surgical Knots and Suturing Techniques. (2024). [online] Available from https://en.wikipedia.org/wiki/Surgical_knot.
20. Wang Y, Thompson C. Innovations in Knot Tying Techniques for Minimally Invasive Surgery. Innovations in Surgery. 2022;18(4): 250-60.
21. Williams NE, Tan JL. Comparative Study of Knot Security in Laparoscopic Surgery. J Surg Res. 2020;245:217-23.
22. Zimmerman KA, Patel ND. Laparoscopic Knotting: A Visual Guide for Surgeons. Philadelphia: Lippincott Williams & Wilkins; 2022.

Starter Knot for Continuous Suturing

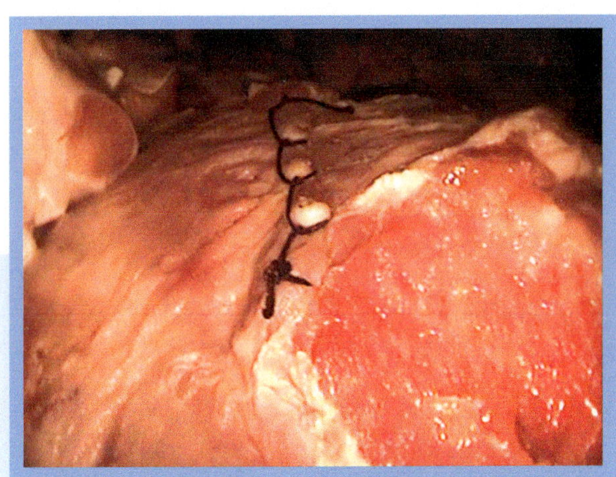

■ INTRODUCTION

Intracorporeal suturing and knot tying rank among the most challenging aspects of laparoscopic procedures. The Dundee Jamming slip knot, an innovation from the University of Dundee, UK, was designed as a user-friendly extracorporeal knot to initiate continuous suturing within the abdominal cavity during laparoscopic surgeries. It has become a common practice to commence continuous sutures in laparoscopic surgery using the Dundee Jamming slip knot.

Our confidence in the simplicity and safety of this knot within the realm of laparoscopic surgery, combined with our goal of teaching the fundamental principles of knot tying and suturing, inspired us to create this book. This effort is especially significant in an era where suturing staple devices have become increasingly prominent in laparoscopic surgery. Through this chapter, our main objective is to elucidate the technique of this knot and its application in laparoscopic procedures.

■ APPLICATIONS

The Dundee slip knot is highly versatile in various surgical scenarios, including the continuous closure of viscera. It is particularly useful for suturing viscerotomes after stapled anastomosis, securing anastomoses such as gastrojejunostomy or ileocolostomy. Additionally, it can be effectively employed for continuous serosal or peritonia closures, where adding an extra one or two hitches in starting the knot is recommended to enhance security.

■ ADVANTAGES

The Dundee slip knot offers simplicity in extracorporeal application, ensuring a secure knot when appropriately locked. This knot's versatility extends to both continuous and interrupted intracorporeal suturing, accommodating both monofilament and braided threads. Additionally, it presents a cost-effective alternative when compared to the expenses associated with stapling devices.

■ DISADVANTAGES

While passing through tissue, the thread can potentially cause abrasion against the anchor eyelet or even lead to cutting as it moves within the tissue. Consequently, it is not regarded as the ideal choice for interrupted sutures.

■ TECHNIQUE

The Dundee slip knot comprises both an extracorporeal and intracorporeal component when employed for continuous suturing within the abdominal cavity.

For this technique, the suture material attached to the Endoski needle should be trimmed to an appropriate length, typically around 15–30 cm. It is crucial to ensure that the thread length does not exceed 40 cm, as this can makes intracorporeal handling extremely challenging.

The knot is initiated in an extracorporeal fashion and is subsequently introduced into the abdominal cavity to initiate the continuous suturing process. To safeguard all ligatures and sutures from potential interference with the cannula valve mechanisms, we strongly recommend the use of an introducer tube.

Extracorporeal Component

Step 1

Start with the formation of an extracorporeal loop by passing the thread around the index finger of one hand allowing the short limb of the thread to pass above and cross over the long limb. The crossover point of the two limbs should be pinched by the ring and middle fingers (**Figs. 1A and B**).

Step 2

A second loop is formed by passing the index and the thumb fingers through the loop to hold the long limb from its proximal part and pull out through the already formed loop to create a new loop and a first sliding hitch, as shown in **Figures 2 and 3**.

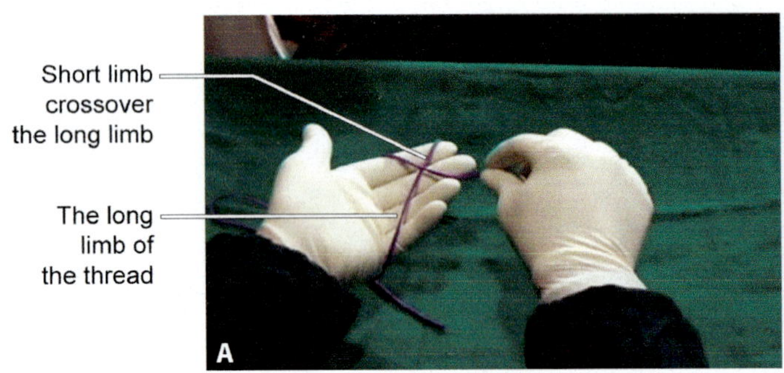

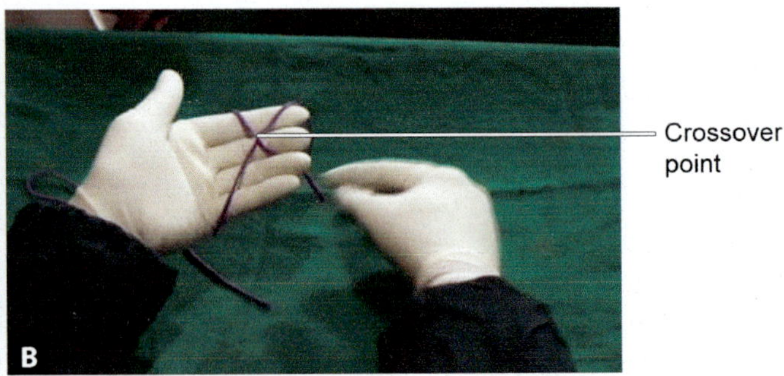

Figs. 1A and B: (A) Beginning of Dundee knot; (B) The short limb of the thread crosses over the long limb.

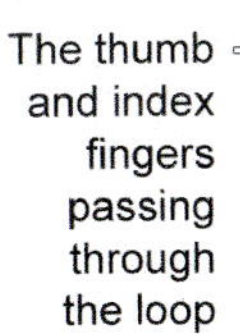

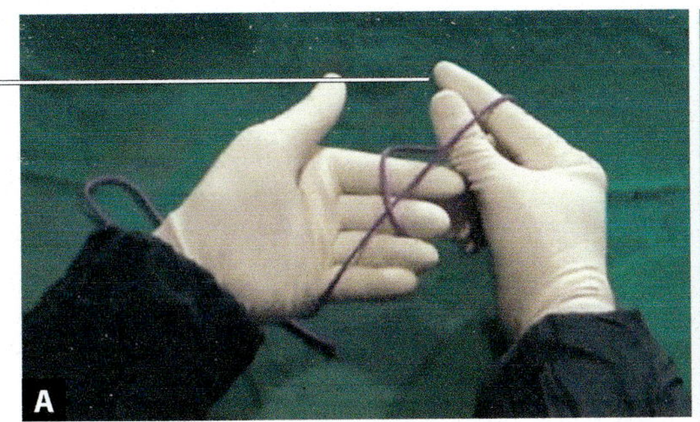

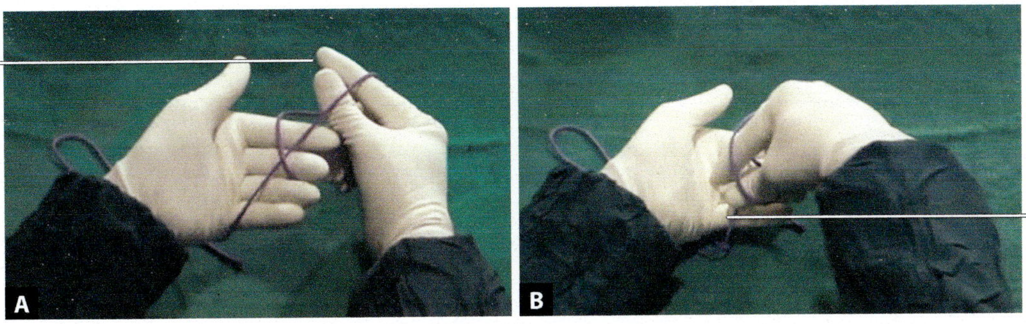

Figs. 2A and B: After passing your index and thumb fingers through the first loop, grasp the long limb of the thread from its proximal part.

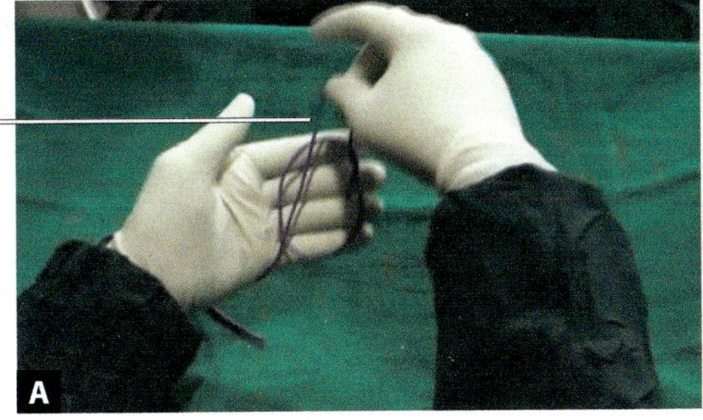
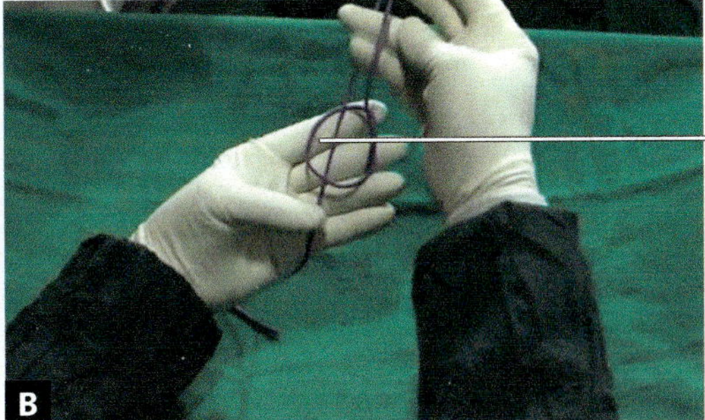

Figs. 3A and B: Demonstrating the formation of the first hitch of the Dundee knot.

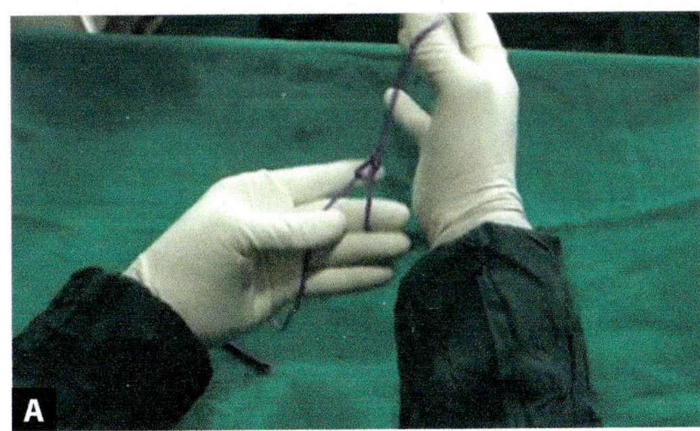
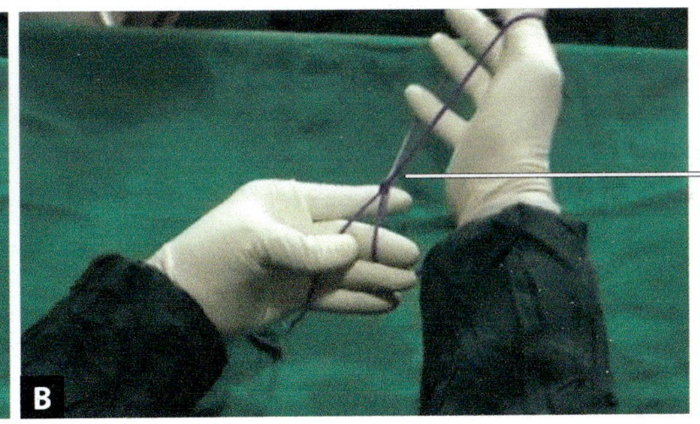

Figs. 4A and B: First hitch being stretched.

Step 3

The sliding hitch should be stretched as shown in **Figures 4A and B**.

Step 4

The maneuver in step 3 is repeated to form the third loop and second slipping hitch **(Figs. 5A to G)**.

Now, Dundee knot is locked and ready to be introduced to the abdominal cavity. The length of both the loop and of the tail should be at least 1 cm. The suture is picked up by the needle holder at its midpoint.

Make sure to test the slippery action of the knot before this maneuver.

Intracorporeal Component

It is the component performed inside the abdominal cavity by locking the Dundee knot, and performing the continuous suture.

Continuous Suture

Once the thread is within the abdominal cavity, the following steps should be followed:

- *Needle placement:* Pass the needle through the tissue that needs to be approximated.
- *Thread pull:* Pull the thread until the Dundee loop is anchored at the level of the tissue eyelet where the needle initially entered.

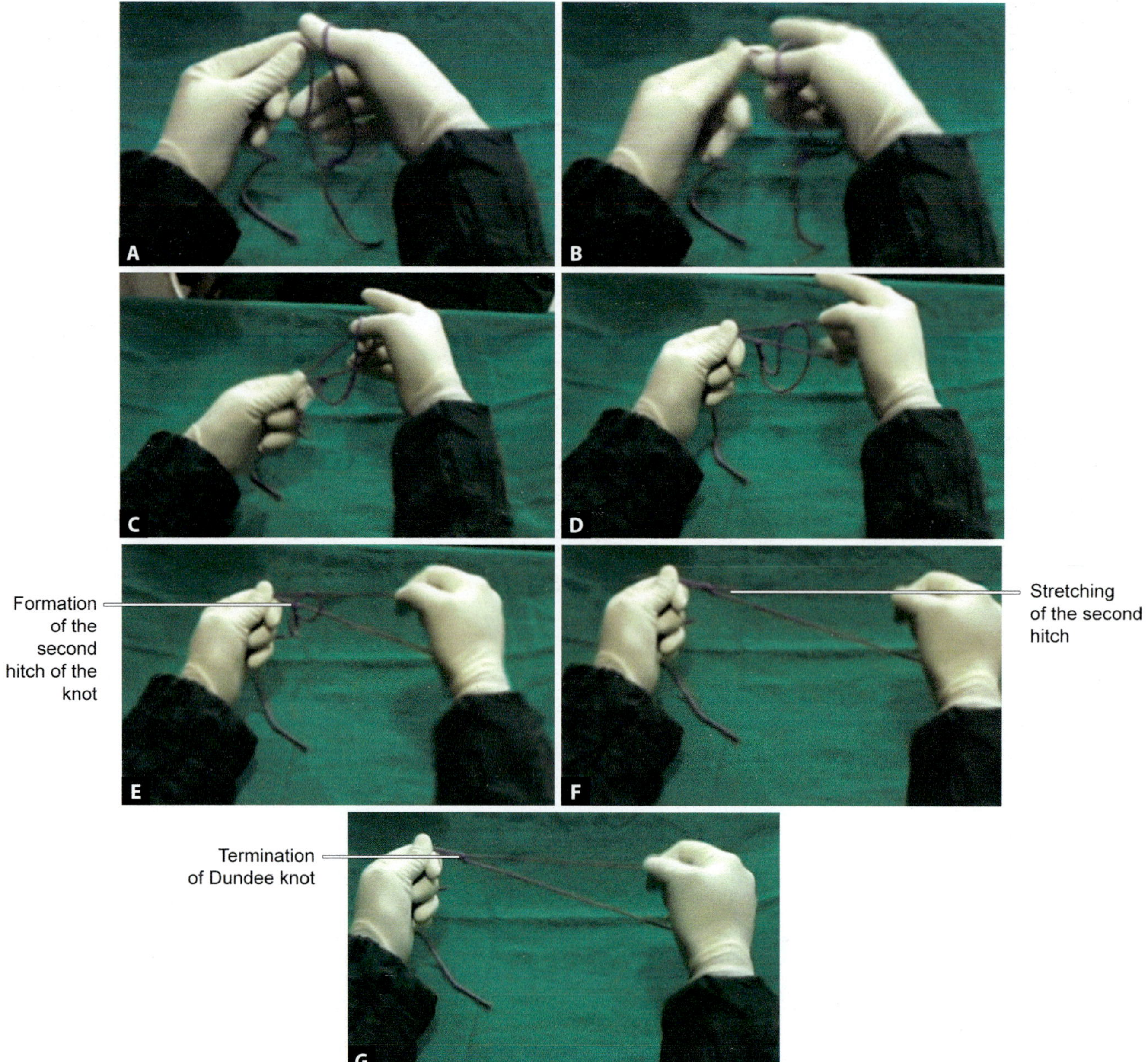

Figs. 5A to G: Termination of Dundee Jamming slip knot by formation of three loops and two sliding hitches.

- *Knot locking:* Before commencing the continuous suture, ensure the knot is locked. This is achieved by passing the needle through the Dundee loop and stretching it until the knot is completely secured.

- *Continuous suturing:* Continue the process by passing the needle through a C-shaped thread before inserting it through the tissue to lock the stitch. Pull the thread to maintain tension during the continuous suturing. Repeat this maneuver as necessary.

- *Termination:* Conclude the continuous suture by utilizing an Aberdeen knot or another appropriate knot, such as the tumble square. Detailed visual demonstrations of these steps are demonstrated below.

These steps illustrate the meticulous technique required for successful intracorporeal suturing with the Dundee slip knot.

- *Step 1:* Thread is introduced to the abdominal cavity, and the needle is held by the needle holder as shown in **Figures 6A and B**.

- *Step 2:* The continuous suturing started by introducing the needle through the tissue as shown in **Figures 7A to C**.

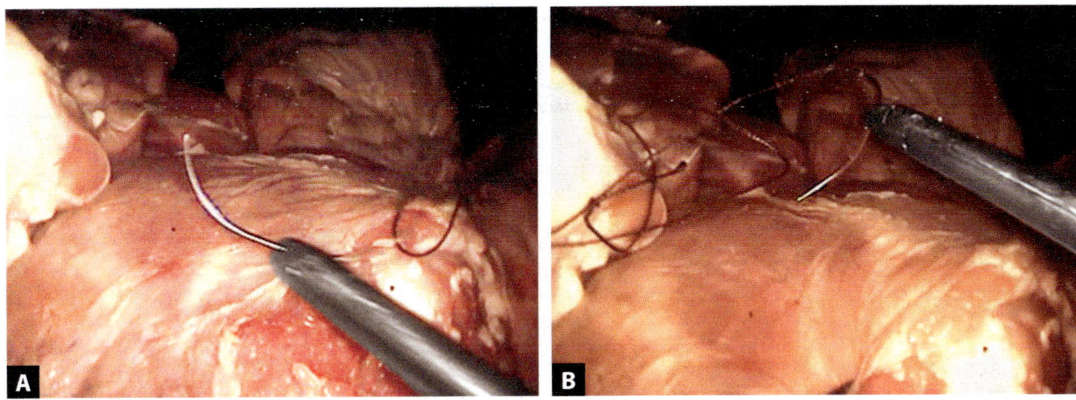

Figs. 6A and B: (A) Intracorporeal Dundee knot; (B) The needle is held by the needle holder to start the continuous suture.

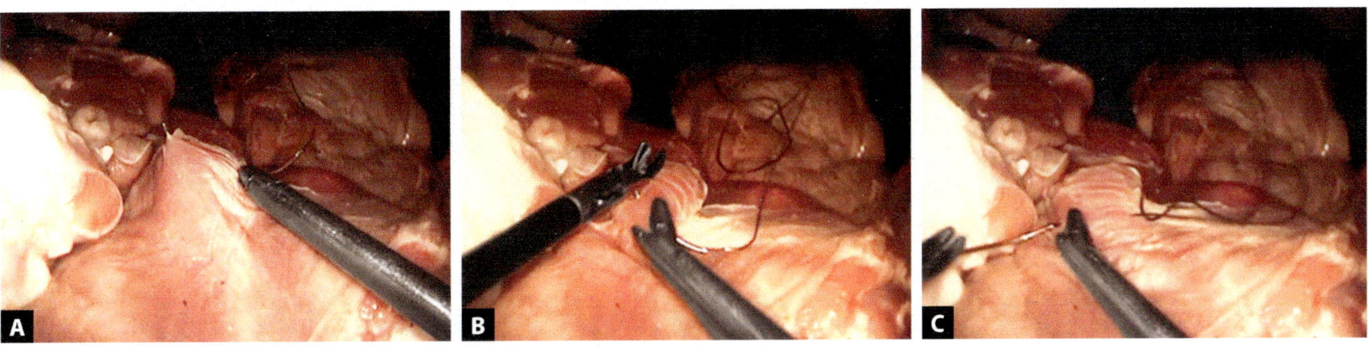

Figs. 7A to C: Starting the continuous suture.

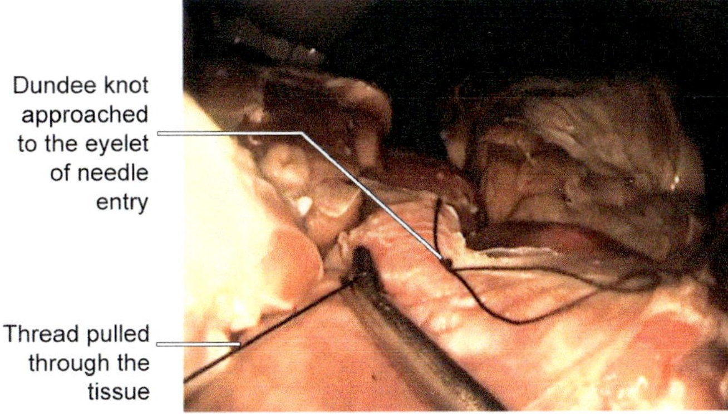

Fig. 8: Thread is pulled through the tissue and the knot is approached to the eyelet of needle entry.

- *Step 3:* Now, the thread should be pulled through the tissue until the Dundee knot reaches the anchor eyelet of needle entry **(Fig. 8)**.
- *Step 4:* The knot should be locked by passing the needle holder through the loop of the knot, holding the thread proximal to the loop and start pulling the thread and the needle out through the knot loop completely then stretch the thread with a force so the knot can be locked with tension safely to the tissue **(Figs. 9A to G)**.

- *Step 5:* Continuous suture is continued by passing the needle through a C-shaped part of the thread before taking other bits of tissue; to lock the stitch in tension as shown in **Figures 10A to G.**

Repeat step 5 as required. The continuous suture then should be terminated by an Aberdeen knot or other knot as below in **Figures 11A to C.**

- *Step 6:* Formation of Aberdeen knot and termination of continuous suture as shown in **Figures 12 and 13.**

Termination of continuous sutures can be performed by Aberdeen knot or any other knot, **Figure 13** demonstrates the end stage of the continuous suture.

■ CONCLUSION

The Dundee Jamming Knot: Revolutionizing Surgical Suturing Techniques

In the precise and evolving world of surgical procedures, the introduction of innovative suturing techniques significantly impacts the efficacy and outcomes of surgeries. Among these innovations, the Dundee Jamming knot stands out as a notable advancement, offering a blend

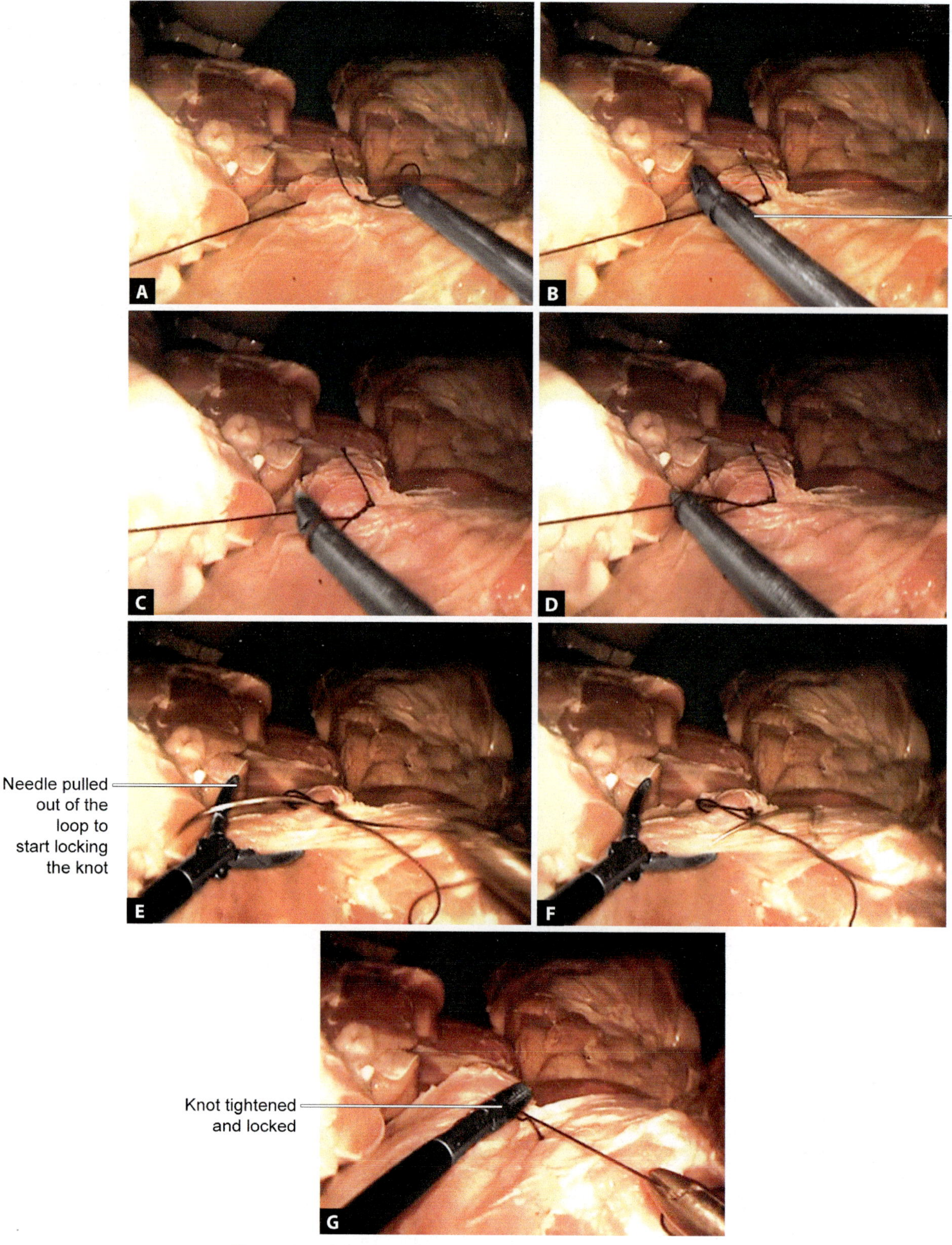

Figs. 9A to G: Locking the Dundee knot before starting continuous suture.

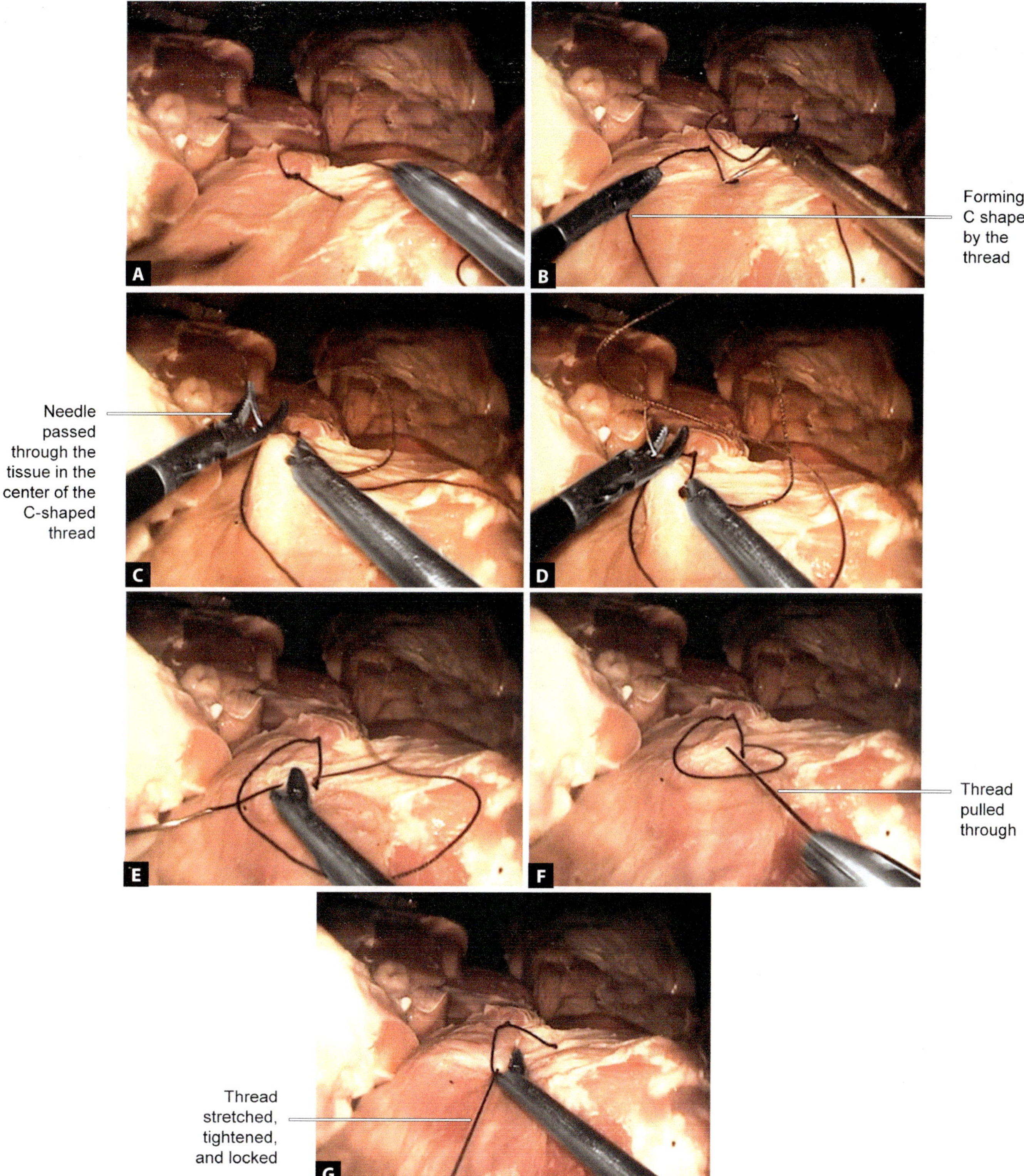

Figs. 10A to G: Forming a C shape by the thread and passing the needle through the tissue at the center of C-shaped thread.

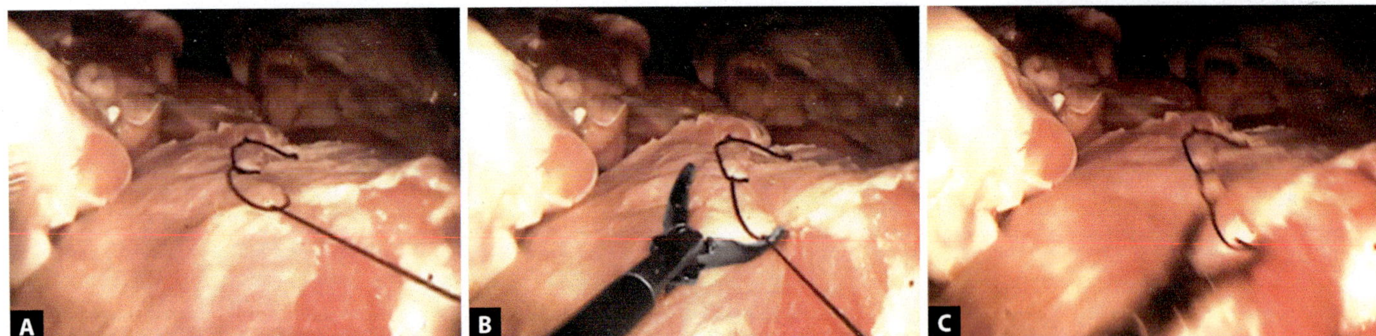

Figs. 11A to C: Continuous suture is performed by forming a C shape by the thread and introducing the needle into the tissue at the center of the C-shaped thread.

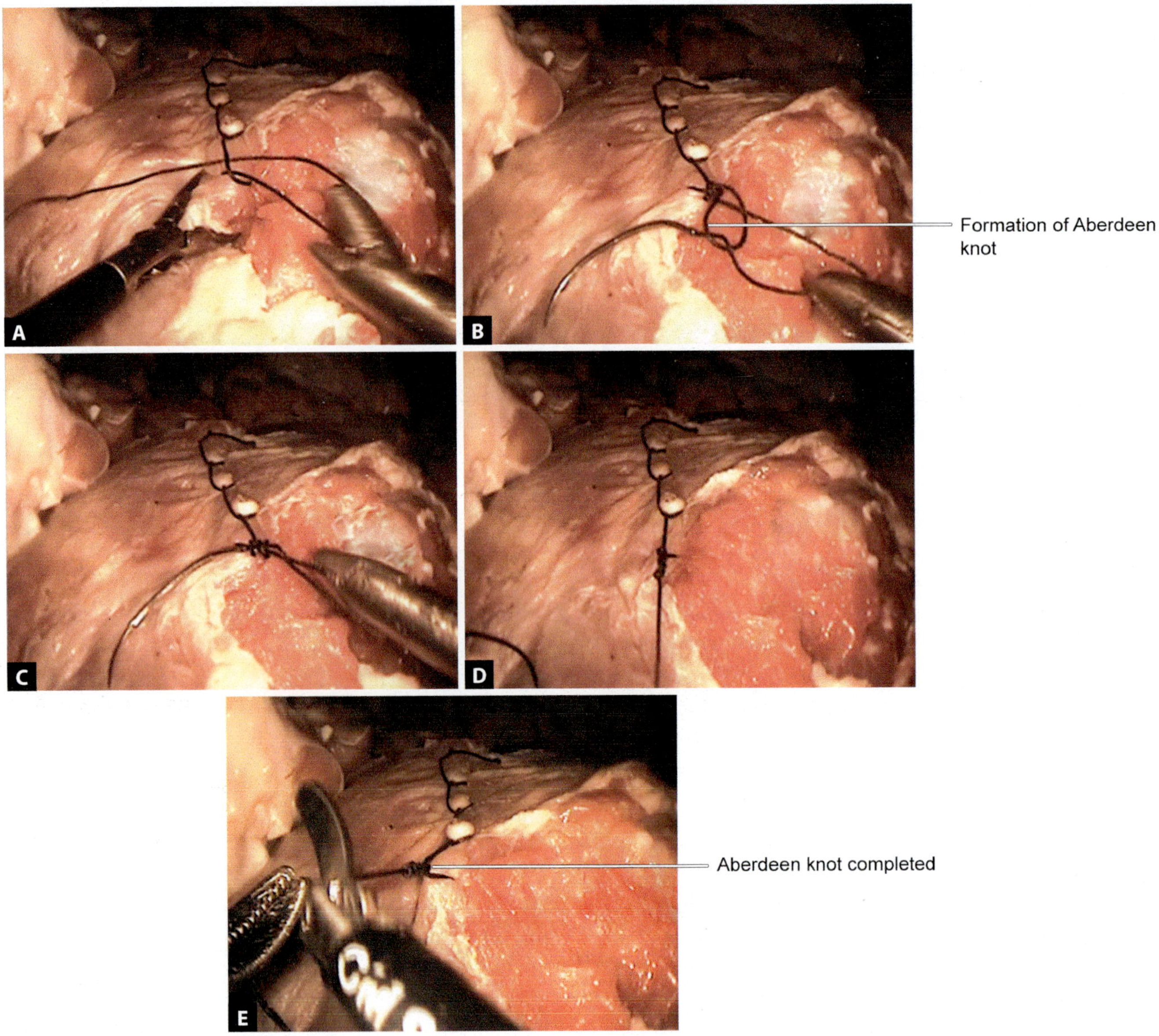

Figs. 12A to E: Formation of Aberdeen knot and cutting the end of the thread.

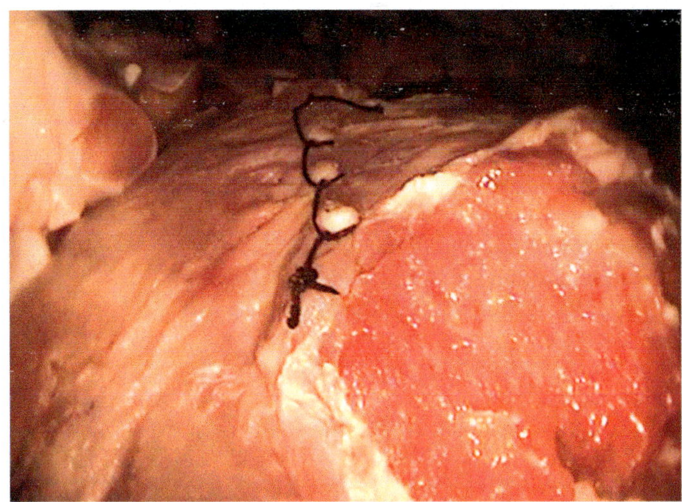

Fig. 13: Termination of the continuous suture.

of simplicity, security, and efficiency that revolutionizes how surgeons approach suturing, particularly in challenging surgical environments.

- *Origins and design:* Originating from the University of Dundee, a leading institution in medical research and education, the Dundee Jamming knot was developed by surgeons seeking a reliable knotting technique that could be easily replicated and would hold securely under various conditions. The design of the knot is ingeniously simple yet highly effective, utilizing the principle of friction and a unique looping mechanism that "jams" the knot into place, preventing slippage and untightening.
- *Application in surgery:* The versatility of the Dundee Jamming knot makes it a valuable addition to the surgeon's toolkit. Its primary application lies in situations where knot security is paramount, and the risk of knot slippage could lead to complications or failure of the surgical procedure. This includes high-tension areas or tissues that are prone to swelling, where traditional knots might loosen over time. The Dundee Jamming knot has found its place in various surgical specialties, from general surgery to orthopedics and even veterinary medicine, demonstrating its adaptability and reliability across different fields.
- Benefits of the Dundee Jamming Knot:
  - *Enhanced security:* The design ensures that once tightened, the knot's tension prevents it from loosening, offering unparalleled security in tissue approximation and healing.
  - *Simplicity in execution:* Despite its effectiveness, the Dundee Jamming knot is relatively simple to perform, even in the constrained spaces typical of minimally invasive surgeries. This simplicity accelerates the learning curve for surgical trainees.
  - *Versatility:* Its application across a range of surgical specialties underscores the knot's versatility, suitable for both internal and external sutures.
  - *Time efficiency:* In surgeries where time is of the essence, the quick execution of the Dundee Jamming knot can significantly reduce suturing time, benefiting both the surgical team and the patient.
- *The future of surgical knotting:* The Dundee Jamming knot exemplifies the continuous innovation in surgical techniques aimed at improving patient care and surgical outcomes. Its development is a testament to the importance of practical innovation in the field of surgery—innovations that may seem minor but can have a profound impact on the success of surgical procedures and the well-being of patients.

As surgical technology progresses, with advancements in robotic surgery and minimally invasive techniques, the principles behind the Dundee Jamming knot will likely inspire future innovations in surgical knotting and suturing devices. The ongoing exploration of materials, knotting techniques, and their applications in surgery promises to further enhance the efficacy, safety, and efficiency of surgical interventions.

■ BIBLIOGRAPHY

1. Chen MH, Khalil H. Laparoscopic Suturing Techniques for Surgeons. Oxford: Oxford University Press; 2022.
2. Choi E, Kim DY. The use of biodegradable sutures in laparoscopic surgery. J Biomed Mater. 2024;15(3):438-45.
3. Fernandez R, Martin CJ. Ergonomics in laparoscopic suturing: minimizing surgeon fatigue. J Ergon Surg. 2023;17(3):145-54.
4. Gomez R, Lee T. Evolution of suturing techniques in laparoscopic surgery. J Minim Invasive Surg. 2021;28(2):123-32.
5. Gupta S, Mehra R. Barriers to learning laparoscopic suturing: a survey of surgical residents. Education in Surgery. 2023;47(1):55-62.
6. Harper D, Lombardi A. Adapting traditional suturing techniques for laparoscopic applications. Surgical Techniques Review. 2021;35(4):320-8.
7. Kumar V, Saxena AK. Advanced Techniques in Laparoscopic Surgery. Berlin: Springer; 2020.
8. Lavelle JF, Sinclair MF. Automated suturing devices in laparoscopic surgery: a comparative analysis. Technology in Surgery. 2020;22(6):789-98.

9. Lee J, Kim S. Innovations in laparoscopic suturing instruments. Int J Med Robot. 2022;18(1):e2210.

10. Mendez C, Gupta A. Laparoscopic suturing: mastery through technique and practice. London: Elsevier Health Sciences; 2023.

11. Mishra RK. Textbook of Laparoscopy for Surgeons and Gynecologists, 4th edition. New Delhi: Jaypee Brothers Medical Publishers (P) Ltd; 2021.

12. Mishra RK. Textbook of Practical Laparoscopic Surgery. New Delhi: Jaypee Brothers Medical Publishers (P) Ltd; 2009.

13. Morrison T, Jacobs LR. Teaching laparoscopic suturing: the role of simulation in medical schools. Medical Teacher. 2021;43(7):778-84.

14. Nguyen L, Ho CP. Impact of suture materials on laparoscopic knot reliability. Materials in Surgery. 2024;9(2):200-10.

15. O'Reilly MP, Saunders BH. Virtual Reality Training for Laparoscopic Surgery. Cambridge: Cambridge University Press; 2022.

16. Patel R, Thompson J. The role of simulation in learning laparoscopic suturing and knotting. Medical Education Online. 2021;26:1857289.

17. Rodriguez A, Davis SS. Robotic-assisted laparoscopic knot tying: methods and efficiency. Surg Innov. 2019; 26(4):459-66.

18. Shimi SM, Lirig M, Vander-Velpen G, Cusehieri A. Comparative study of holding strength of slipknot using absorbable and nonabsorbable ligature materials. Surg Endosc. 1994;11:1285-91.

19. Smith JA, Patel VR (Eds). Principles of Laparoscopic Suturing and Knotting. New York: Springer; 2023.

20. Surgical Knots and Suturing Techniques. (2024). [online] Available from: https://en.wikipedia.org/wiki/Surgical_suture. [Last accessed]

21. Wang Y, Thompson C. Innovations in knot tying techniques for minimally invasive surgery. Innova Surg. 2022;18(4):250-60.

22. Williams NE, Tan JL. Comparative study of knot security in laparoscopic surgery. J Surg Res. 2020;245:217-23.

23. Zimmerman KA, Patel ND. Laparoscopic Knotting: A Visual Guide for Surgeons. Philadelphia: Lippincott Williams & Wilkins; 2022.

Aberdeen Termination

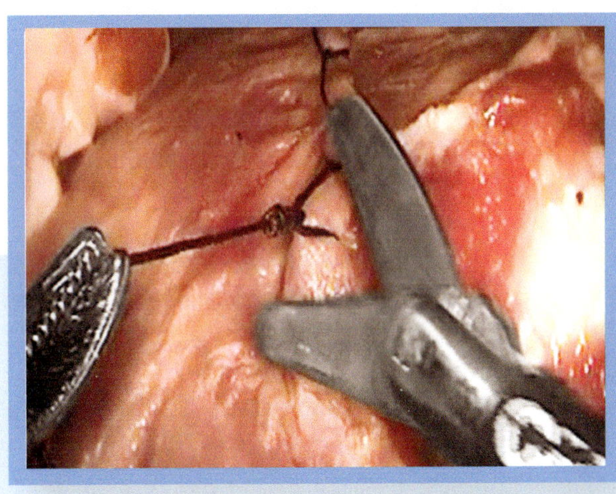

■ INTRODUCTION

Why every laparoscopic surgeon should learn how to approximate tissues by traditional means?

Over the past three decades, gynecologic laparoscopy has undergone a remarkable transformation. Initially limited to diagnostic purposes and tubal ligation, it has evolved into a crucial surgical tool for treating various gynecologic conditions. Today, laparoscopy ranks among the most frequently performed surgical procedures by gynecologists.

Laparoscopy represents a unique surgical approach, combining characteristics of both minor and major surgeries. From the patient's perspective, laparoscopic procedures often appear minor due to the small incisions, relatively low postoperative pain levels, and short recovery times. In cases where laparoscopy involves minimal intra-abdominal surgery, such as diagnostic procedures or tubal fulguration, the postoperative discomfort and risk of complications can resemble those of minor procedures.

However, it is essential to remember that at its core, laparoscopy remains an intra-abdominal procedure, carrying all the intraoperative and postoperative risks associated with laparotomy. These risks include infection and potential injury to neighboring intra-abdominal structures. Even when major intra-abdominal surgeries are performed laparoscopically, such as hysterectomies, there is still notable postoperative pain and morbidity. Nevertheless, the absence of a large abdominal incision ensures that postoperative pain and morbidity are consistently less severe than with similar major surgeries performed through laparotomy.

As laparoscopy has gained prominence in gynecology, various techniques have been developed to facilitate the efficient tying and cutting of large vessels. Traditional methods involving intracorporeal or extracorporeal knot tying have proven effective in this regard. More recently, innovative instruments have emerged to assist in the suturing process.

The ability to suture and tie knots has long been a fundamental skill for surgeons. While the introduction of advanced laparoscopic equipment for suturing, tying, and knotting is undoubtedly valuable, it should not entirely replace traditional suturing and tying techniques.

In the vast and intricate world of surgical knot tying, the Aberdeen termination knot stands out as a paramount technique, particularly favored for its strength, security, and efficiency. This chapter delves into the Aberdeen termination knot, exploring its origins, methodology, applications, and the pivotal role it plays in ensuring the safety and effectiveness of surgical procedures.

■ ORIGIN AND IMPORTANCE

The Aberdeen termination knot has its roots in the maritime and fishing industries, where knot security is critical. Adapted for surgical use, this knot has become a cornerstone in closing sutures with a focus on minimizing knot failure and promoting optimal healing. Its application spans a variety of surgical disciplines, showcasing its versatility and reliability.

■ THE TECHNIQUE EXPLAINED

The Aberdeen termination knot is particularly noted for its ability to securely finish continuous suturing sequences, providing an effective means of preventing suture slippage at the termination point. The technique involves the following key steps:

- *Suture advancement:* After the continuous suture line is placed, the surgeon leaves a small loop at the last stitch.
- *Knot formation:* The free end of the suture is threaded back through this loop and then weaved in and out of the preceding suture line several times.
- *Securing the knot:* As the free end is pulled tight, it locks into place, forming a secure and low-profile knot that minimally interferes with tissue healing.

■ ADVANTAGES OF THE ABERDEEN TERMINATION KNOT

The Aberdeen termination knot offers several significant benefits in surgical settings:

Security: It provides a highly secure method of finishing a continuous suture line, significantly reducing the risk of knot failure.

Tissue safety: Its low-profile nature and secure locking mechanism minimize tissue irritation and promote healing.

Efficiency: This knot can be tied relatively quickly and easily, enhancing surgical efficiency without compromising safety or effectiveness.

■ APPLICATIONS IN LAPAROSCOPIC SURGERY

The Aberdeen termination knot is versatile, finding utility in various surgical procedures where continuous suturing is employed. It is particularly beneficial in areas where suture integrity is paramount, such as in the closure of peritoneum and serosal incisions or in suturing internal organs where a secure, nonbulky knot is required to minimize tissue disruption.

CHALLENGES AND MASTERY

While the Aberdeen termination knot is highly effective, mastering it requires practice and understanding of its underlying principles. Surgeons often utilize simulation-based training to develop the dexterity and precision needed to execute this knot confidently in a clinical setting.

The Aberdeen termination knot is a testament to the ongoing evolution of surgical techniques, embodying a blend of tradition, innovation, and precision. Its adoption in surgical practice underscores the continuous quest for enhancing patient safety, surgical efficiency, and optimal healing outcomes. As the field of surgery progresses, mastering such advanced knotting techniques remains crucial for surgeons dedicated to providing the highest standard of care, making the Aberdeen termination knot an indispensable part of the surgical toolkit.

COST-EFFECTIVENESS

Low-income countries have often been reluctant to adopt this innovative surgical approach, reserving it exclusively for the affluent population. This hesitancy stems from the introduction of costly and sometimes unnecessary techniques, driven by profit motives. Expensive methods like lasers, disposable clip applicators, and pretied loop ligatures, which charge a fee for each tie, while beneficial in specific procedures, have overshadowed the simplicity of suturing and tying. The latter, when used alongside electrocautery, achieves similar surgical outcomes at a significantly lower cost. However, this has increased the overall expense of surgery, undermining the benefits of reduced morbidity and shorter hospital stays. As a result, these costly and sophisticated methods have made operative laparoscopy less accessible to economically disadvantaged countries, where these advantages are most needed.

Building on Clarke's original concept, it is worth noting that all procedures suitable for laparoscopic surgery in developing nations can be accomplished through suturing and tying. The instruments required for these techniques are much more cost-effective than their high-tech counterparts. This set of instruments includes a ligator, suture needle forceps, tissue forceps, and reusable scissors. As far back as 1972, Clarke suggested the use of electrocautery to complement suturing and tying techniques.

In many third-world countries, laparoscopic surgery is still colloquially referred to as Light Amplification by Stimulated Emission of Radiation (LASER) surgery. This terminology emerged from the aggressive marketing efforts of powerful surgical instrument corporations. However, this expensive technology was largely unnecessary in these regions. The consequence has been the emergence of glamorous surgery primarily accessible to the wealthy elite. Clarke's vision of operative laparoscopy, on the other hand, was rooted in providing a cost-effective surgical approach with shorter hospital stays and faster recoveries, directly benefiting underprivileged patients.

BENEFIT FOR THE PATIENT

In many third-world countries, patients express concerns when metal clips are inadvertently left inside their abdomens. Survival rates after complications like hematomas, bile duct drainage following cholecystectomy, or unintended ureter damage during hysterectomy, often associated with clip-guns, can be significantly lower in poorly equipped hospitals. Some of these complications can be either prevented or effectively treated during laparoscopic procedures by surgeons skilled in suturing and tying techniques.

Tubal interruption through electrocauterization has led to premature menopause, dysfunctional uterine bleeding, and even hysterectomy in younger women. In third-world regions, sterilization is typically considered a definitive procedure. The use of plastic clips for temporary sterilization necessitates a second operation, which many patients cannot afford. On the other hand, suturing and tying for tubal interruption is a more localized procedure with fewer effects on the ovaries. In women from third-world countries, the complications arising from extensive electrical burns in the adnexa can have catastrophic consequences. Moreover, follow-up care is often nonexistent in these regions.

SIMPLE INSTRUMENTS: CAN BE MADE AND MAINTAINED IN THE THIRD WORLD

The essential instruments needed for suturing and tying in laparoscopy include the suture needle forceps, ligature, and laparoscopic scissors. The suture needle forceps are straightforward, locally repairable, and can be manufactured in some third-world countries. Needles can be replaced when they become dull and can also be sharpened. Any suitable suture material can be utilized, eliminating the need for more expensive, nonreusable needles with fused-on sutures, as required by laparoscopic needle holders. The Clarke ligator, which has proven its value worldwide, is a simple rod with a grooved distal end. Laparoscopic scissors have long been manufactured in third-world countries. These simple instruments and techniques are well-suited for the often poorly equipped and isolated hospitals in our third-world regions.

Knots have been used since the time of primitive humans for trapping animals and crafting weapons. Today's laparoscopic knots are essentially adaptations of knots used by seamen, fishermen, weavers, or hangmen. In much of the literature on laparoscopic surgery, the learning curve for mastering this technique is described as steep.

Indeed, laparoscopy represents more than just a new technique; it represents an entirely different approach to tissue approximation. The visualization is distinct, the instruments are different, and the tactile aspects are markedly different. The skill of laparoscopic suturing and knotting requires extensive practice. As a young surgeon in training, you often spend countless nights tying knots repeatedly until perfection is achieved.

Several techniques for laparoscopic tissue approximation are available, with the most commonly used including:
- Laparoscopic extracorporeal and intracorporeal knots
- Surgical glues that act as tissue adhesives
- Laparoscopic clips
- Laparoscopic staplers
- Laser welding

■ LAPAROSCOPIC SUTURING AND KNOTTING

It is essential to keep in mind that a knot is either precisely correct or fundamentally incorrect; there is no middle ground. The process of knot tying involves three distinct steps:
1. Configuration (tying)
2. Shaping (drawing)
3. Securing (locking or snuggling)

Choice of Suture Material

Ideal Suture Characteristics

The selection of suture material significantly impacts wound healing. Desirable suture characteristics include:
- Good knot security
- Adequate tensile strength

- Flexibility and ease of handling
- Inertness and nonallergenic nature
- Resistance to infection
- Smooth passage through tissue
- Absorbability (when needed)

Surgeons should opt for sutures they are comfortable working with and appropriate for the specific surgical purpose. This decision should take into account the expected duration of tensile strength.

For internal sutures, it is advisable to minimize the number of knots used to ensure knot security, avoid excessive knot-related issues, and prevent foreign body reactions.

Knots

The knot plays a paramount role in in vivo suture closure. In fact, it is the key determinant of suture strength in a substantial 95% of suture tests. Complex knots, although offering greater security, can introduce complications that weaken the overall suture strength.

Moreover, the size of the knot is a critical consideration. For instance, transitioning from 3 to 5 throws with the same suture increases the foreign body volume by 50%.

■ ABERDEEN TERMINATION

This technique is an adaptation of a commonly used method for concluding abdominal closure in open surgery. To complete the continuous suture, three interlocking loops are formed. To facilitate tension maintenance in the suture line, the penultimate stitch can be locked. Subsequently, another bite is taken, and the suture is partially drawn through, leaving a small loop. This loop is large enough for a needle holder to pass through and grasp the standing part of the suture. Then, a loop is drawn through the first loop and tightened onto the tissues. This process is repeated three times, with each loop being tightened as you progress. To tighten each loop, tension should be applied to the leg of the loop exiting from the tissues or the preceding loop.

Finally, the standing part and needle are pulled entirely through the last loop. The standing part is elevated, and the suture is tensioned with counter pressure from the jaws of the needle holder, which are placed on either side of the suture. The excess suture is cut off, leaving a reasonable length of approximately 1 cm.

■ STEPS OF ABERDEEN TERMINATION KNOT

- *Step 1:* At the end of continuous suturing, the last stitch should be taken unlocked (**Figs. 1A and B**).
- *Step 2:* A loop at the needle end is passed under the last stitch entering the tissue (**Figs. 2A and B**).

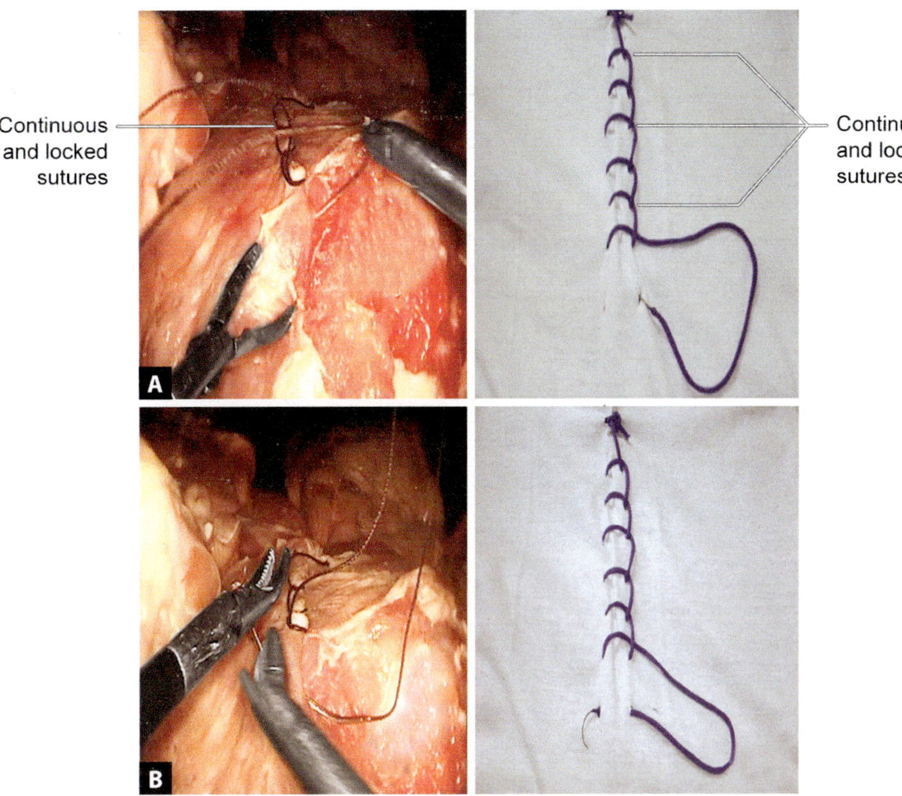

Figs. 1A and B: Aberdeen termination knot—step 1.

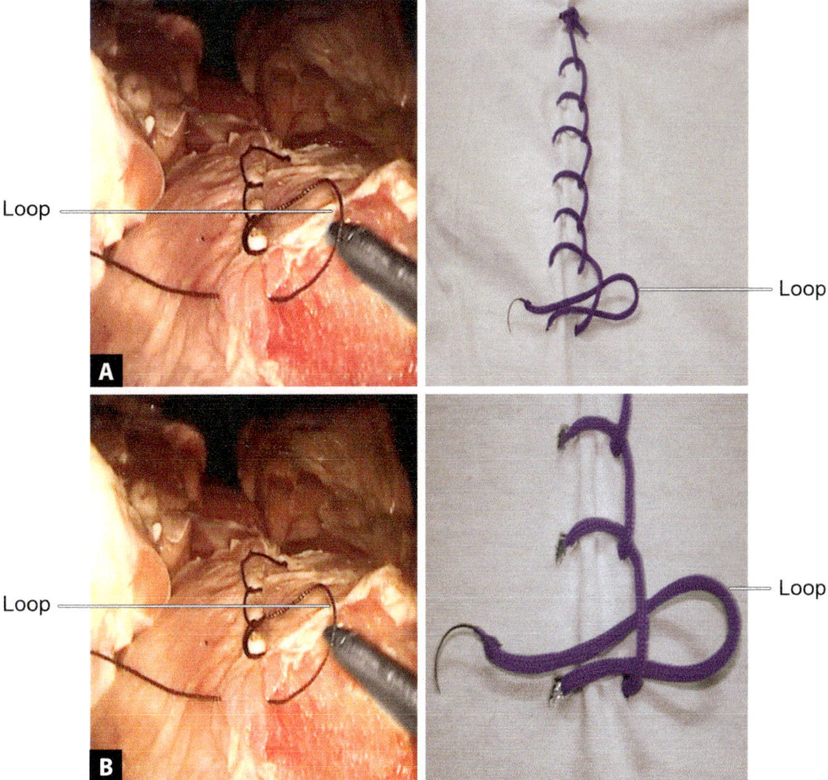

Figs. 2A and B: Aberdeen termination knot—step 2.

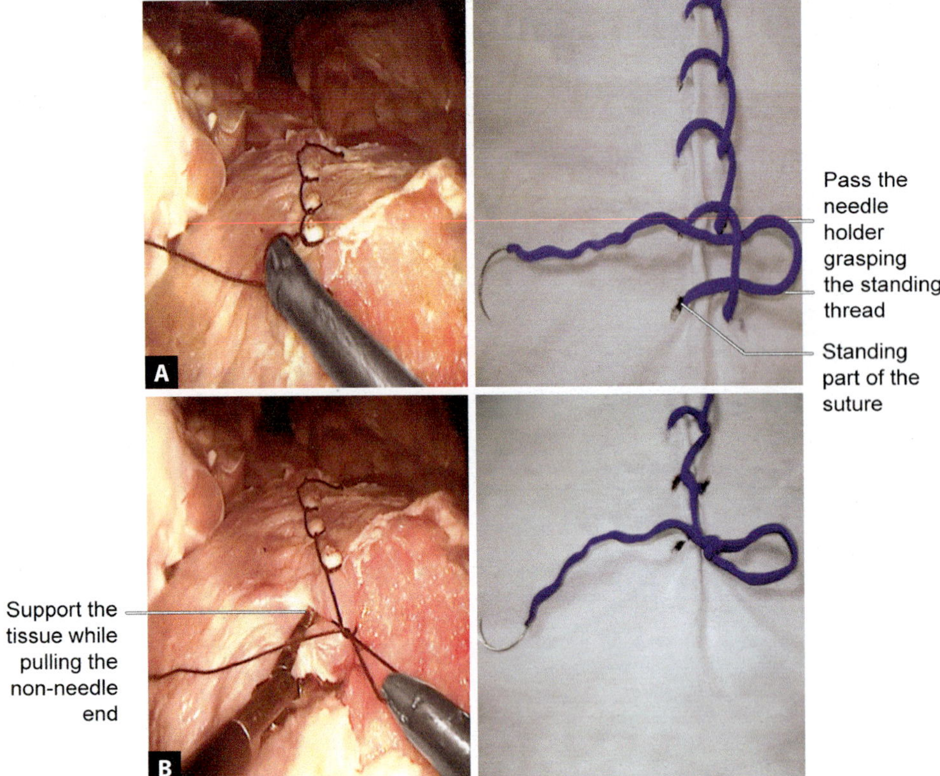

Figs. 3A and B: Aberdeen termination knot—step 3.

- *Step 3:* The needle holder is now introduced through the loop and the standing part of the suture is picked up and pulled, this makes tension on the continuous suturing above and finishes the first knot (**Figs. 3A and B**).
- *Step 4:* After finishing tying the first knot, pull the suture toward the needle end to decrease the size of the loop, and introduce the needle holder through it grasping the non-needle end, this will complete the second knot (**Figs. 4A and B**).
- *Step 5:* The standing end of the thread is pulled by the needle holder while supporting the tissue with the Maryland forceps (**Fig. 5**).
- *Step 6:* The needle holder is introduced through the loop and the needle end of the thread is grasped and pulled through the needle, this will form the third knot (**Figs. 6A to C**).
- *Step 7:* The needle thread is pulled by the needle holder while supporting the tissue with Maryland forceps to tighten the knot (**Fig. 7**).
- *Step 8:* The remaining part of the thread is pulled by Maryland forceps and cut using scissors (**Figs. 8A and B**).

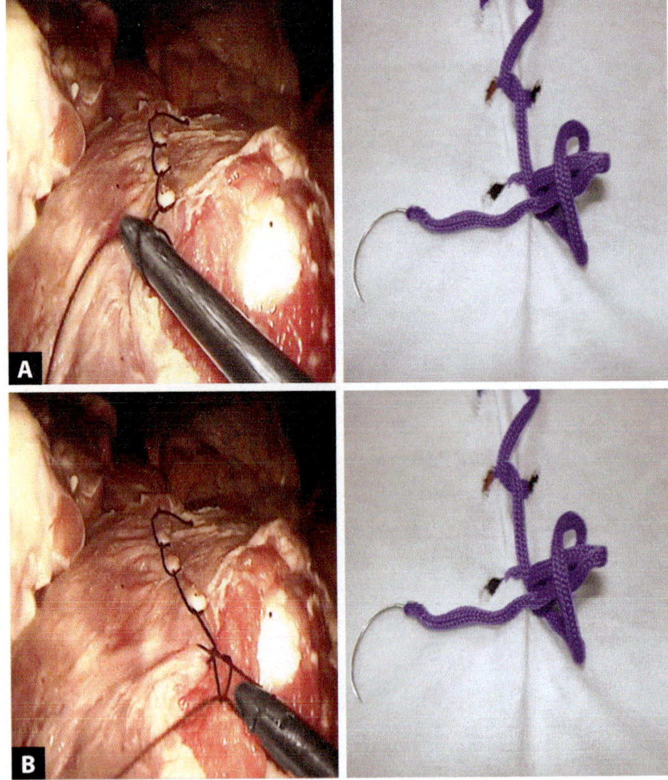

Figs. 4A and B: Aberdeen termination knot—step 4.

■ USES OF ABERDEEN TERMINATION KNOT

Aberdeen termination knot is used in situations where the tension on the tissue is not desired or required, like the closure of the peritoneum.

It is better to use Vicryl suture material in this type of knot because Polydioxanone (PDS) suture is difficult to tie.

■ ADVANTAGES OF ABERDEEN TERMINATION KNOT

- It is an easy knot, does not require special instruments or extraordinary skills to perform, and can be tied using a single port.

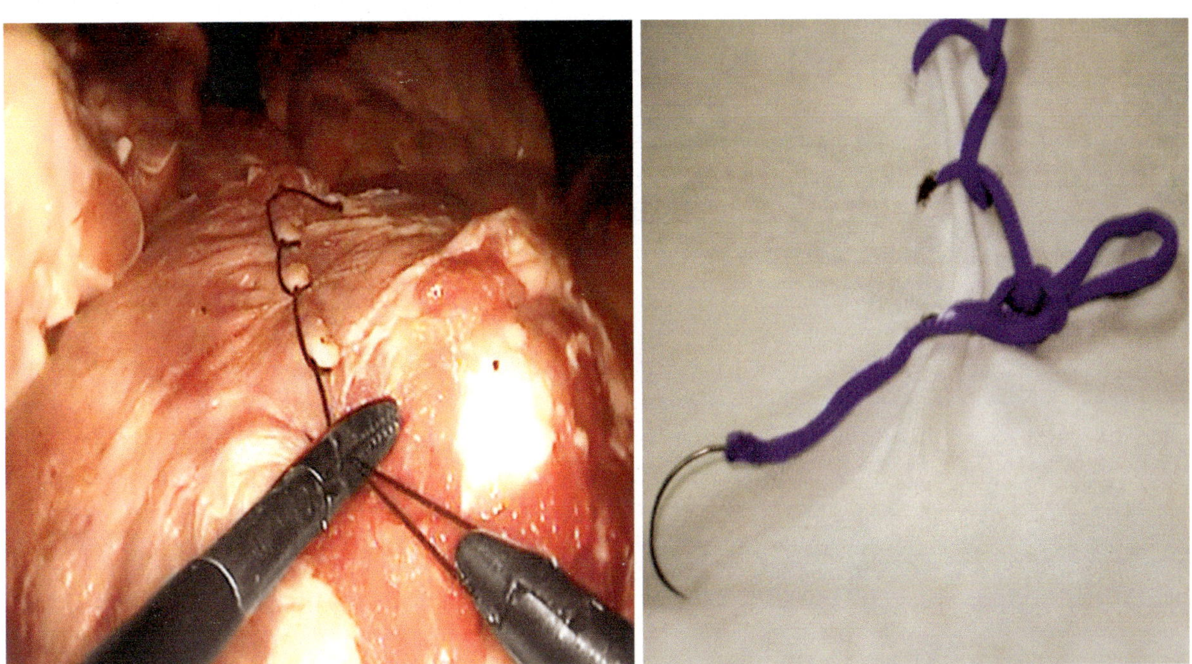

Fig. 5: Aberdeen termination knot—step 5.

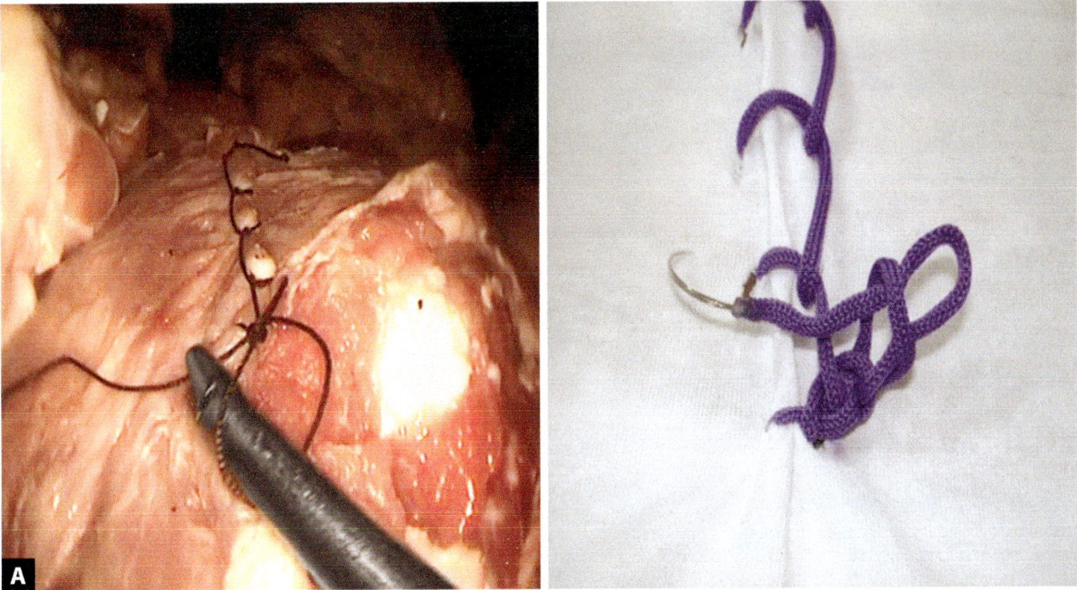

Fig. 6A: Pulling suture loop within loop to terminate the knot.

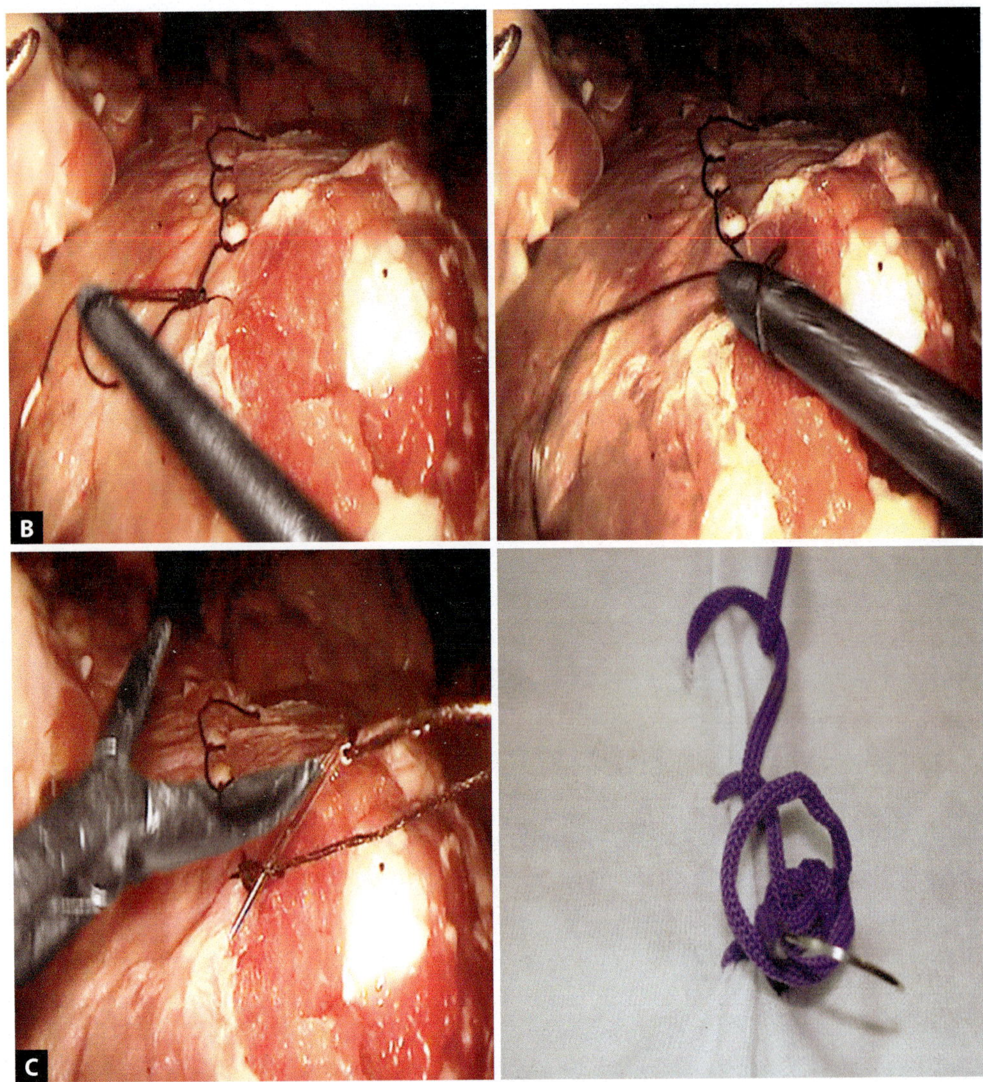

Figs. 6B and C: Last loop of Aberdeen termination knot—step 6.

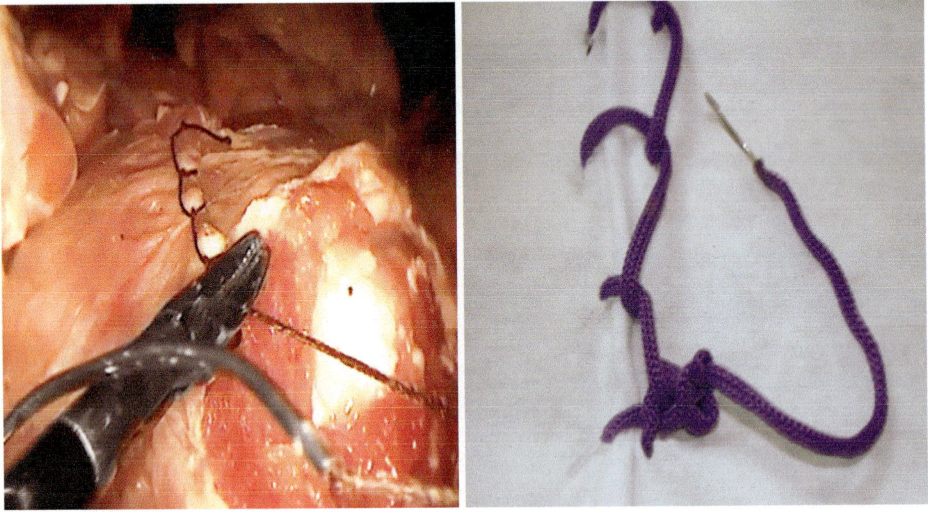

Fig. 7: Aberdeen termination knot—step 7.

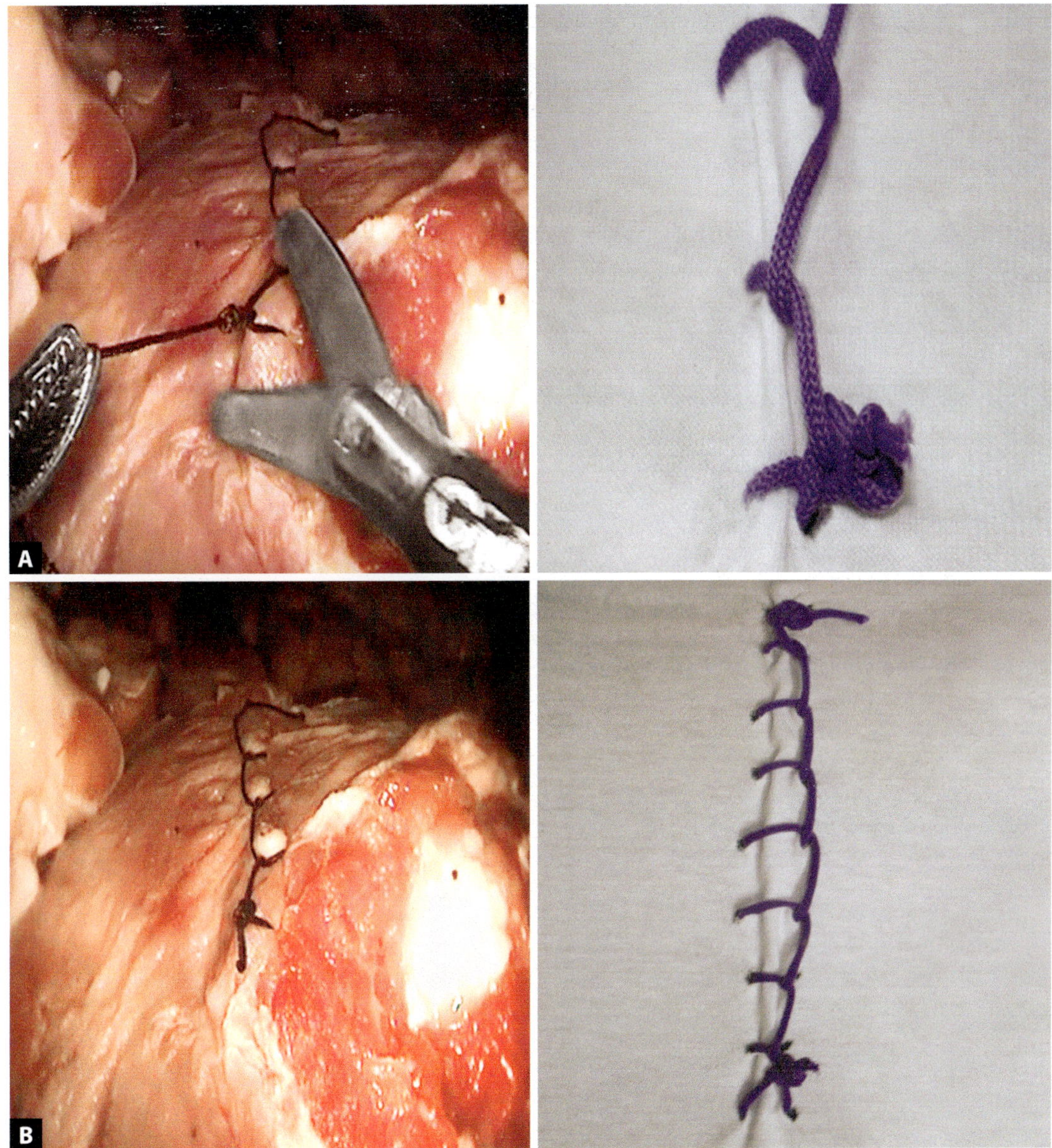

Figs. 8A and B: Aberdeen termination knot—step 8.

- Can be tied much easily than the square knot in difficult sites like anterior abdominal wall and at sites where the working space is limited.
- Is preferred in sites where the tension is not needed.

DISADVANTAGES OF ABERDEEN TERMINATION KNOT

- It consists of three ties around a loop making it relatively large which may lead to foreign body reactions and infections.
- It is a loose knot and should not be used in sites where tension is required, such as in closing the myoma bed in which tumble square knot is preferred

RECOMMENDATION

Laparoscopic suturing constitutes a vital component of advanced laparoscopic surgery training.

Only through regular training and practice can a surgeon develop the necessary suturing and knot-tying skills. The Aberdeen termination knot is best employed in peritoneal closure and in scenarios where tension is not a requisite.

CONCLUSION

Every laparoscopic surgeon should be well-versed in the fundamentals of traditional suturing and knot-tying. While the new techniques for tissue approximation represent progress and should be incorporated into practice, they should complement, rather than replace, traditional methods.

The Aberdeen termination knot is a straightforward and easily acquired intracorporeal knot. However, it produces a relatively large knot and is best employed with nonslippery suture material and a rounded needle for closing the peritoneum when tension is not necessary. It is not suitable for situations where tension is required, such as controlling bleeding or obliterating dead spaces or the myoma bed.

■ BIBLIOGRAPHY

1. Chen MH, Khalil H. Laparoscopic Suturing Techniques for Surgeons. Oxford: Oxford University Press; 2022.
2. Choi E, Kim DY. The use of biodegradable sutures in laparoscopic surgery. J Biomed Mater. 2024;15(3):438-45.
3. Clarke HC. Laparoscopy—new instruments for suturing and ligation. Fertil Steril. 1972;23(4):274-7.
4. Fernandez R, Martin CJ. Ergonomics in laparoscopic suturing: minimizing surgeon fatigue. J Ergono Surg. 2023;17(3):145-54.
5. Gomez R, Lee T. Evolution of suturing techniques in laparoscopic surgery. J Minim Invasive Surg. 2021;28(2):123-32.
6. Gupta S, Mehra R. Barriers to learning laparoscopic suturing: a survey of surgical residents. Education in Surgery. 2023;47(1):55-62.
7. Harper D, Lombardi A. Adapting traditional suturing techniques for laparoscopic applications. Surgical Techniques Review. 2021;35(4):320-8.
8. Kumar V, Saxena AK. Advanced Techniques in Laparoscopic Surgery. Berlin: Springer; 2020.
9. Lavelle JF, Sinclair MF. Automated suturing devices in laparoscopic surgery: a comparative analysis. Technology in Surgery. 2020;22(6):789-98.
10. Lee J, Kim S. Innovations in laparoscopic suturing instruments. Int J Med Robot. 2022;18(1):e2210.
11. Mendez C, Gupta A. Laparoscopic Suturing: Mastery Through Technique and Practice. London: Elsevier Health Sciences; 2023.
12. Mishra RK. Textbook of Laparoscopy for Surgeons and Gynecologists, 4th edition. New Delhi: Jaypee Brothers Medical Publishers (P) Ltd; 2021.
13. Mishra RK. Textbook of Practical Laparoscopic Surgery. New Delhi: Jaypee Brothers Medical Publishers (P) Ltd; 2008.
14. Morrison T, Jacobs LR. Teaching laparoscopic suturing: the role of simulation in medical schools. Medical Teacher. 2021;43(7):778-84.
15. Najmaldin A, Guillou P. Documented history of modern laparoscopic surgery A Guide to Laparoscopic Surgery. Hoboken, New Jersey: Wiley–Blackwell; 2000.
16. Nguyen L, Ho CP. Impact of suture materials on laparoscopic knot reliability. Materials in Surgery. 2024;9(2):200-10.
17. O'Donovan PJ, Downes EGR, McGurgan P. Textbook of Advances in Gynaecological Surgery. London: Greenwich Medical Media Ltd; 2002.
18. O'Reilly MP, Saunders BH. Virtual Reality Training for Laparoscopic Surgery. Cambridge: Cambridge University Press; 2022.
19. Patel R, Thompson J. The Role of Simulation in Learning Laparoscopic Suturing and Knotting. Medical Education Online. 2021;26:1857289.
20. Rodriguez A, Davis SS. Robotic-assisted laparoscopic knot tying: methods and efficiency. Surgical Innovation. 2019;26(4):459-66.
21. Shimi SM, Lirig M, Vander-Velpen G, Cusehieri A. Comparative study of holding strength of slipknot using absorbable and nonabsorbable ligature materials. Surg Endosc. 1994;11:1285-91.
22. Smith JA, Patel VR (Eds). Principles of Laparoscopic Suturing and Knotting. New York: Springer; 2023.
23. Surgical Knots and Suturing Techniques. (2024). [online] Available from https://en.wikipedia.org/wiki/Surgical_suture
24. Wang Y, Thompson C. Innovations in knot tying techniques for minimally invasive surgery. Innov Surg. 2022;18(4):250-60.
25. Williams NE, Tan JL. Comparative study of knot security in laparoscopic surgery. J Surg Res. 2020;245:217-23.
26. Zimmerman KA, Patel ND. Laparoscopic Knotting: A Visual Guide for Surgeons. Philadelphia: Lippincott Williams & Wilkins; 2022.

Role of Clip and Staplers in Laparoscopic Surgery

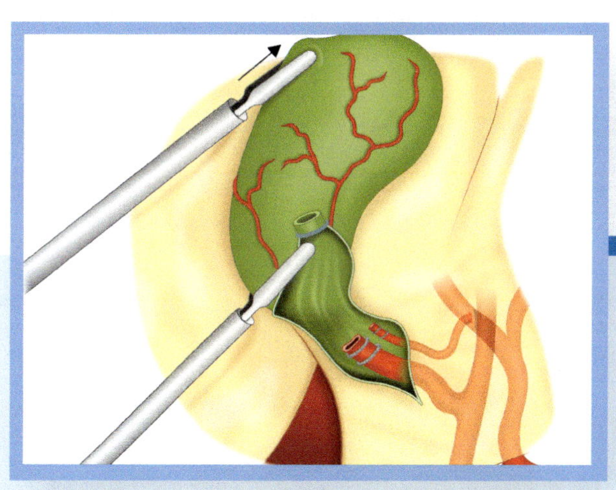

■ INTRODUCTION

The technique for stapling for surgery is said to have been influenced by the Roman use of ants for wound closure. This technique was pioneered by Hungarian surgeon Hümér Hültl, known as the father of surgical stapling (1908).

Staplers are instruments that deliver several rows of staples in a prearranged fashion. Depending on the purpose of the device, the staples are deployed either in linear geometry over a distance of 30–60 mm (linear stapler) or as concentric rings (circular staplers).

Delivery of three rows of staples without cutting the tissue is used to close defects such as an enterotomy.

Combined with a cutting knife in between two to three stapler rows, the staplers allow one to cut and close off the tissue on both cutting edges at the same time.

Spillage of luminal contents (blood, stool, etc.) can therefore be avoided.

The staples come in different sizes and are preloaded into the stapling device itself and the reload cartridges.

Different cartridge colors are used by the manufacturers to highlight different indications, e.g., white cartridge for vascular and blue cartridge for bowel.

The optimal staple size and depth vary according to the tissue that it is being used for. Vascular staplers have a tighter design and exert more hemostatic compression on the vascular structures in order to prevent bleeding.

Laparoscopic staplers are longer, thinner and may be articulated to allow for access from a restricted number of trocar ports.

Staplers for hollow viscous organs (bowel, stomach, etc.), on the other hand, are designed to avoid ischemia at the cut edge and thus at the site of the anastomosis. The stapling procedure for both situations is the same. However, the impact of a potential stapling failure is much higher for high-flow vascular pedicles than for low-pressure bowels.

In order to develop safe habits for vascular stapling, it is therefore advisable to:
- Keep the staple closed after firing for few minutes to allow for intrinsic homeostasis to take effect.
- Maintain stapling site control on both vascular ends by means of instruments. This prevents the vessels from retracting and permits one to easily reapply another staple row or to use clips to control a bleeding should it occur.

The risk of creating arteriovenous fistulae after mass occlusion of vascular pedicle is anecdotal.

Nowadays, staplers are frequently used in many kinds of procedures, from simple appendectomy to more advanced gastrointestinal (GI), thoracic, or vascular surgery.

Autosuture surgical stapler has wide application in surgery and facilitating many kinds of procedures such as:
- Gastrectomy and gastrojejunostomy
- Gastric bypass
- Resection and anastomosis
- Splenectomy
- Biliopancreatic diversion
- Colorectal surgery

Nowadays, staplers are usually B shaped and made from titanium. The advantages of noncrushing, B-shaped titanium staplers are:
- Provide excellent tissue resection
- Provide hemostasis
- Permit nutrition to pass through staple line to the cut edge of tissue
- Promote healing and reduce possibility of necrosis
- Are placed in two (three) rows over suture line
- Are essentially inert, reducing inflammation
- Are applied mechanically so that equal tension is created all along the staple lines, eliminating any potential weak spots
- Reduced starburst or shadows on computed tomography (CT) or magnetic resonance imaging (MRI)
- Can reduce operating time (and time under anesthesia)
- Reduce blood loss
- Reduce manipulation of tissue and also tissue trauma

■ INSTRUMENTATIONS

Laparoscopic Clip Applicator

Disposable preloaded clip applicators are available in 5 and 10 mm diameter. These are expensive but nice to use because the loading time of clip can be minimized. Disposable clip applier comes with 20 preloaded clips. In case of emergency when bleeding has to be stopped immediately, one after another clip can be applied rapidly with the help of these clip applicators **(Figs. 1 to 4)**.

Titanium is the most widely used metal in minimal access surgery for tissue approximation. It rarely reacts with human body and this is why it is popular. It is easy to apply and can be left inside abdominal cavity. After few weeks, it is covered by fibrous tissue. Titanium clip

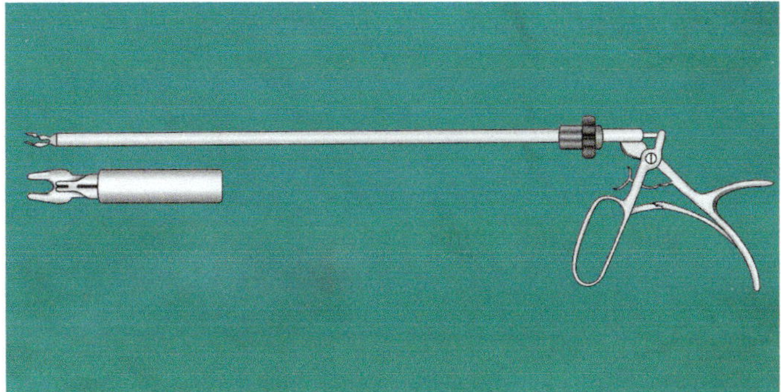

Fig. 1: Laparoscopic titanium clip applicator.

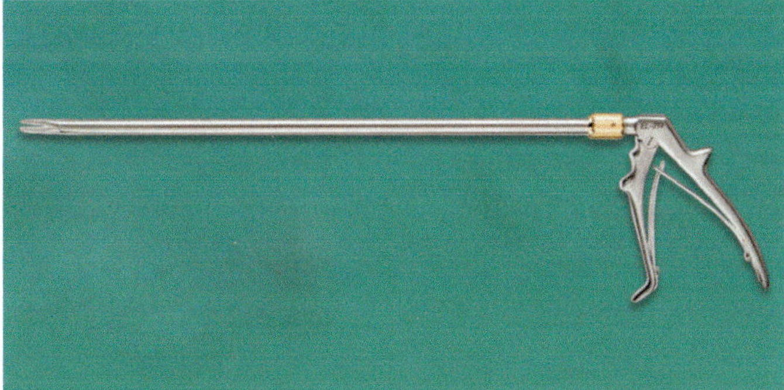

Fig. 2: Laparoscopic reusable clip applicator.

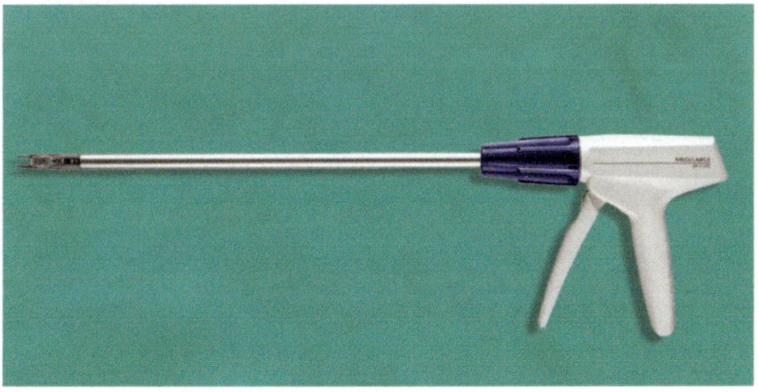

Fig. 3: Laparoscopic disposable clip applicator.

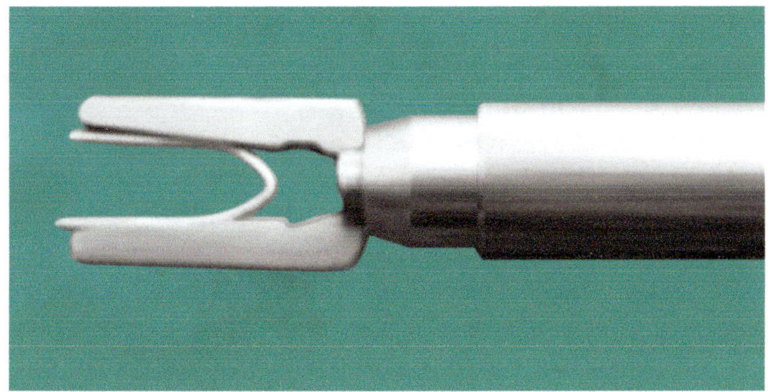

Fig. 4: Clips loaded over laparoscopic clip applicator.

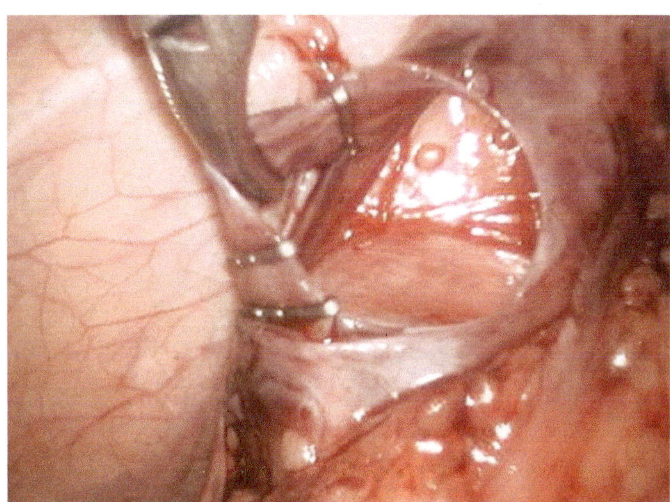

Fig. 5: Clips applied around spermatic vein.

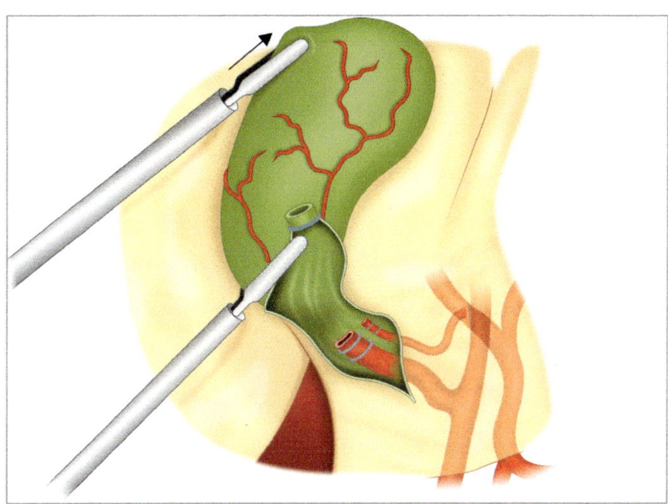

Fig. 6: Clip on cystic duct and artery.

is used by 99% of surgeons for clipping cystic duct and cystic artery at the time of laparoscopic cholecystectomy. Recently, silicon clips have been launched. Absorbable clips (Absolok, Ethicon) are preferred to clip cystic ducts nowadays. It adds to safety by working at the tip and it does not have chance to form cystic duct clip stone.

The absorbable soft clips can also be used in running stitches at the beginning and at the termination of knotting. The clip can be applied over spermatic vessels for the treatment of varicose vessels **(Fig. 5)**.

Medium–large-sized clip is of 9 mm and used most frequently for cystic duct and cystic artery **(Fig. 6)**. The medium-sized clip is 7 mm in length and can be used to clip cystic artery or thin cystic duct. The large-sized clip is 11 mm in length and it is used to control thick wide cystic ducts or large mesenteric vessels. The jaw of clip applicator should be at right angle to the structure and before clipping surgeon should take care that both the jaws are seen.

If one of the jaws is hidden, there is always a possibility that some tissue will get entrapped between the jaw of clip and clip will be loose. At the time of securing any duct or artery with titanium clip, three clips are generally applied. Two clips are left toward the structure which is secured and one clip is toward the tissue which surgeon wants to remove to prevent spillage of fluid. The distance between first and second clip should be 3 mm and distance between second and third clip should be 6 mm so that after cutting in between second and third clip, there will be 3 mm stump both the side. The clip should not be applied very near to each other, because clips are held in position by dumbbell formation and if they are very near to each other, they will nullify the dumbbell formation of each other and both the clips will be loose.

Titanium clip **(Fig. 7)** is most widely used tissue approximation technique used by general laparoscopic surgeon.

- Double clip should be applied over important structures.
- Always confirm the dumbbell effect after clipping.
- Dumbbell effect after clipping confirms the tension on tissue **(Fig. 8)**.
- Do not clip fatty pedicles and clip applicator should be at right angle to the clip **(Fig. 9)**.
- Check positioning of jaws, the tips, and content before clipping.
- Beware of cross clipping.

Cat Eye Stone

Sometimes, clip applied on cystic duct may internalize and act as foreign body. In rare cases, cat eye stone has been reported with the use of titanium clips. After many years, it stimulates stone formation by deposition of bile. It is called cat eye stone because after taking a cross-section of these stone, the titanium clips look like pupil of a cat seen in dark **(Fig. 10)**.

Hernia Stapler, Endoanchor, and Tacker

For fixing mesh in hernia surgery, many preloaded devices are available. Currently, three popular brands of implants to fix the mesh are available. These are Tacker, Protack, or Anchor **(Figs. 11 and 12)**. The comparative chart of these implants is shown in **Table 1**.

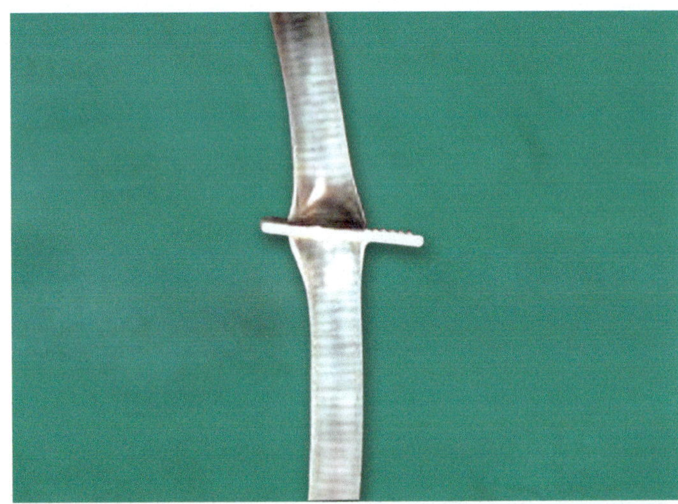

Fig. 8: Dumbbell formation is necessary to prevent slippage of clip.

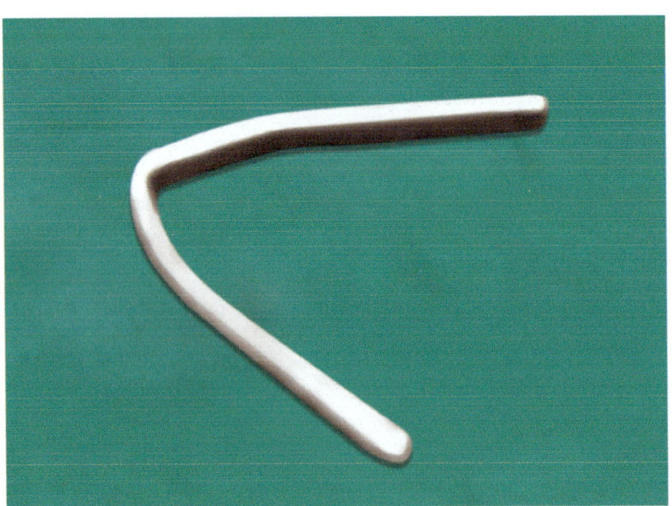

Fig. 7: Titanium clip.

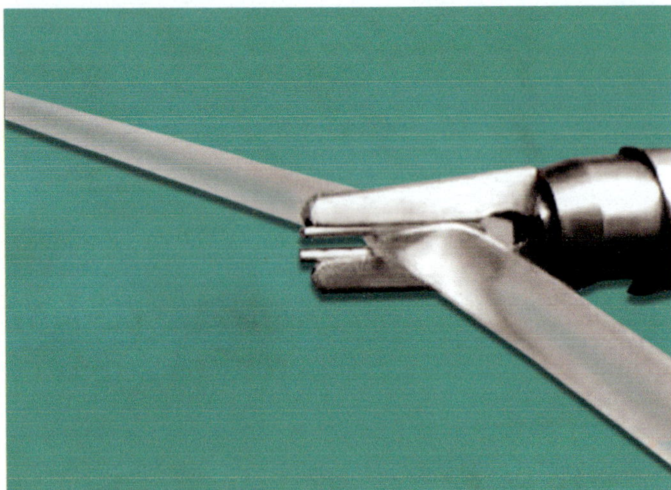

Fig. 9: Clip applicator should be kept at right angle to the structure which the surgeon wants to clip.

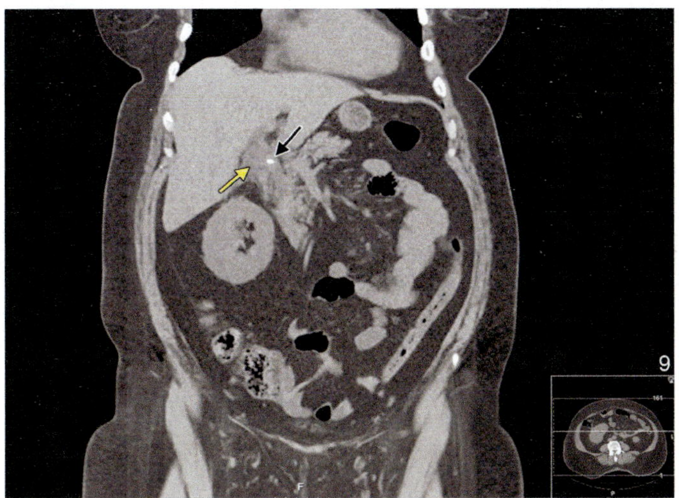

Fig. 10: Cat eye stone.

Different Types of Endo Gastrointestinal Linear Staplers Used in Laparoscopic Surgery

Laparoscopic surgery, also known as minimally invasive surgery, has revolutionized the field of GI surgery. One of the essential tools in laparoscopic GI procedures is the linear stapler. These devices are crucial for creating secure and efficient anastomoses (connections) and closures within the GI tract. In this chapter, we will explore the different types of endo GI linear staplers commonly used in laparoscopic surgery and their applications:

- *Disposable linear staplers:* They are designed for single use and they come preloaded with staples and a cutting mechanism. These staplers are often used in procedures where precision and ease of use are critical. They are particularly valuable in creating secure anastomoses in the GI tract.

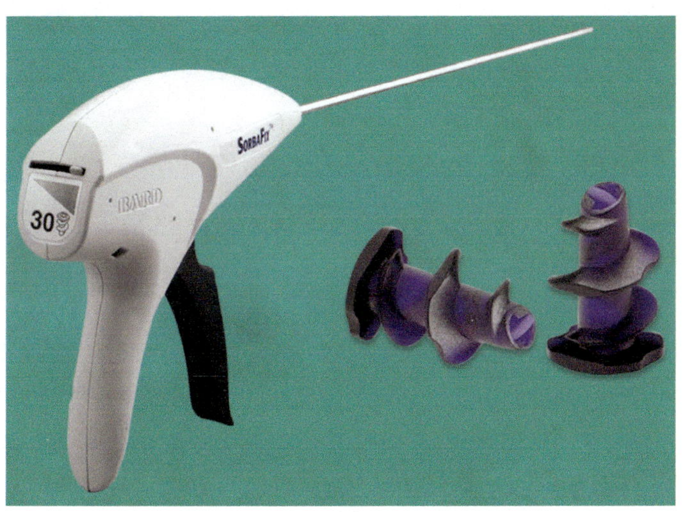

Fig. 11: Endoancher and tacker.

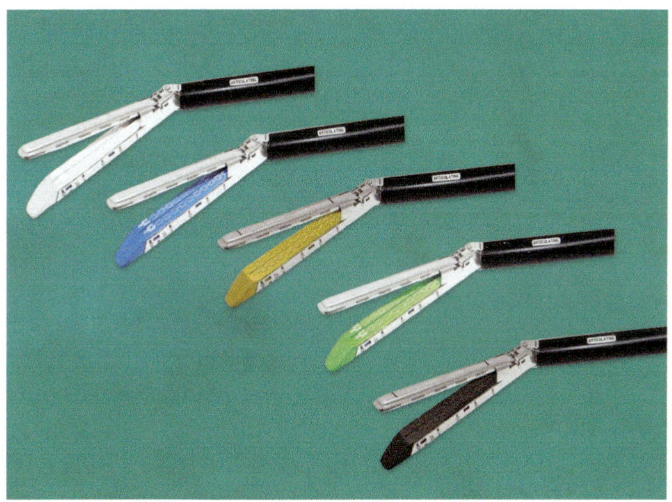

Fig. 12: Jaw and cartridge of stapler.

TABLE 1: Difference in implants for fixing mesh.

Feature	ESS endoanchor	Tyco protack	Tyco tacker
Number of implants	20	30	20
Geometry of implant	Anchor	Helical fastener	Helical fastener
Implant material	Nitinol	Titanium	Titanium
Implant length	5.9 mm	3.8 mm	3.6 mm
Implant width	6.7 mm	4 mm	3.4 mm
Port size required	5 mm	5 mm	5 mm
Shaft length	360 mm	356 mm	356 mm
Trigger fire orientation	Release to deploy	Depress to deploy	Depress to deploy

- *Applications:* Disposable linear staplers are frequently used in colorectal surgeries, such as bowel resections and anastomoses. They are also employed in gastric bypass surgery and esophageal procedures.
- *Reloadable linear staplers:* They are designed for multiple uses within a single surgical procedure. Surgeons can reload these staplers with fresh cartridges as needed. They offer cost-efficiency and versatility in surgeries with various stapling requirements.
  - *Applications:* Reloadable linear staplers are often used in complex laparoscopic procedures, including multilayered anastomoses and tissue transections.
- *Endo GI articulating linear staplers:* They have a flexible head that can be adjusted to different angles, allowing for increased maneuverability in challenging anatomical locations. This flexibility is advantageous in procedures where precise alignment is crucial.
  - *Applications:* Articulating linear staplers are frequently used in bariatric surgeries, such as gastric bypass, where the stapler needs to access tight spaces.
- *Endo GI curved linear staplers:* Curved linear staplers have a curved design that enables them to conform to the natural curvature of the GI tract. This feature allows for better tissue alignment and can reduce the risk of postoperative complications.
  - *Applications:* Curved linear staplers are often used in surgeries involving the esophagus, where a curved staple line is needed to create secure connections.
- *Powered linear staplers:* They are equipped with a motorized mechanism that facilitates staple deployment and tissue cutting. These staplers are known for their speed and precision in creating anastomoses.
  - *Applications:* Powered linear staplers are frequently used in surgeries that require rapid stapling, such as laparoscopic gastric bypass procedures.
- *Endo gastrointestinal buttress material:* Buttress material can be used in conjunction with linear staplers to reinforce staple lines, reducing the risk of leaks and bleeding. These materials can be absorbable or nonabsorbable.
  - *Applications:* Buttress material is often employed in surgeries where secure and leak-proof anastomoses are crucial, such as colorectal and esophageal procedures.

Endo GI linear staplers are essential tools in laparoscopic surgery, enabling surgeons to create secure and efficient anastomoses and closures within the GI tract. The choice of stapler type depends on the specific surgical procedure and the surgeon's preferences. With various stapler options available, laparoscopic surgeons can tailor their approach to each patient's unique needs, ensuring safer and more effective GI surgeries. As technology continues to advance, we can expect further innovations in the field of endo GI linear staplers, further improving surgical outcomes.

There are many varieties of laparoscopic stapler. The LONG45A Endocutter manufactured by Ethicon has a shaft that is 10 cm and it allows easier access during laparoscopic weight loss surgery, such as gastric bypass, where longer instruments are needed for morbidly obese patients. The ETS45 and ETS-FLEX45 Endoscopic Linear Cutters provide a 45 mm staple and cut line **(Fig. 13)**. The 34 cm shaft length makes the device suitable for many minimally invasive surgical procedures. The cutters are intended for transaction, resection, and/or creation of anastomosis in minimally access surgical procedures.

Complications related to the use of laparoscopic instruments are numerous and varied, surgeon must understand and look for two types of complications.

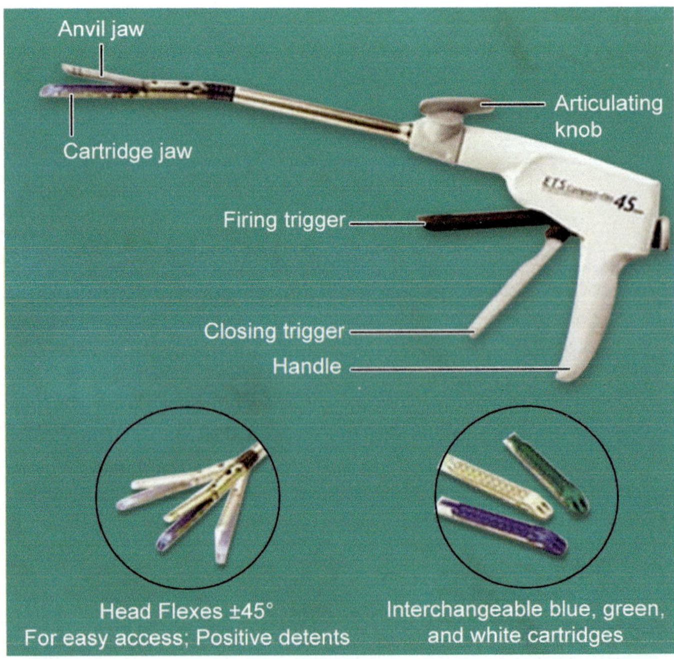

Fig. 13: Endopath ETS compact-Flex 45 articulating endoscopic linear cutters.

- *Electrical insulation:* The use of monopolar current through the hooks, graspers, and scissors requires that instruments have perfectly insulated sheath. Repeated cleaning and sterilization can lead to insulation failure and leakage of current.
- *Instrument breakage:* Repeated exposure to high pressure and high temperature sterilization can degrade the mechanism of instrument. Considerable mechanical strain applied on the instrument articulation can cause these to break. If mechanical part gets lost in the abdominal cavity, then they must be retrieved. If laparoscopic retrieval of lost part of instrument is not possible, conversion to open surgery may be necessary.

Laparoscopic surgical instruments are extremely variable and increasing number of instruments is being designed for specific application. Instruments are getting complex with greater functionality and freedom of movement. Such instruments reflect the trend toward the automation of procedure. In the future, such developments ultimately will lead to full robotization.

Linears and circulars are of many types of staplers used in laparoscopic surgery, as shown in **Figures 14 to 16**.

More recent studies have shown that with current suturing techniques, there is no significant difference in outcome between hand suture and mechanical anastomosis, but mechanical anastomosis is significantly quicker to perform.

Stapling is much faster than suturing by hand and also more accurate and consistent; in bowel and lung surgery, stapler is primarily used because staple lines are less likely to leak blood, air, or bowel content.

Following figures show after insertion of staplers in proper position and approximation of two edge of bowel and firing, titanium staple moved forward and changed to form B-shape, as described in **Figures 17A to C**.

Turn the screw on the tail of circular stapler body—the clockwise direction will approximate two-bowel edge and control tissue compression and finally in green area, devices are capable to fire **(Figs. 17A to C)**.

With turning screw in the clockwise direction, two bowel edges are approximated and attached to each other completely under direct vision **(Figs. 18A and B)**.

Arrow in green area shows device is ready for firing **(Figs. 18C and D)**.

After firing, B-shape staple in concentric two rows anastomosed adjacent bowel edges **(Figs. 18E to G)**.

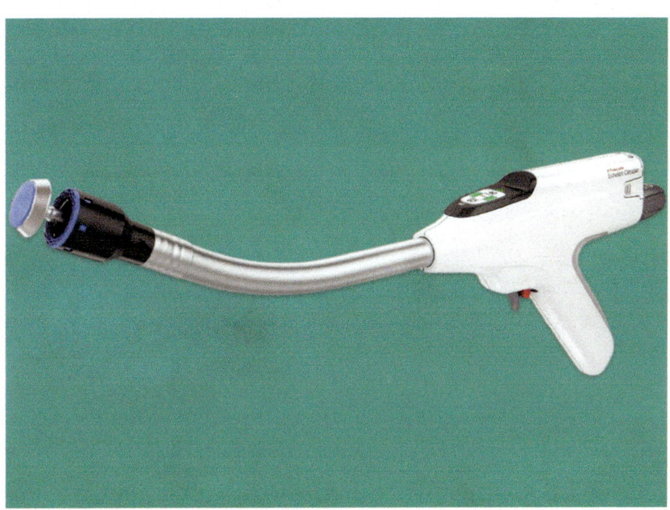

Fig. 15: Circular stapler.

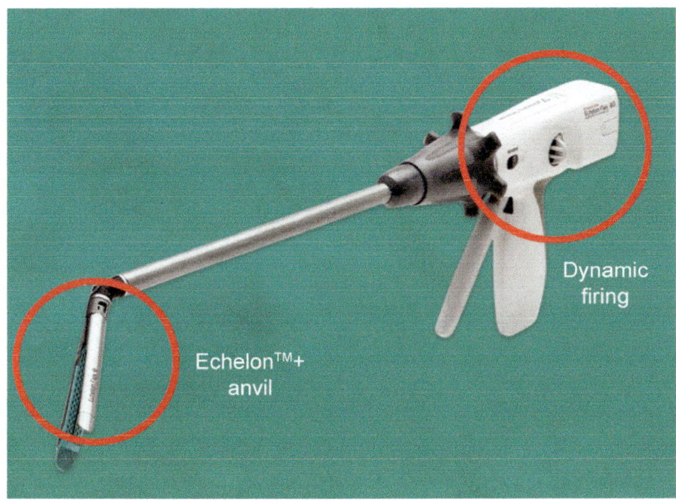

Fig. 14: Linear stapler.

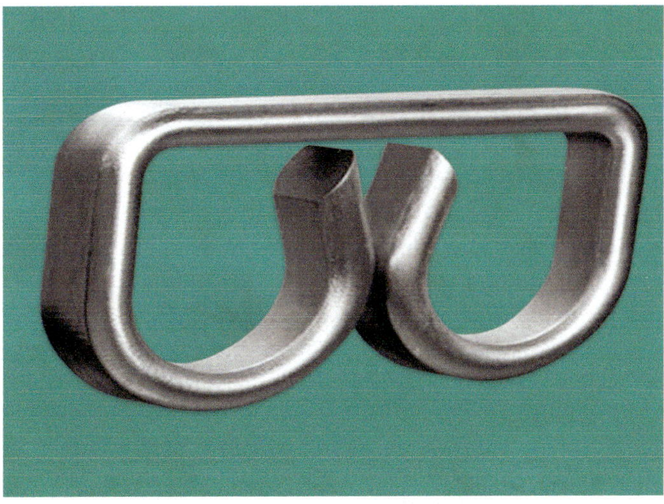

Fig. 16: B-shaped titanium stapler.

Pressure of about 30 seconds should be kept and then released **(Fig. 19A)**.

Then one must return screw in the counterclockwise direction (1/2–3/4 circle, **Fig. 19B**).

Next, with brief movement (up and down), slowly remove the stapler from bowel **(Figs. 19C to F)**.

In following pictures, the vascular stapler has been used (white cartridge) during colorectal surgery for closure and transection of infectious mesenteric vessels **(Figs. 20A to C)**.

Figures 21A to D show that linear stapler (blue cartridge) performed side-to-side anastomosis of bowel. Stay suture approximated two loop of bowels **(Fig. 21A)**.

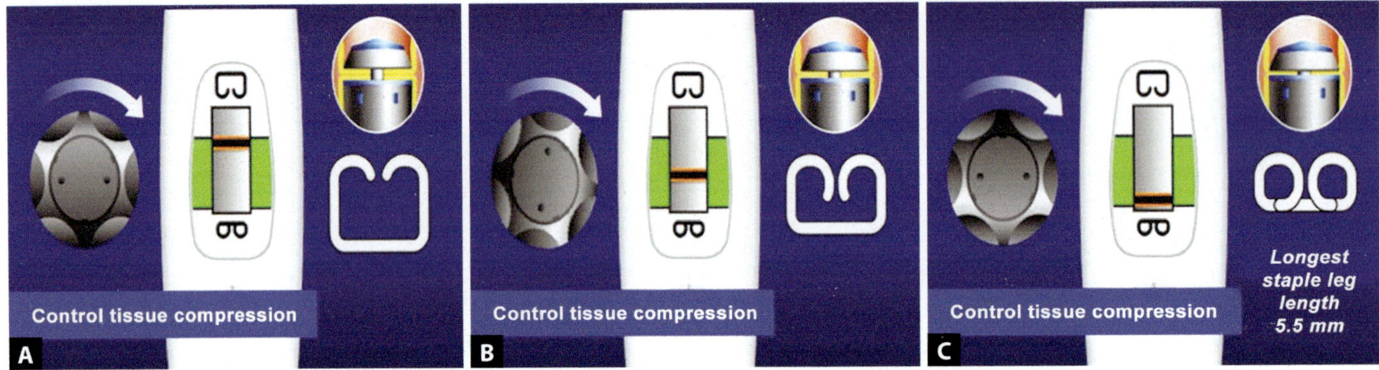

Figs. 17A to C: Insertion of staplers and approximation of two edge of bowel and firing.

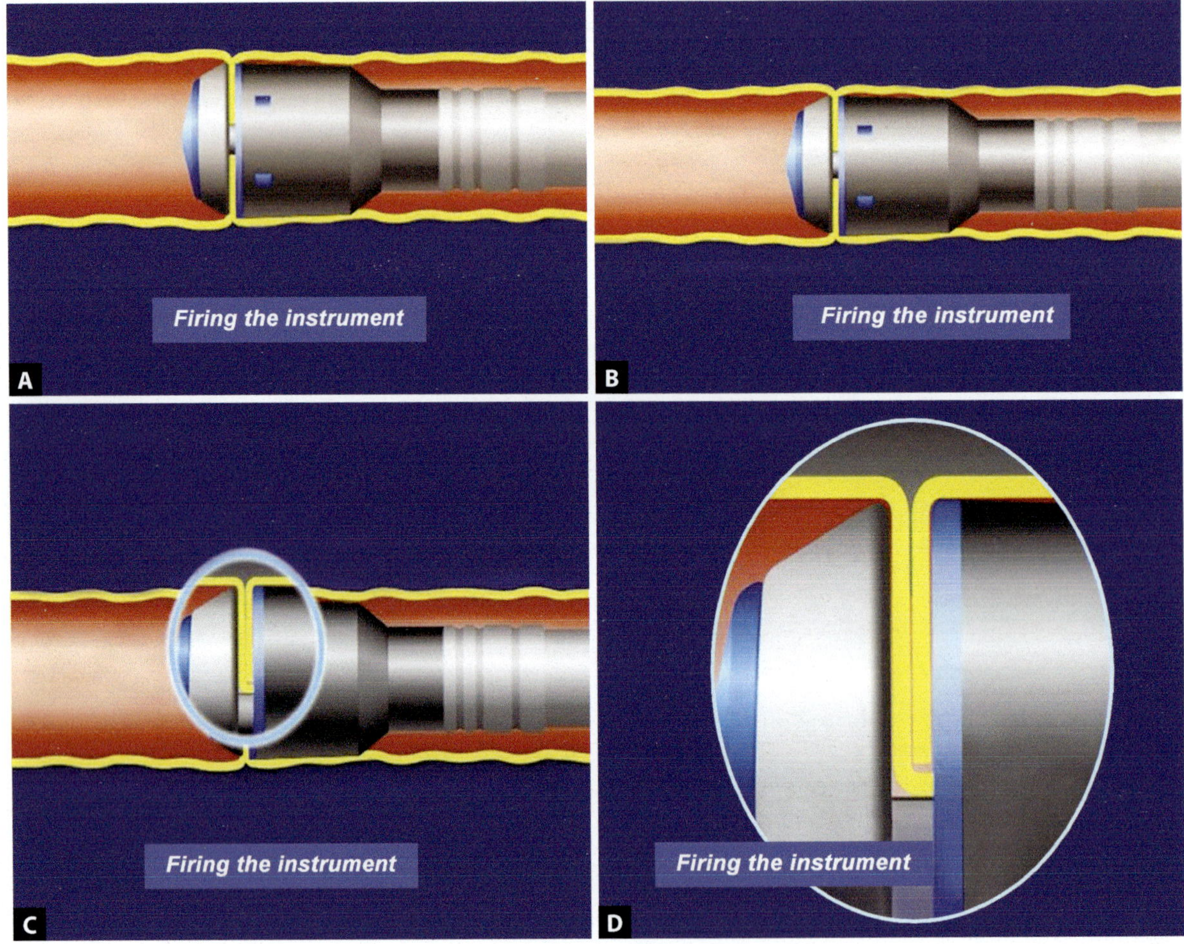

Figs. 18A to D

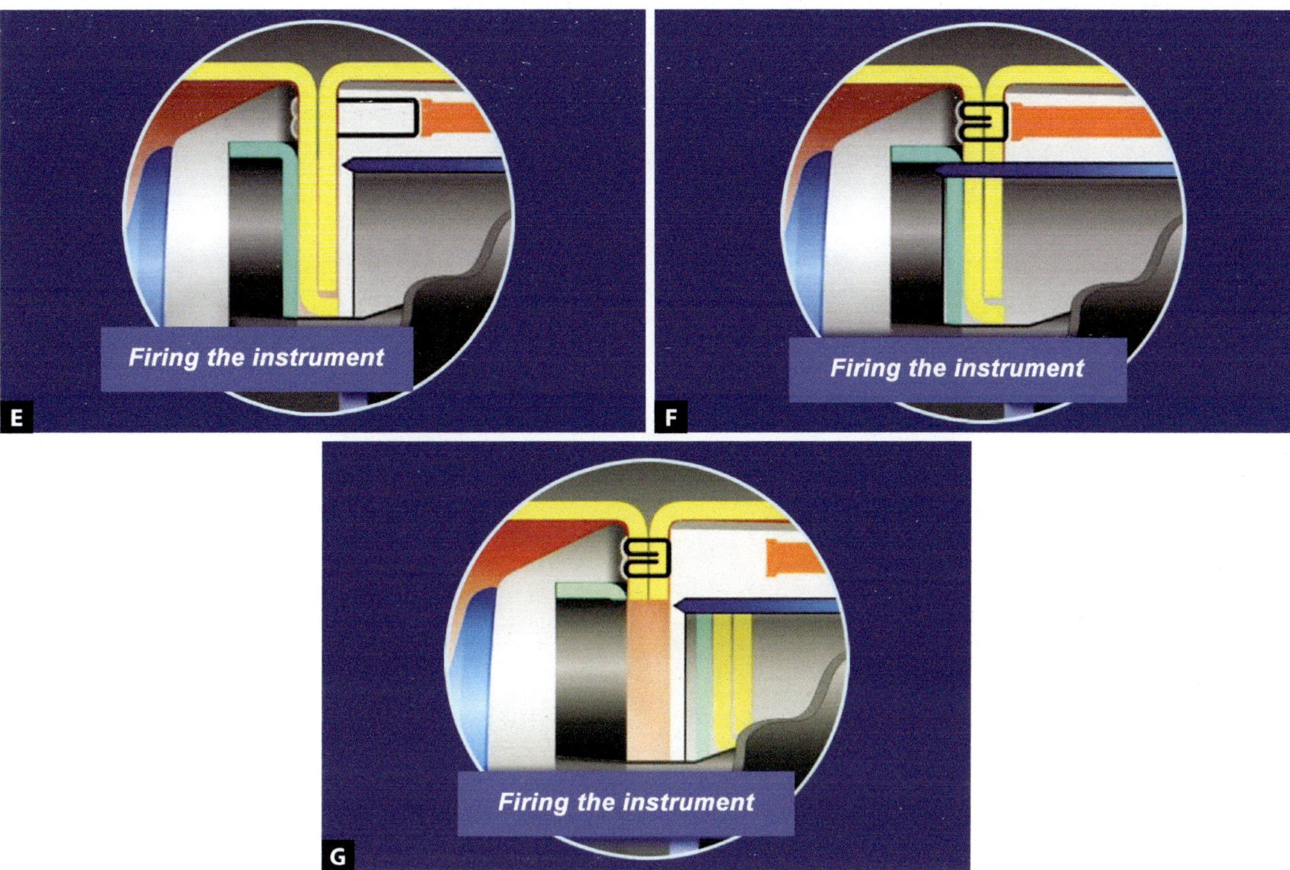

Figs. 18A to G: (A and B) Turning the screw on the tail of circular stapler body in clockwise direction; (C and D) Stapler is ready for firing; (E to G) Stapler after firing.

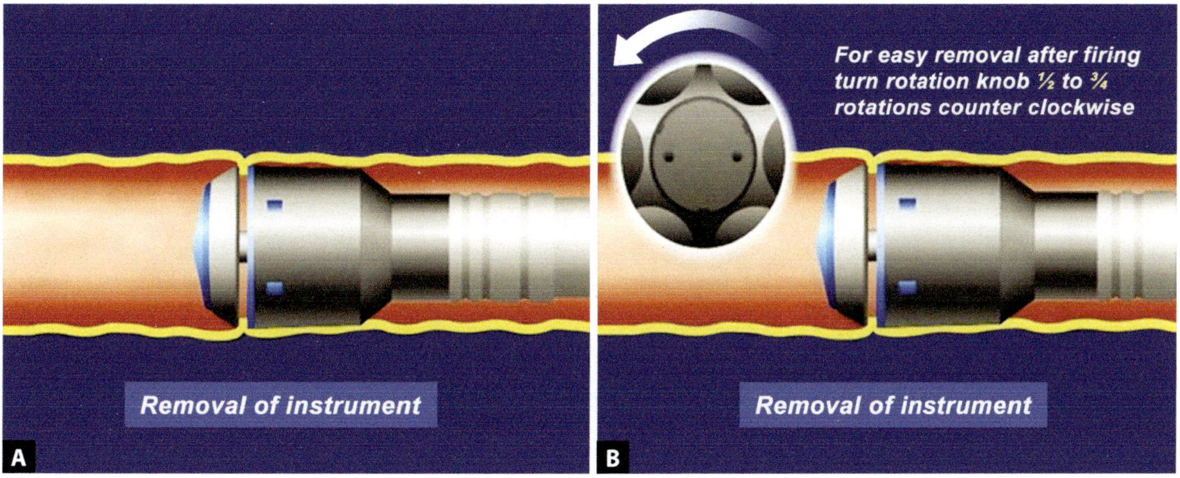

Figs. 19A and B

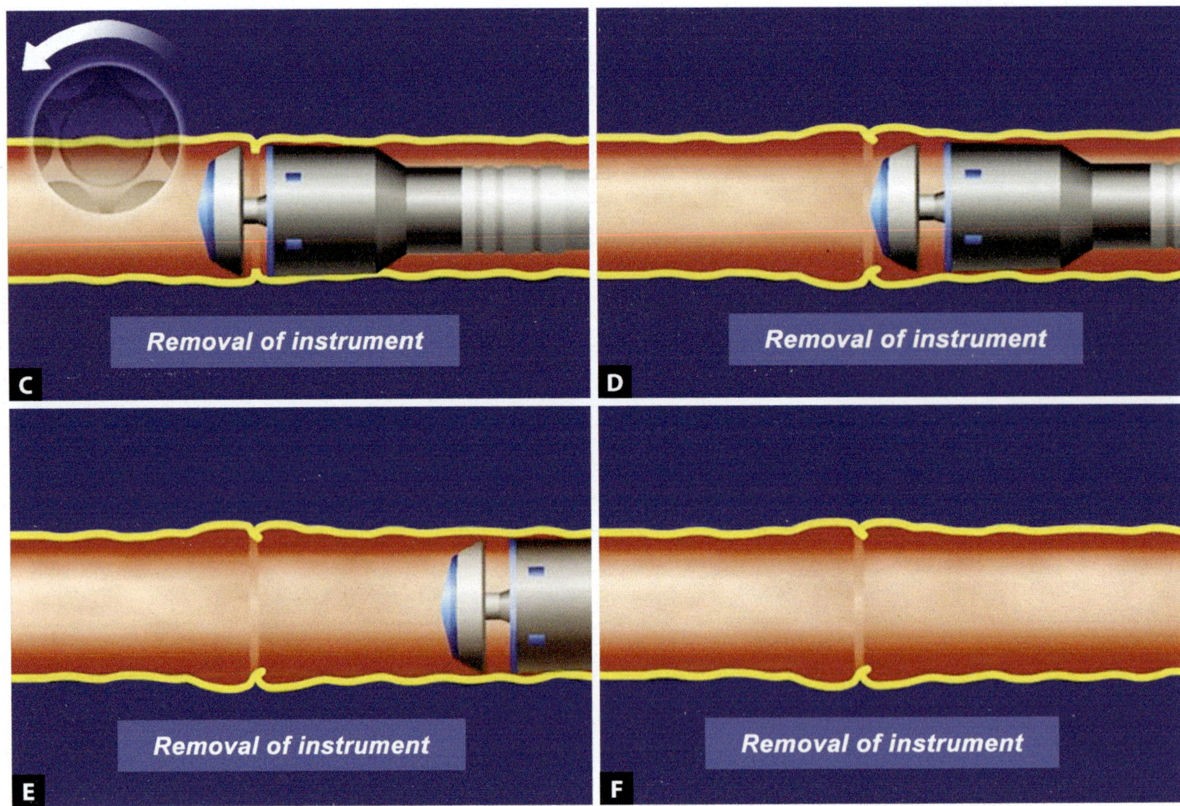

Figs. 19A to F: (A and B) Removal of instrument; (C to F) Removal of instrument from bowel.

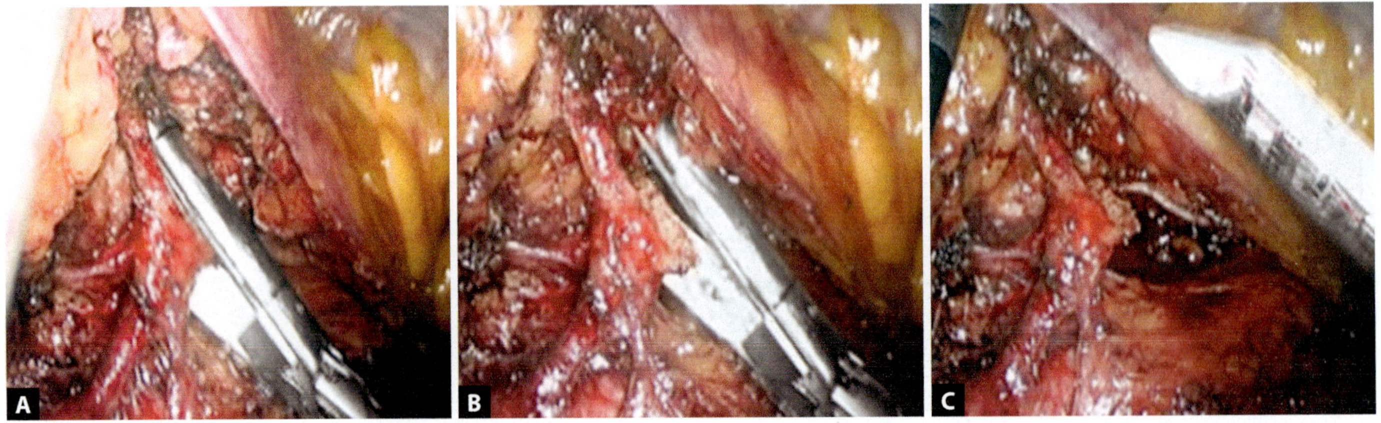

Figs. 20A to C: Use of vascular stapler in colorectal surgery.

Making a small enterotomy in antimesenteric border of each loop **(Fig. 21B)**.

Insert jaw of linear stapler one by one from small enterotomy **(Figs. 22A and B)**. Approximate jaws of stapler in proper position and now it is ready for firing **(Fig. 22C)**.

Remove stapler after completion of anastomosis **(Fig. 23)**. Enterotomy window is closed by hand suturing **(Figs. 24A to G)**.

Rectosigmoid Resection and Anastomosis with Staplers

- Linear staplers make two rows of staple in each side of descending colon and at the same time cut in between **(Figs. 25A to C)**.
- With special device or by handmade purse string, suture in descending colon at the site of transection **(Figs. 26A and B)**.

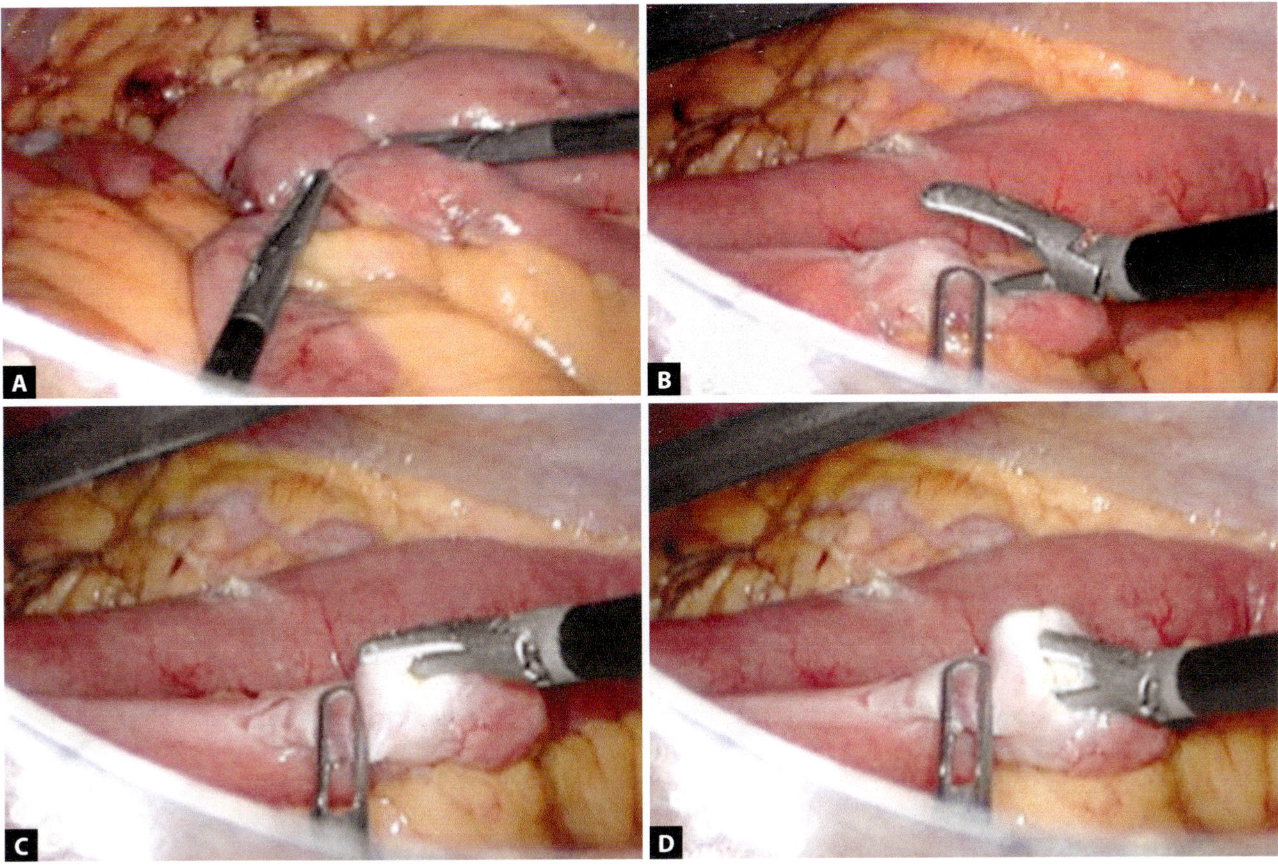

Figs. 21A to D: Linear stapler (side-to-side anastomosis of bowel).

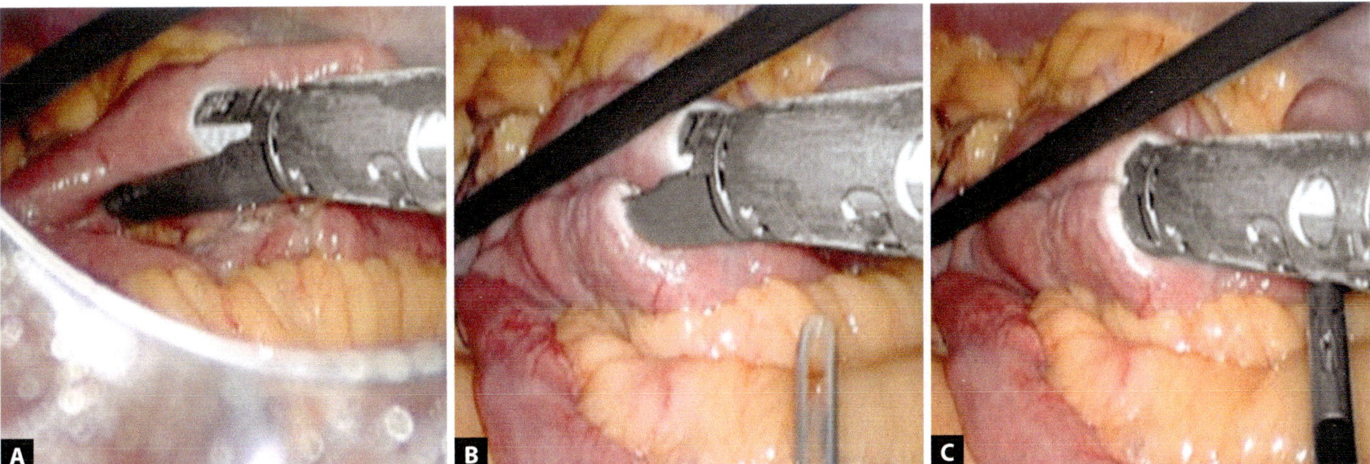

Figs. 22A to C: (A and B) Insertion of jaw of linear stapler from small enterotomy and (C) is ready for firing.

- The stapler head (anvil) is inserted into the proximal bowel end and purse is tightened **(Figs. 27A and B)**. After resection of the specimen, the bowel is subsequently returned into the peritoneal cavity.

- The long and curved stapler body is inserted transanally and the anvil is centrally deployed under direct vision next to the staple line on the rectal stump **(Fig. 27C)**.

- Anvils of stapler head and body are connected with an audible click either in hand-assisted or in purely laparoscopic technique after reestablishing the pneumoperitoneum.

- Firing the stapler results in an inverting anastomosis and should result in two intact tissue rings (doughnuts) and an airtight anastomosis.

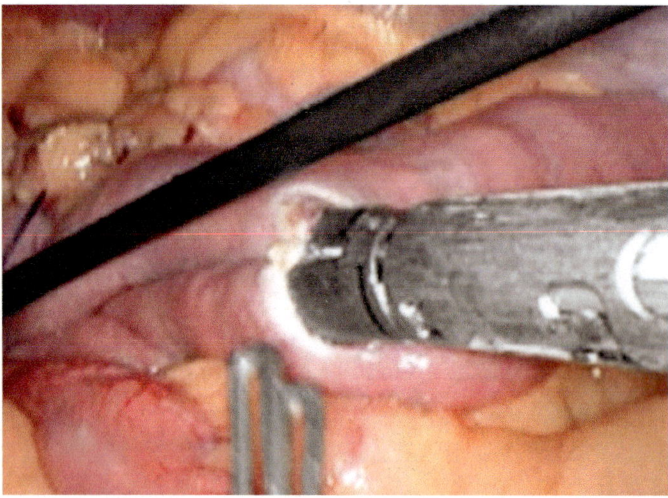

Fig. 23: Removal of stapler after completion of anastomosis.

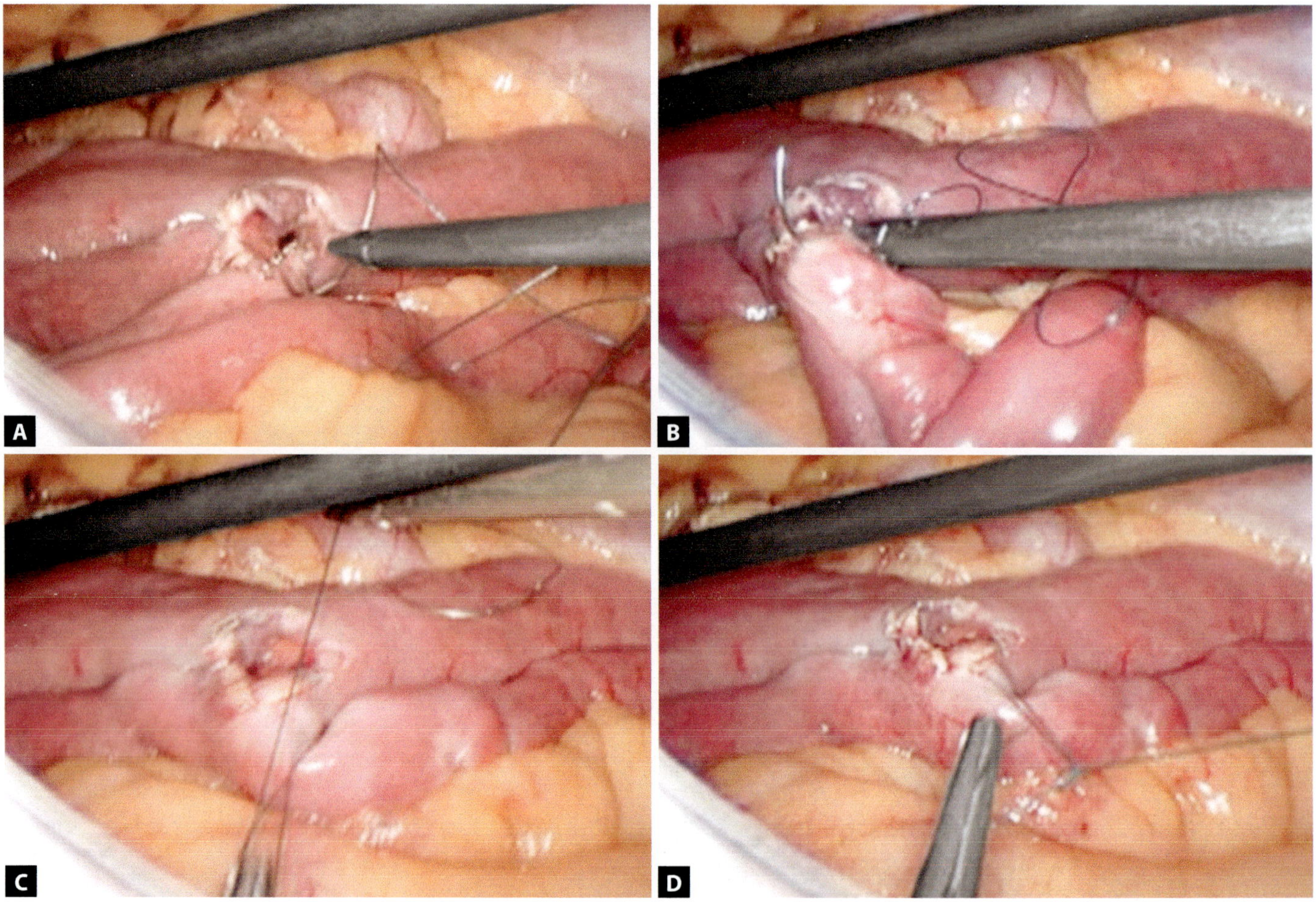

Figs. 24A to D

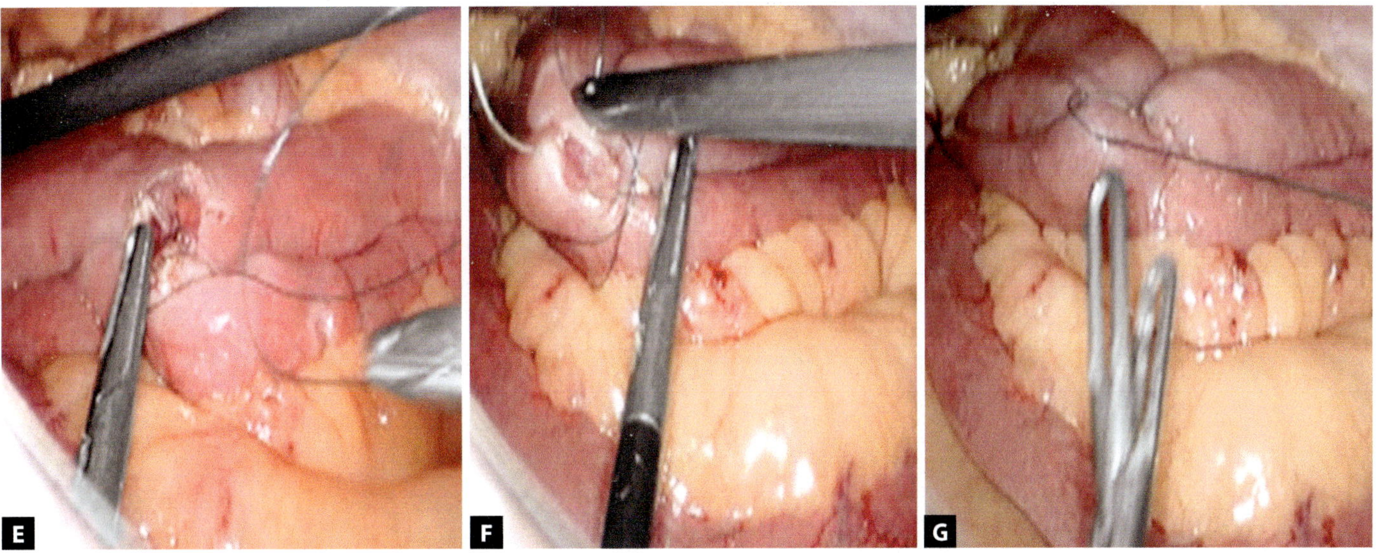

Figs. 24A to G: Closing enterotomy window by hand suturing.

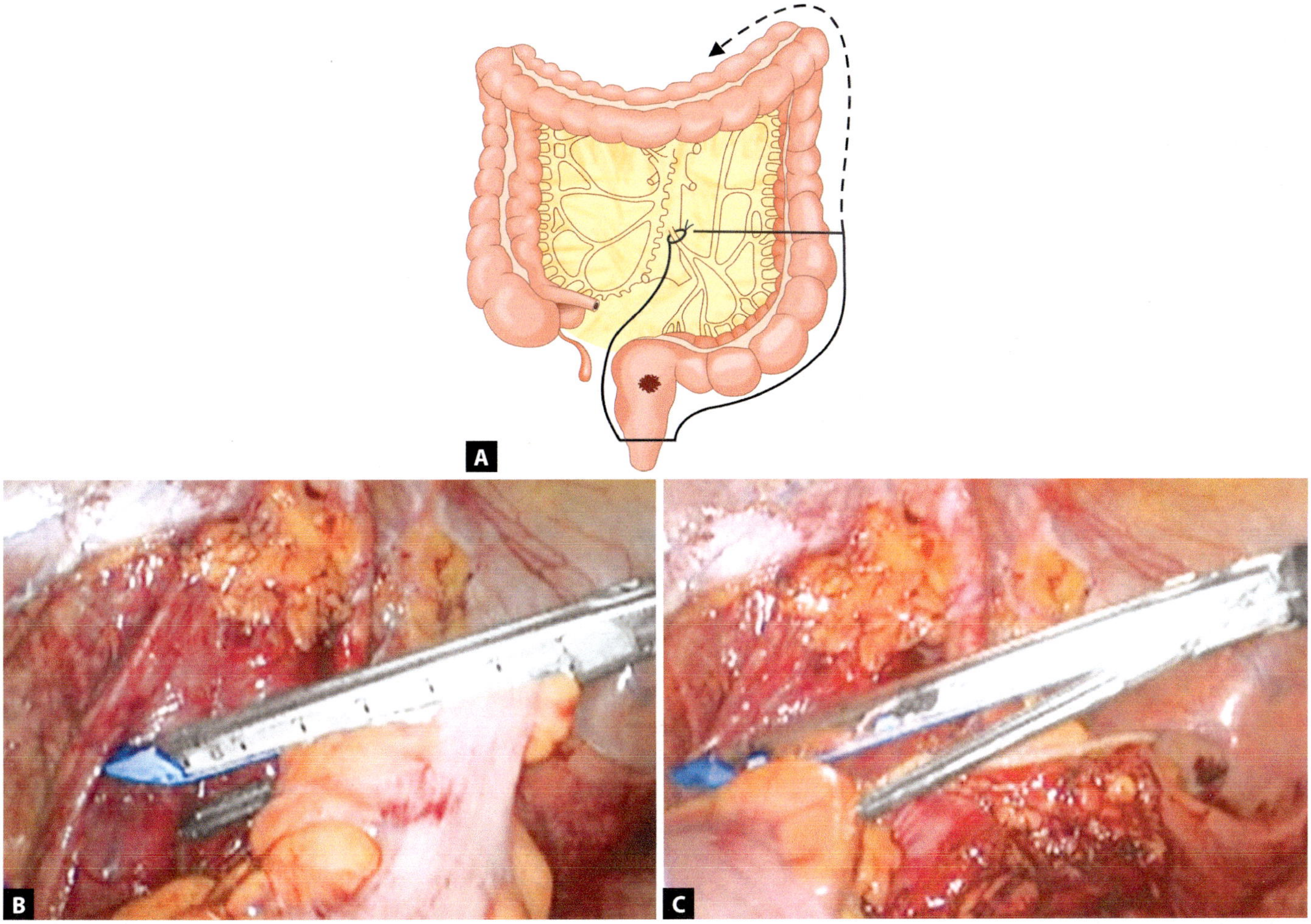

Figs. 25A to C: Rectosigmoid resection and anastomosis with staplers.

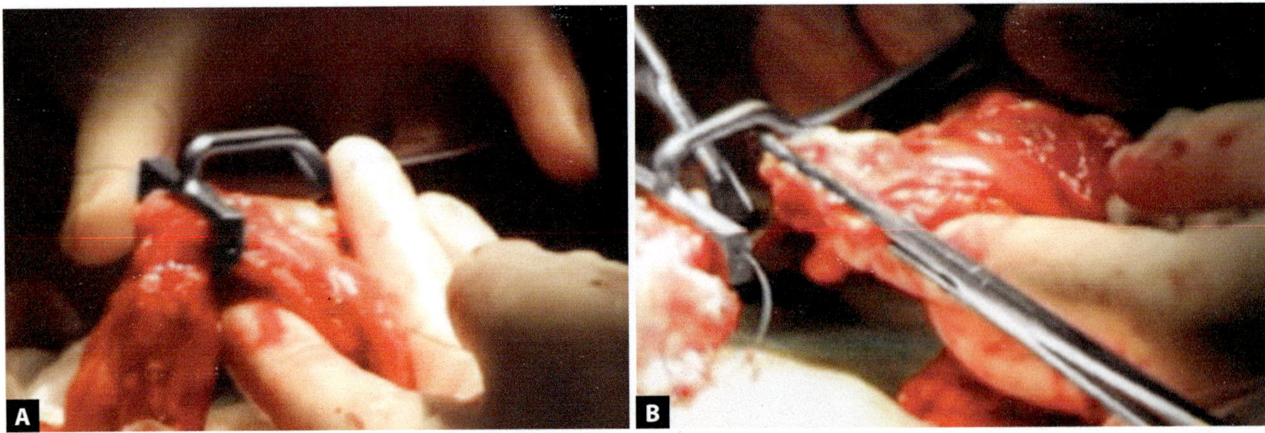

Figs. 26A and B: Removal of diseases part of colon

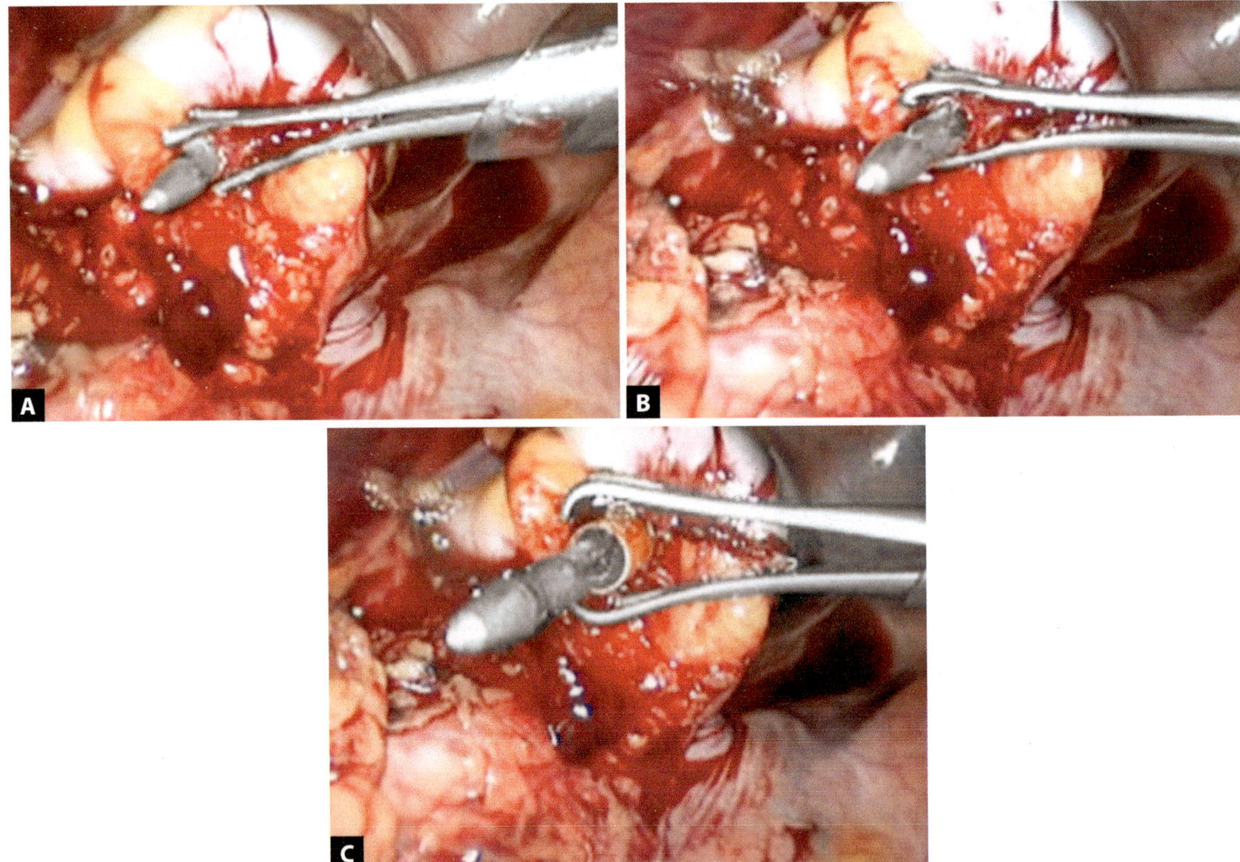

Figs. 27A to C: (A and B) After rectosigmoid resection ready for anastomosis with staplers; (C) Rectal stump.

Anvils of stapler head and body are connected with an audible click **(Figs. 28A and B)**.

Under vision bowel edge approximated by means of turning the screw of stapler body in clockwise direction **(Fig. 28C)**.

Stapler is ready for fire and resulting in anastomosis **(Fig. 28D)**.

Laparoscopic Circular Stapler

Laparoscopic colorectal surgery has become a widely accepted approach for various conditions, including colorectal cancer, diverticular disease, and inflammatory bowel disease. One of the critical aspects of these surgeries is the creation of secure and precise anastomoses, which connect different sections of the colon or rectum. Circular staplers play a crucial role in achieving this, ensuring optimal outcomes for patients. In this chapter, we will explore the different types of circular staplers used in laparoscopic colorectal surgery and their applications.

Different types of circular staplers in laparoscopic colorectal surgery:

- *Disposable circular staplers:* They are designed for single use and come preloaded with staples. They are known for their ease of use and reliability. These staplers offer the advantage of reduced risk of cross-contamination between patients.
  - *Applications:* Disposable circular staplers are frequently used in laparoscopic low anterior resections and ileocolic anastomoses for conditions such as colorectal cancer and Crohn's disease.
- *Reloadable circular staplers:* They can be used for multiple anastomoses within a single procedure. Surgeons can replace the cartridges with fresh ones as needed. These staplers offer cost-efficiency and flexibility.
  - *Applications:* Reloadable circular staplers are often employed in complex laparoscopic colorectal surgeries that require multiple anastomoses, such as segmental colectomies.
- *Powered circular staplers:* They feature a motorized mechanism that simplifies the process of stapling and tissue cutting. These staplers are known for their speed and precision, reducing the risk of errors during anastomosis.
  - *Applications:* Powered circular staplers are commonly used in laparoscopic colorectal surgeries, especially when creating end-to-end anastomoses. They are particularly valuable in procedures where time is a critical factor, such as in emergencies.
- *Curved circular staplers*: They have a unique curved design that allows them to conform to the natural curvature of the colorectal anatomy. This design facilitates better alignment and can reduce the risk of complications.

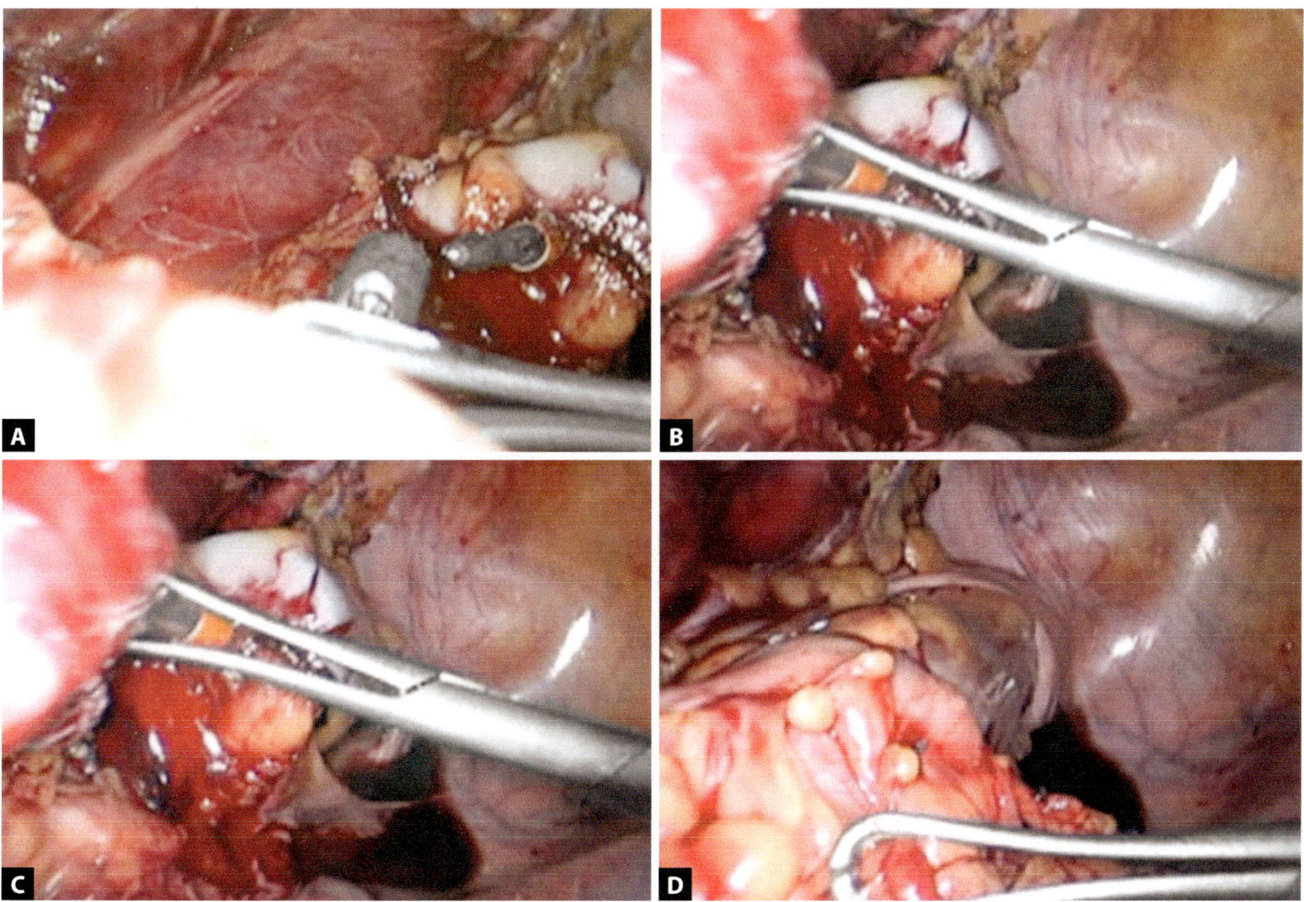

Figs. 28A to D: Rectosigmoid resection and anastomosis with staplers.

- *Applications:* Curved circular staplers are often preferred in laparoscopic colorectal surgeries involving the rectum, where a curved staple line is necessary for optimal anastomosis.
- *Articulating circular staplers:* They have a flexible head that can be adjusted to different angles, enhancing maneuverability during surgery. This flexibility is advantageous in procedures where precise alignment is crucial.
  - *Applications:* Articulating circular staplers are commonly used in laparoscopic colorectal surgery when the anastomosis site is challenging to access.
- *Circular staplers with buttress material:* Circular staplers can be used in conjunction with buttress material, which helps reinforce the staple line. This reduces the risk of leaks and complications in the postoperative period.
  - *Applications:* Circular staplers with buttress material are frequently employed in laparoscopic surgeries where secure and leak-proof anastomoses are vital, such as low anterior resections.

Circular staplers are indispensable tools in laparoscopic colorectal surgery, enabling surgeons to create precise and secure anastomoses. The choice of stapler type depends on the specific surgical procedure, the patient's anatomy, and the surgeon's preferences. Each type of circular stapler offers unique advantages, allowing laparoscopic surgeons to tailor their approach to achieve the best possible outcomes for their patients. As technology continues to advance, we can anticipate further innovations in circular stapler design, enhancing the safety and effectiveness of laparoscopic colorectal surgeries.

■ DISCUSSION

Although most surgical staples are made of titanium, stainless steel is more often used in some skin staples and clips.

Titanium produces less reaction with the immune system and being on ferrous does not interfere significantly with MRI scanners, although some imaging artifacts may result.

Synthetic absorbable (bioabsorbable) staples are also now becoming available, based on polyglycolic acid, as with many synthetic absorbable sutures. Based on above evidence, staplers are safe and effective.

■ HEM-O-LOK

One critical aspect of laparoscopic surgery is securing blood vessels and other tissues, which is typically achieved using various techniques and instruments. One such instrument is the Hem-o-Lok clip, a versatile and widely used device in minimally invasive procedures. In this chapter, we will explore the use of Hem-o-Lok clips in laparoscopic surgery, including their advantages and common applications.

What are Hem-o-Lok Clips?

Hem-o-Lok clips are small, nonabsorbable polymer clips that are designed to securely occlude or ligate blood vessels, tissue structures, and other anatomical components during laparoscopic surgery. These clips are available in various sizes to accommodate different vessel or tissue diameters **(Fig. 29A)**. There are different sizes of applicators also available **(Fig. 29B)**. They are typically made from biocompatible materials, such as a mixture of polycarbonate and acrylonitrile–butadiene–styrene (ABS) resin, ensuring that they do not elicit an immune response or cause adverse reactions in the body.

Hem-o-Lok clips, or Hem-o-Lok ligating clips, are commonly used in laparoscopic surgery to secure and ligate blood vessels, tissues, or structures. These clips come in various sizes to accommodate different vessel or tissue diameters. The sizes of Hem-o-Lok clips typically include:

- *Medium–large (ML) or medium (M):* This size is commonly used for sealing and ligating medium-sized vessels or structures in laparoscopic procedures. The approximate range for this size is around 7.0–12.0 mm when fully closed.
- *Large (L):* This size of Hem-o-Lok clips are used for ligating larger vessels or tissues. The approximate range for this size is around 9.0–15.0 mm when fully closed.
- *Extra-large (XL):* This size of Hem-o-Lok clips are the largest and are used for securing very large vessels or structures. The approximate range for this size is around 11.0–18.0 mm when fully closed.

The choice of clip size depends on the specific vessel or tissue being secured during surgery. Surgeons typically select a clip size that matches the diameter of the structure they are ligating. Using the appropriate clip size ensures a secure and effective closure without damaging the tissue or causing undue compression **(Figs. 30A and B)**.

It is important for the surgical team to have a variety of clip sizes available during laparoscopic procedures to accommodate different anatomical variations and surgical needs. The precise sizing may vary depending on the manufacturer of the clips, so surgeons should refer to the product information provided by the manufacturer for specific sizing details.

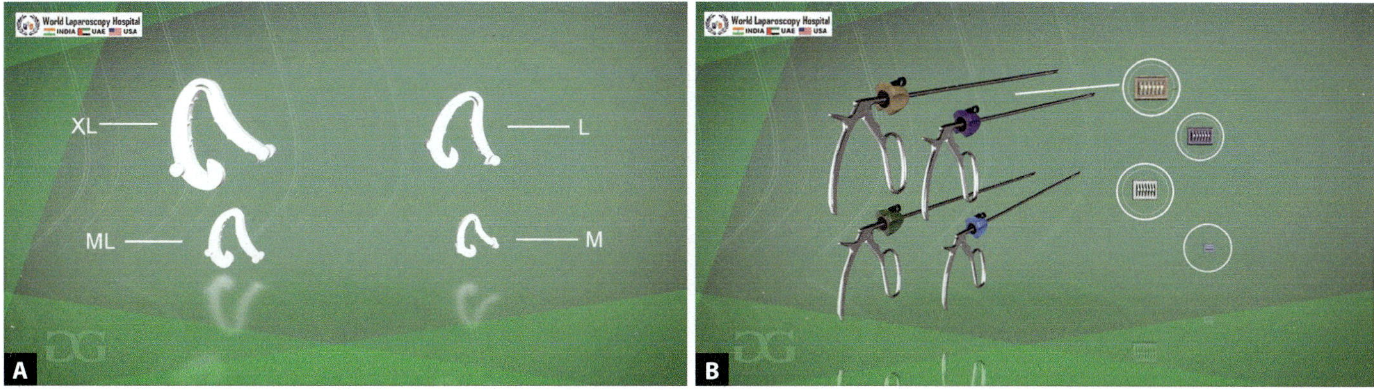

Figs. 29A and B: (A) Different sizes of Hem-o-Lok clips; (B) Different sizes of Hem-o-Lok clips applicator. (L: large; M: medium; ML: medium–large; XL: extra-large)

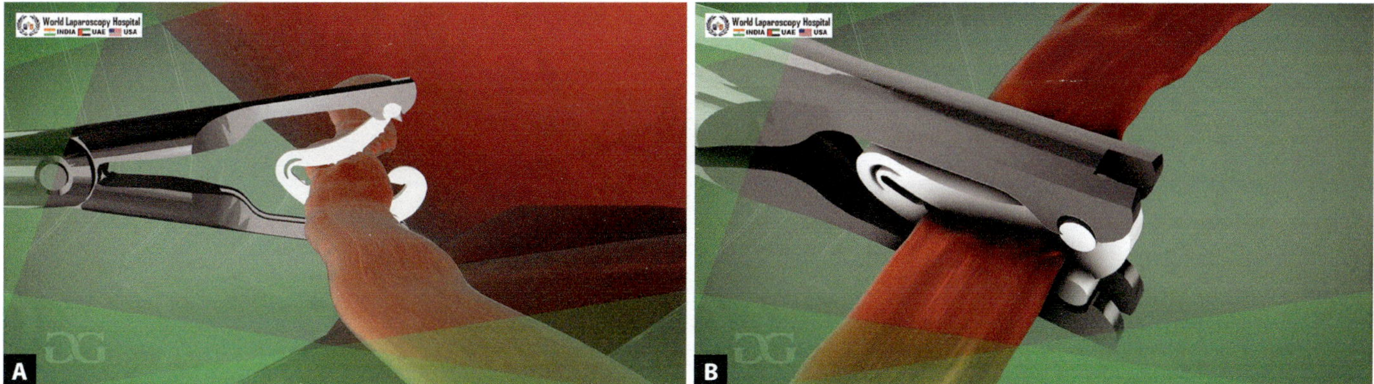

Figs. 30A and B: (A) Hem-o-Lok clips on artery; (B) Hem-o-Lok clips holding artery.

Advantages of Using Hem-o-Lok Clips

- *Precision and control:* Hem-o-Lok clips provide surgeons with precise control over the vessels or tissues being secured. This precision is crucial in laparoscopic surgery, where limited visibility and restricted movement require accurate and efficient instruments.
- *Safety:* Hem-o-Lok clips are designed to be atraumatic, meaning they minimize tissue damage during application. They have a smooth inner surface that prevents vessel damage while ensuring a secure closure.
- *Durability:* These clips are robust and durable, maintaining their integrity once applied. Their strong grip ensures that they stay in place until the targeted tissue or vessel has healed.
- *Consistency:* Hem-o-Lok clips offer consistency in their performance, reducing the risk of complications associated with variations in technique or suture quality.
- *Time efficiency:* The ease of applying Hem-o-Lok clips makes them a time-efficient option in laparoscopic surgery. Surgeons can quickly and confidently secure vessels or tissues, contributing to shorter operating times.
- *MRI safe:* Hem-o-Lok clips are not affected by MRI, so it is safe if MRI is required just after surgery **(Fig. 31)**.

Applications of Hem-o-Lok Clips in Laparoscopic Surgery

- *Hysterectomy:* During laparoscopic hysterectomy, surgeons use Hem-o-Lok clips to secure the uterine arteries. This minimizes blood loss and ensures the safe removal of the uterus.
- *Cholecystectomy:* In laparoscopic gallbladder removal (cholecystectomy), Hem-o-Lok clips are used to ligate the cystic duct and artery, preventing bile leakage and bleeding.
- *Nephrectomy:* Hem-o-Lok clips play a crucial role in laparoscopic nephrectomy, where they are used to seal blood vessels and secure the renal hilum before kidney removal.
- *Bariatric surgery:* Hem-o-Lok clips are employed in various bariatric procedures to control blood vessels

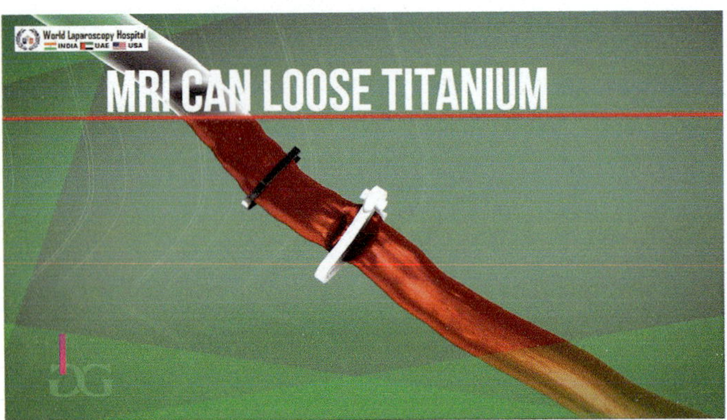

Fig. 31: Hem-o-Lok clips safe during magnetic resonance imaging (MRI).

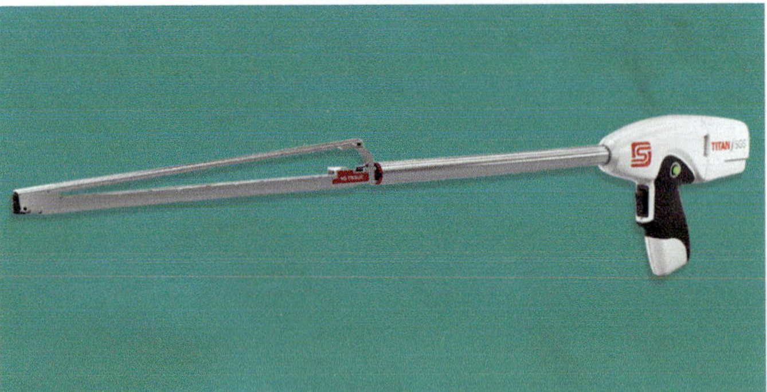

Fig. 32: Single fire stapler of Standard Bariatrics.

and ensure a secure closure in gastric bypass, sleeve gastrectomy, and other weight loss surgeries.

- *Colon resection:* Laparoscopic colon resections often involve the use of Hem-o-Lok clips to secure the mesenteric vessels and ensure proper tissue approximation.
- *Prostate surgery:* In laparoscopic prostatectomy, Hem-o-Lok clips are used to control the dorsal venous complex (DVC) and other vessels around the prostate.

Hem-o-Lok clips have become indispensable tools in laparoscopic surgery due to their precision, safety, and efficiency. These clips provide surgeons with a reliable means of securing blood vessels and tissues, reducing the risk of complications and improving patient outcomes. As technology continues to advance, the use of Hem-o-Lok clips and similar devices will likely evolve, further enhancing the field of minimally invasive surgery. Surgeons and medical professionals should stay updated on the latest developments and best practices related to the use of Hem-o-Lok clips in laparoscopic procedures to ensure optimal patient care.

ADVANCED SINGLE FIRE STAPLER

The single fire stapler of Standard Bariatrics: A new tool for sleeve gastrectomy **(Fig. 32)**.

Traditionally, sleeve gastrectomy has been performed using a linear stapler. This type of stapler fires multiple staples in a row, creating a long, continuous line of tissue transection. However, this approach can be time-consuming and can lead to inconsistent results **(Fig. 33)**.

The single fire stapler of Standard Bariatrics is a new device that is designed to simplify and improve the sleeve gastrectomy procedure. This stapler fires a single cartridge of staples, which creates a seamless, continuous staple line.

The single fire stapler has several advantages over traditional linear staplers. First, it is faster and easier to use. Second, it creates a more consistent staple line, which can help to reduce the risk of complications. Third, it allows the surgeon to visualize the entire staple line in a single plane, which can help to ensure that the procedure is performed correctly.

The single fire stapler of Standard Bariatrics is a promising new tool for sleeve gastrectomy. It has the potential to simplify the procedure, improve outcomes, and reduce the risk of complications.

Following are some of the specific benefits of the single fire stapler of Standard Bariatrics:

- It is faster and easier to use than traditional linear staplers.
- It creates a more consistent staple line, which can help to reduce the risk of complications.
- It allows the surgeon to visualize the entire staple line in a single plane, which can help to ensure that the procedure is performed correctly.
- It can be used to create a variety of staple lines, including straight, curved, and angulated lines.
- It is safe and effective and has been used in over 12,000 surgical procedures till today.

The single fire stapler of Standard Bariatrics is a valuable tool for bariatric surgeons. It can help to simplify and improve the sleeve gastrectomy procedure and can help to reduce the risk of complications.

POWER STAPLER USED IN LAPAROSCOPIC SURGERY

One of the critical components of laparoscopic surgery is ensuring secure and precise tissue closure.

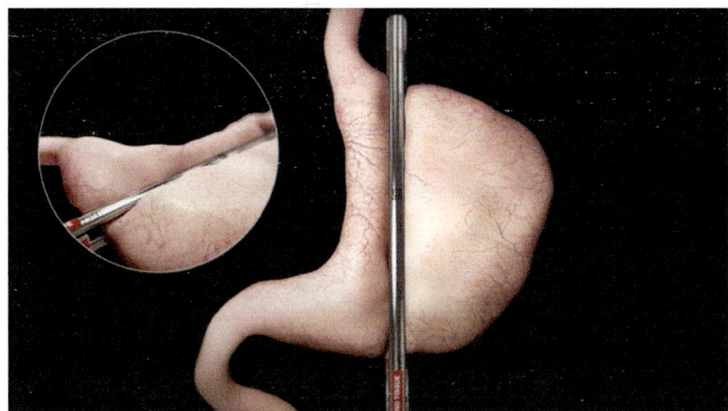

Fig. 33: Single fire stapler used in sleeve gastrectomy.

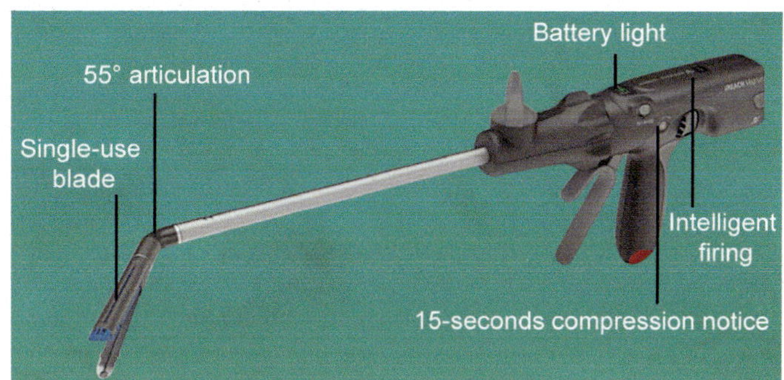

Fig. 34: Power staplers in laparoscopic surgery.

Traditional methods of suturing and stapling have been augmented with technological advancements, including the introduction of power staplers. In this chapter, we will explore the advantages of using power staplers in laparoscopic surgery **(Fig. 34)**:

- *Speed and efficiency:* One of the most significant advantages of power staplers in laparoscopic surgery is the speed and efficiency they offer. These devices can rapidly deploy multiple rows of staples and simultaneously cut tissue, significantly reducing operative time. Speed is especially crucial in laparoscopic surgery as it helps minimize anesthesia exposure and improve patient outcomes.
- *Precision:* Power staplers are engineered to create precise anastomoses (the connection of tubular structures like the intestines) and secure tissue closure. The automated process ensures uniform staple placement, reducing the risk of human error. This precision is vital in achieving leak-proof and tension-free anastomoses, which are critical for patient safety.
- *Consistency:* Consistency in staple formation is essential in laparoscopic surgery as it directly impacts the integrity of tissue closure. Power staplers consistently deliver the same results, staple after staple, ensuring that each anastomosis is of high quality. Surgeons can trust that the staple lines are uniform and reliable.
- *Reduced tissue trauma:* Power staplers are designed to minimize tissue trauma during the stapling process. They exert even pressure along the staple line, reducing the risk of tissue damage or tearing. This is particularly valuable when working with delicate tissues or in patients with compromised tissue integrity.
- *Enhanced visibility:* Many power staplers are equipped with advanced features, such as integrated cameras and lighting systems. These features improve visibility in the surgical field, allowing surgeons to make precise decisions during the procedure. Enhanced visualization contributes to safer and more accurate surgeries.
- *Reduced postoperative complications:* The secure and uniform staple lines created by power staplers reduce the risk of postoperative complications, such as leaks, bleeding, and infections. This can lead to shorter hospital stays, faster recovery times, and improved patient satisfaction.
- *Versatility:* Power staplers come in various types and sizes, allowing surgeons to choose the most suitable stapler for the specific procedure. Whether it is GI, thoracic, or vascular surgery, there is a power stapler designed to meet the unique demands of each operation.
- *Ergonomics:* Many power staplers are ergonomically designed to minimize surgeon fatigue and discomfort during long procedures. Comfortable grip handles and intuitive controls enhance the surgeon's experience and precision.
- *Minimal learning curve:* While power staplers offer advanced capabilities, they are designed to be user-friendly, minimizing the learning curve for surgeons and operating room staff. Surgeons can quickly adapt to these devices and incorporate them into their surgical practice. The use of power staplers in laparoscopic surgery has significantly advanced the field, offering numerous advantages that benefit both surgeons and patients. Their speed, precision, and consistency contribute to safer surgeries with reduced postoperative complications. As technology continues to evolve, power staplers are likely to become even more sophisticated, further enhancing their role in the field

of laparoscopic surgery. Surgeons can look forward to improved patient outcomes and enhanced procedural efficiency through the continued integration of power staplers into their practice.

■ CONCLUSION

Clip and staplers offer several advantages in surgery. They are faster, save time, and help preserve tissue vascularization. Additionally, they cause less trauma to tissues, reduce the risk of contamination with luminal contents, and are less likely to result in staple line leaks of blood, air, or bowel contents. Staplers are also less reactive with the immune system due to their nonferrous nature and do not significantly interfere with MRI scanners, although some imaging artifacts may still occur. Furthermore, there are now synthetic absorbable types of staplers available, further expanding their utility in surgical procedures.

■ BIBLIOGRAPHY

1. Chen MH, Khalil H (Eds). Laparoscopic Suturing Techniques for Surgeons. Oxford: Oxford University Press; 2022.
2. Choi E, Kim DY. The Use of Biodegradable Sutures in Laparoscopic Surgery. J Biomed Mat. 2024;15(3): 438-45.
3. Fernandez R, Martin CJ. Ergonomics in Laparoscopic Suturing: Minimizing Surgeon Fatigue. J Ergonomics Surg. 2023;17(3):145-54.
4. Gomez R, Lee T. Evolution of Suturing Techniques in Laparoscopic Surgery. J Minim Invasive Sur. 2021;28(2):123-32.
5. Gupta S, Mehra R. Barriers to Learning Laparoscopic Suturing: A Survey of Surgical Residents. Education Surg. 2023;47(1):55-62.
6. Hamilton EC, Sims TL, Hamilton TT, Mullican MA, Jones DB, Provost DA. Clinical predictors of leak after laparoscopic Roux-en-Y gastric bypass for morbid obesity. Surg Endosc. 2003;17(5):679-84.
7. Harper D, Lombardi A. Adapting Traditional Suturing Techniques for Laparoscopic Applications. Surg Techniques Rev. 2021;35(4):320-8.
8. Jones DB, Wu JS, Soper NJ (Eds). Laparoscopic Surgery: Principles and Procedures, 2nd edition, revised and expanded. Switzerland: Taylor & Francis; 2004.
9. Kumar V, Saxena AK (Eds). Advanced Techniques in Laparoscopic Surgery. Berlin: Springer; 2020.
10. Lavelle JF, Sinclair MF. Automated Suturing Devices in Laparoscopic Surgery: A Comparative Analysis. Technol Surg. 2020;22(6):789-98.
11. Lee J, Kim S. Innovations in Laparoscopic Suturing Instruments. Int J Med Robot. 2022;18(1):e2210.
12. Mendez C, Gupta A. Laparoscopic Suturing: Mastery Through Technique and Practice. London: Elsevier Health Sciences; 2023.
13. Mishra RK (Ed). Textbook of Laparoscopy for Surgeons and Gynecologists, 4th edition. New Delhi: Jaypee Brothers Medical Publishers (P) Ltd.; 2021. p. 900.
14. Mishra RK (Ed). Textbook of Practical Laparoscopic Surgery, 1st edition. New Delhi: Jaypee Brothers Medical Publishers (P) Ltd.; 2008.
15. Morrison T, Jacobs LR. Teaching Laparoscopic Suturing: The Role of Simulation in Medical Schools. Med Teacher. 2021;43(7):778-84.
16. Nguyen L, Ho CP. Impact of Suture Materials on Laparoscopic Knot Reliability. Mat Surg. 2024;9(2):200-10.
17. O'Reilly MP, Saunders BH (Eds). Virtual Reality Training for Laparoscopic Surgery. Cambridge: Cambridge University Press; 2022.
18. Patel R, Thompson J. The Role of Simulation in Learning Laparoscopic Suturing and Knotting. Med Education Online. 2021;26:1857289.
19. Rodriguez A, Davis SS. Robotic-Assisted Laparoscopic Knot Tying: Methods and Efficiency. Surg Innov. 2019;26(4):459-66.
20. Sauerland S, Neugebauer E. Laparoscopy for Every Acute Appendicitis? Surg Endosc. 2007;21:342.
21. Shimi SM, Lirici MM, Vander Velpen G, Cuschieri A. Comparative study of holding strength of slipknot using absorbable and nonabsorbable ligature materials. Surg Endosc. 1994;11:1285-91.
22. Smith JA, Patel VR (Eds). Principles of Laparoscopic Suturing and Knotting. New York: Springer; 2023.
23. Surgical Knots and Suturing Techniques. (2024). Available from https://en.wikipedia.org/wiki/Surgical_knot.
24. Targarona EM, Balagué C, Berindoague R, Pey A, Martinez C, Hernandez P, et al. Low section of the rectum during laparoscopic total mesorectal excision using the Contour device. Technical report. Surg Endosc. 2007;21(2):327-9.
25. Wang Y, Thompson C. Innovations in Knot Tying Techniques for Minimally Invasive Surgery. Innov Surg. 2022;18(4):250-60.
26. Williams NE, Tan JL. Comparative Study of Knot Security in Laparoscopic Surgery. J Surg Res. 2020;245:217-23.
27. Zimmerman KA, Patel ND. Laparoscopic Knotting: A Visual Guide for Surgeons. Philadelphia: Lippincott Williams & Wilkins; 2022.

Role of Correct Port Position in Laparoscopic Suturing and Knotting

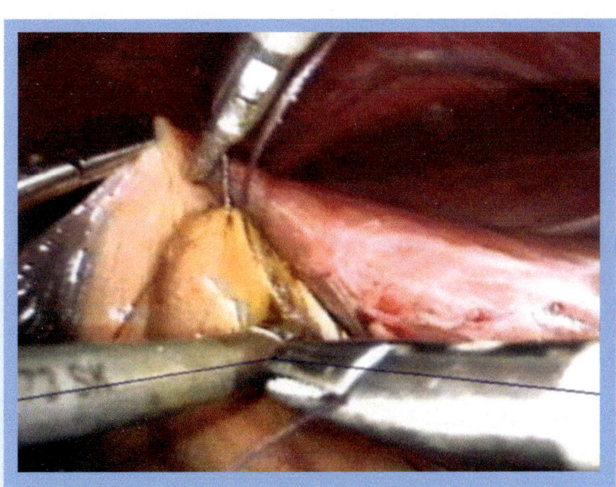

INTRODUCTION

The relative position of the instrument ports is very important in the performance of surgical procedures endoscopically. The angle, the instruments make with the operative site and to each other should mimic, as far as possible, the natural relationship of the hands and eyes during conventional surgery. It is proved that the most common cause of stressful minimal access surgery is the wrong port position. 95% of surgeons and gynecologists use umbilicus as the primary port, but at the time of inserting the secondary port there is controversy among operators and they lack the principles behind the secondary port position.

LAPAROSCOPIC INSTRUMENTS SHOULD BEHAVE LIKE FIRST-CLASS LEVER

A lever is a simple machine that usually consists of a rigid bar or rod that rotates about a fixed pivot point called the fulcrum. If you apply a force to a lever, it will rotate about the fulcrum. Common examples of levers are seesaws, wheelbarrows, crowbars, and nutcrackers. The advantage of using a lever is that with a small amount of effort, you can move a very big load. For example, with a crowbar, a relatively small effort is applied at the end farthest from the fulcrum to lift a heavy weight that is close to the fulcrum. Many other common tools and instruments utilize the principle of the lever. Laparoscopic instruments also behave like a lever and they are supported by a cannula in the middle.

A lever has two related forces associated with it called load and effort. In the third century BC, the Greek mathematician Archimedes first described the principle of the lever that can be expressed as:

The effort × Its distance from the fulcrum = The load × Its distance from the fulcrum

TYPES OF LEVER

Types of levers are as follows **(Figs. 1A to C)**.

- A first-class lever is one where the fulcrum is between the effort and the load just like a seesaw or crowbar. A laparoscopic instrument behaves like a first-class

lever when half of the instrument is inside the abdominal cavity and half of the instrument is outside the abdomen.

- In the second-class lever, such as a wheelbarrow, the load is placed between the effort and the fulcrum.
- In the third-class lever, such as a fishing rod, the effort is placed between the load and the fulcrum.

Examples of common tools (and other items) that use a first-class lever are given in **Table 1**.

If only little length of the laparoscopic instrument is inside and the maximum length is outside there will be the following difficulties:

- All the movement will be rectified; i.e., if the surgeon moves his/her hand 3 cm outside, the inside movement will be only 1 cm.
- The force applied will be magnified; i.e., very gentle force applied over handle of the instrument will exert a great force at the tip of the instrument inside.
- The elevation angle of the instrument will increase <30°, which is ergonomically not suitable to perform surgery (elevation angle is the angle between the instrument and the body of the patient).

If more length of the laparoscopic instrument is inside and only a little is outside, there will be the following difficulties:

- All the movement will be magnified; i.e., if a surgeon moves his/her hand 1 cm outside, the inside movement will be 3 cm.
- The force applied will be rectified; i.e., moderate force applied over the instrument will exert a little force at the tip of the instrument inside.
- The elevation angle of the instrument will increase >30°, which is ergonomically not suitable to perform surgery (the optimum working elevation angle should be 15– 30 degree).

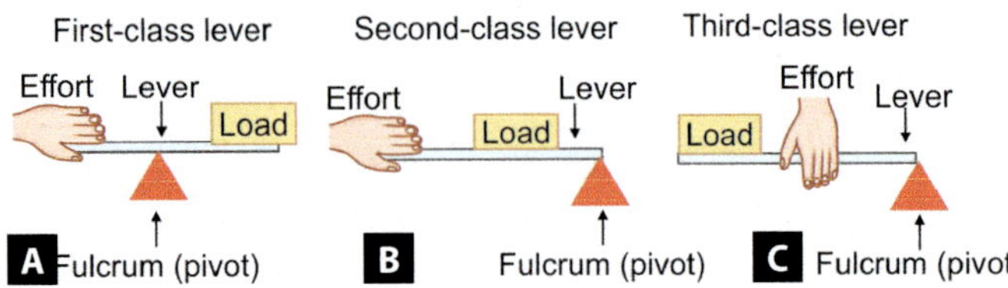

Figs. 1A to C: Types of lever.

Item		Number of class-first levers used
See-saw		A single class-first lever
Hammer's claws		A single class-first lever
Scissors		2 class-first lever
Pliers		2 class-first lever

TABLE 1: Common tools and first-class levers used.

PRIMARY PORT POSITION

The central location and ability of the umbilicus to camouflage scars make it an attractive primary port site for laparoscopic surgery. There are many drawbacks with the umbilicus as well. The umbilicus is a naturally weak area due to the absence of all the layers. Weakness is also due to its location at the midpoint of the abdomen's greatest diameter.

It is easy to believe that there is a difference between the umbilicus and other trocar sites in both susceptibility to infection and postoperative incisional herniation. 873 operations were studied, 561 cholecystectomies, 190 inguinal hernia repairs, 71 Nissen fundoplications, and 51 ventral hernia repairs. The study showed that the increased infection rate at the umbilicus seems to be related to retrieval of infected organs through the umbilicus and not to the umbilicus itself. When umbilicus was used to retrieve the gallbladder after cholecystectomy, the rate of infection was high due to port contamination with the infected gallbladder. Excluding cholecystectomy, the umbilical infection rate was 2%, similar to that of any alternative site. The postoperative ventral hernia rate was 0.8%, the same at the umbilicus as elsewhere if the port more than 10 mm in size is not repaired. It is now proved that the wound infection at the umbilicus is similar to that at other sites; postoperative ventral hernia at the umbilicus is similar to that at other sites and most of the infection after laparoscopic cholecystectomy is due to the contamination of wound due to infected gallbladder.

SECONDARY PORT POSITION

The obligatory passage of the laparoscopic instruments through the abdominal wall generates a fixed point after which all movements are reversed. For instance, when the hand moves to the left, the end of the instrument moves right, and when the hand moves downward, the end of the instrument moves upward. For some surgeons the fulcrum effect is not a problem, but for others, it is an insurmountable obstacle to the performance of advanced laparoscopy.

Because the handling of laparoscopic instruments is through the fixed point at the abdominal wall, the force feedback felt by the surgeon will depend on the length of the instrument inferior to this fixed point.

A satisfactory relationship includes the following **(Fig. 2)**.

- An angle of 60° between the two instruments tips

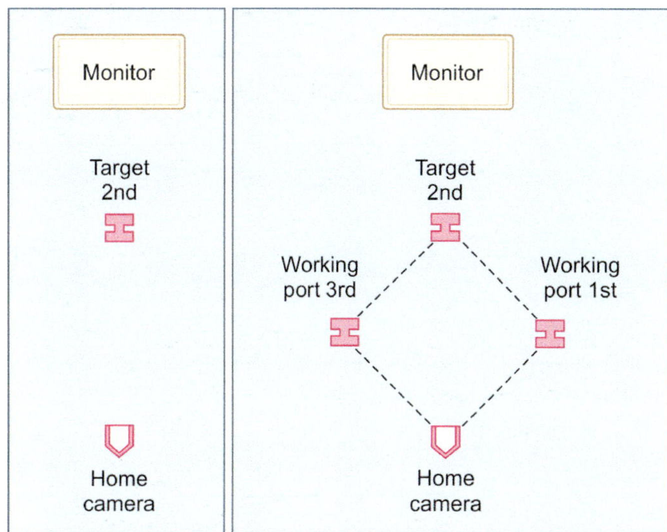

Fig. 2: Baseball diamond concept of port position.

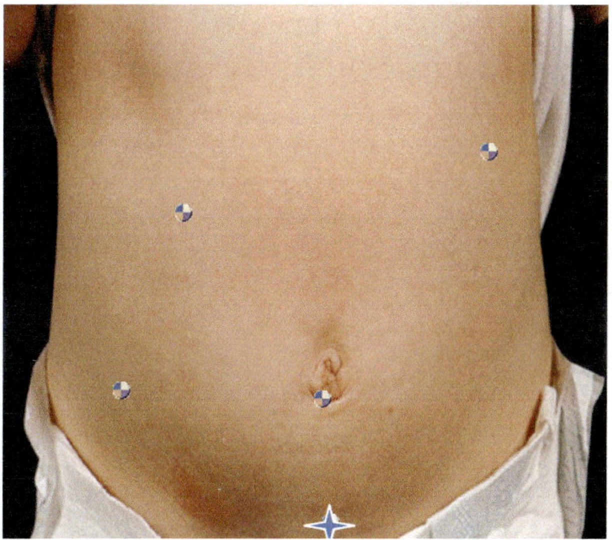

Fig. 3: Deciding the target first.

- Tangential approach to the site
- Appropriate working distance

First Decide the Target

Target may be in suprapubic region for laparoscopically assisted vaginal hysterectomy (LAVH), right iliac fossa for appendectomy, right upper quadrant for laparoscopic cholecystectomy or left upper quadrant for fundoplication **(Fig. 3)**.

Draw the Line of Optimum Area

For optimum task performance, half to two-third instrument should be inside the abdomen. The size

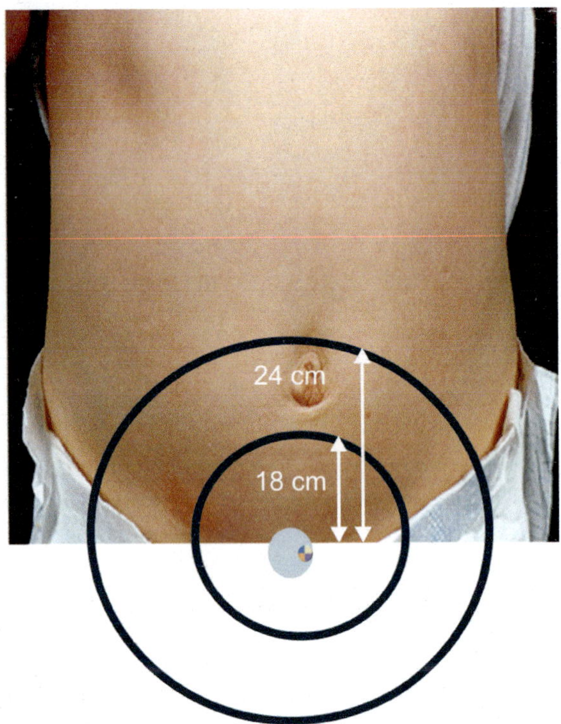

Fig. 4: Draw two arcs on the abdominal wall at 18 and 24 cm from that point and note the area in between.

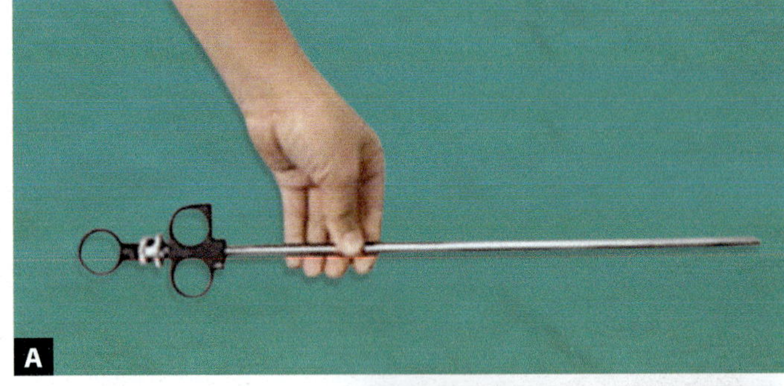

- Telescope should be in the middle of working instruments

- Manipulation angle of instruments should be 60°

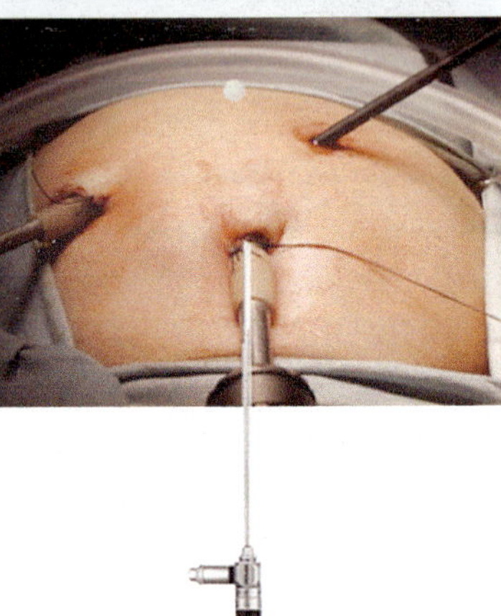

Figs. 5A and B: (A) Instrument; (B) Telescope.

of an adult laparoscopic instrument is 36 cm and a pediatrics instrument is 28 cm. For optimal ergonomics in laparoscopy, the telescope should be positioned between 18 and 24 cm **(Fig. 4)** from the dissection target, and the working instruments should maintain a distance of 18 cm from the target **(Figs. 5A and B)**.

Rule of Diamond for Laparoscopically Assisted Vaginal Hysterectomy

These factors combined with the specific anatomy will determine individual port sites. For standard operations like cholecystectomy, standard port sites related to surface marking may suffice but as more advanced or varied situations are tackled, we recommend that you master the skill of individual port placement using the internal view **(Fig. 6)**.

The manipulation angle of 60° is considered optimal in laparoscopic surgery for several reasons, all of which contribute to enhancing surgical efficiency, precision, and the surgeon's comfort during procedures **(Fig. 7)**. This angle allows for a more natural hand–eye coordination and ergonomic positioning for the surgeon, which is essential for minimizing fatigue and the risk of strain injuries during prolonged surgeries.

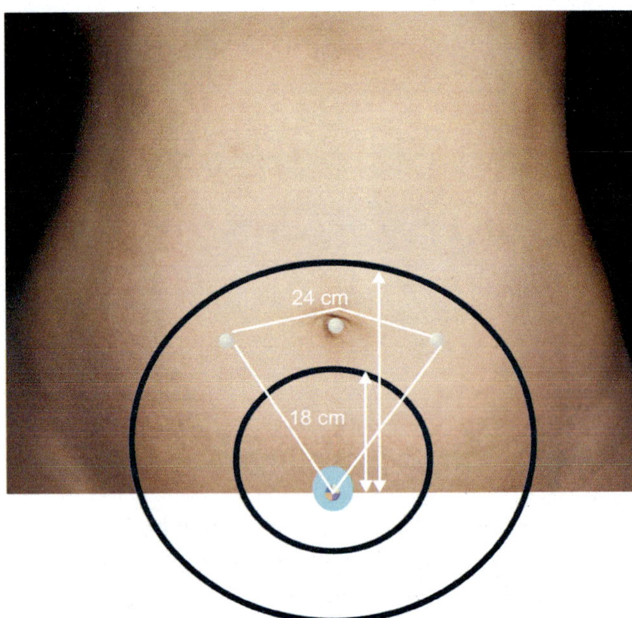

Fig. 6: Rule of diamond for laparoscopically assisted vaginal hysterectomy (LAVH).

- *Ergonomic efficiency:* A 60° angle between the instruments and the visual axis helps mimic the natural movements of the human hands and wrists, making

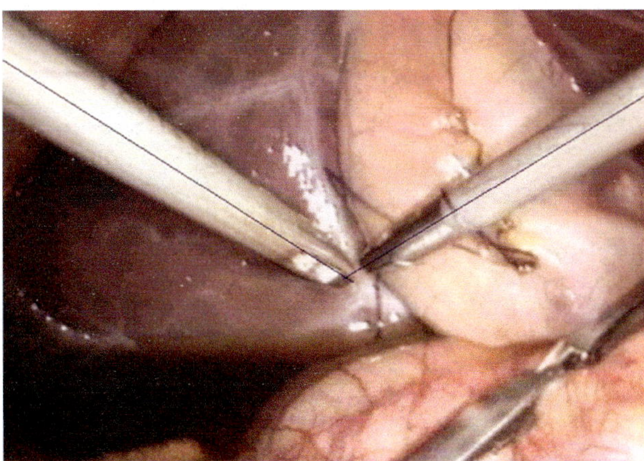

Fig. 7: Manipulation angle of 60° provides superior ergonomic benefits.

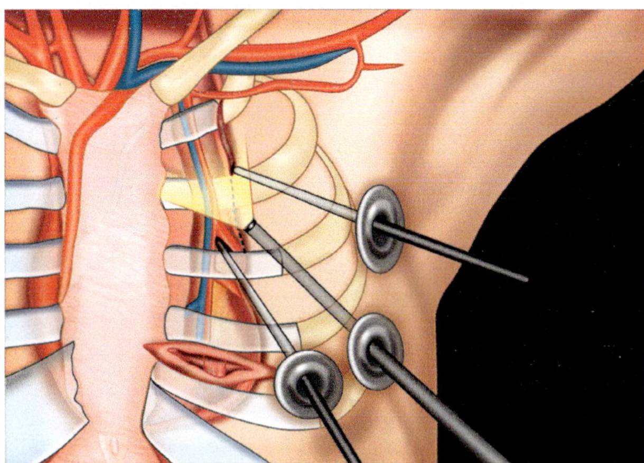

Fig. 8: Manipulation angle 60° is the angle between tips of the instrument.

surgical manipulations more intuitive and reducing the physical stress on the surgeon. This angle enables surgeons to perform complex tasks with greater precision and less effort.

- *Optimal visualization and precision:* This angle provides an optimal view of the surgical field, ensuring that the instruments are in the surgeon's direct line of sight. It enhances depth perception and spatial orientation, allowing for more precise dissection, suturing, and manipulation of tissues. Better visualization directly impacts the accuracy of the procedure and can reduce operative time.
- *Reduction of instrument conflict:* By maintaining a 60° manipulation angle, there is a decrease in the likelihood of instrument crowding and conflict within the limited workspace of laparoscopic surgery. This arrangement facilitates smoother instrument navigation and manipulation, allowing for more efficient tissue handling and reducing the risk of accidental tissue damage.
- *Enhanced dexterity:* The optimal manipulation angle allows for a wider range of motion with the instruments, improving dexterity. Surgeons can achieve more complex maneuvers without the need for excessive force or awkward hand positions, which can lead to fatigue and reduce the effectiveness of the procedure.
- *Reduced physical strain:* Maintaining an ergonomic working posture is crucial in laparoscopic surgery to prevent musculoskeletal strain and injuries over time. The 60° angle helps in aligning the surgeon's hands, wrists, and shoulders comfortably, minimizing the risk of repetitive strain injuries associated with long surgical procedures.

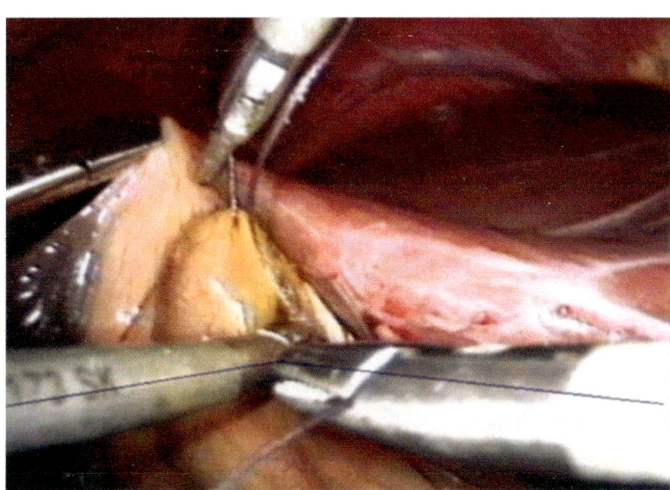

Fig. 9: Manipulation angle of 60° is essential for optimum task performance in laparoscopic surgery.

In summary, the manipulation angle of 60° is a key component of ergonomic principles in laparoscopic surgery, contributing to improved surgeon comfort, reduced fatigue, and enhanced procedural efficiency and safety.

In general, the optic and the two main operating ports usually lie at the points of a flattened triangle, the optic being centrally and more distally placed. Try to keep ports at least 5 cm apart.

The manipulation angle of 60° is angle between the tips of instruments (**Fig. 8**).

A manipulation angle of 60° is essential for optimum task performance in laparoscopic surgery (**Fig. 9**). A manipulation angle of 60° is essential for better instrument control (**Fig. 10**).

■ PORT POSITION IN VARIOUS SURGERIES

Port positions in various surgeries are shown in **Figures 11 to 15**.

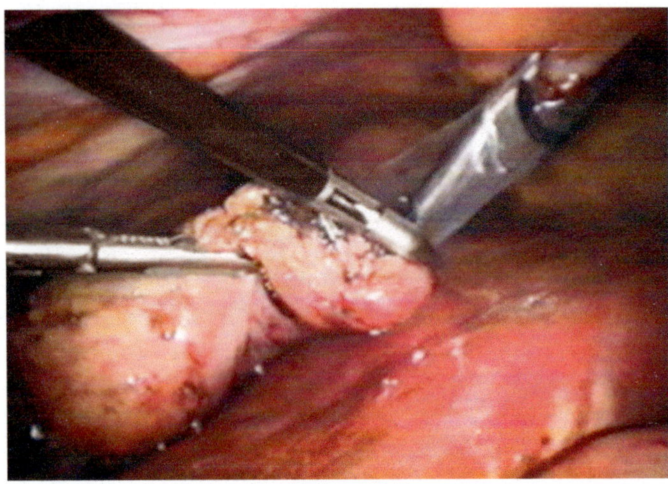

Fig. 10: A manipulation angle of 60° is essential for better instrument control.

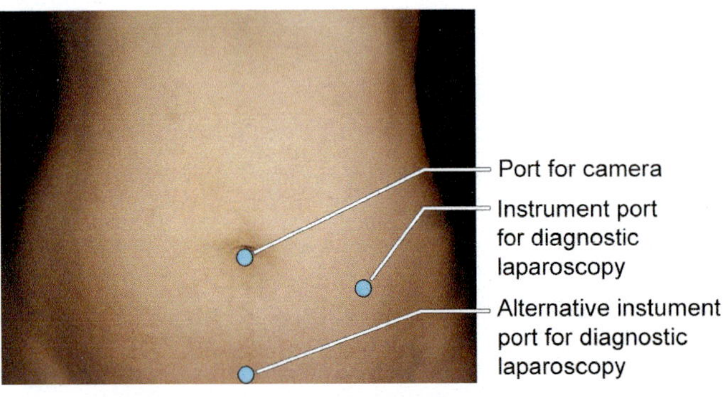

Fig. 11: Port position for diagnostic laparoscopy.

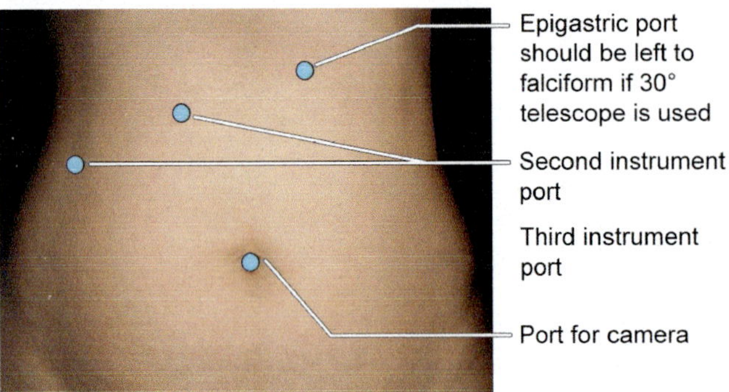

Fig. 12: Port position for cholecystectomy.

■ DRAWBACKS OF INCORRECT PORT POSITION

Swording

Swording occurs when the telescope or the shaft of the assistant's instrument obstructs the operator's instruments. If this occurs you may need to consider:

- Repositioning retracting instruments

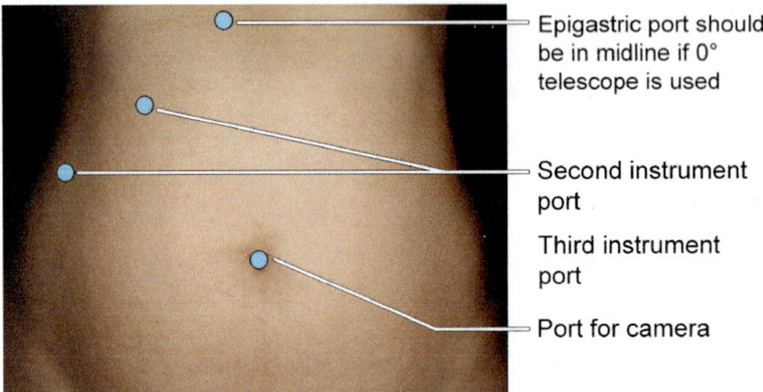

Fig. 13: Alternative port position for cholecystectomy.

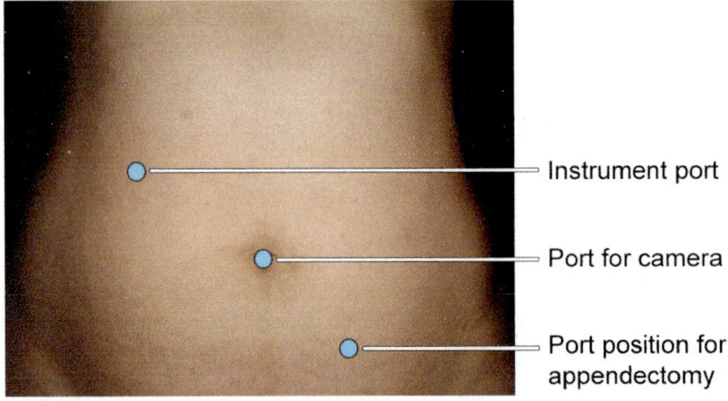

Fig. 14: Port position for appendectomy.

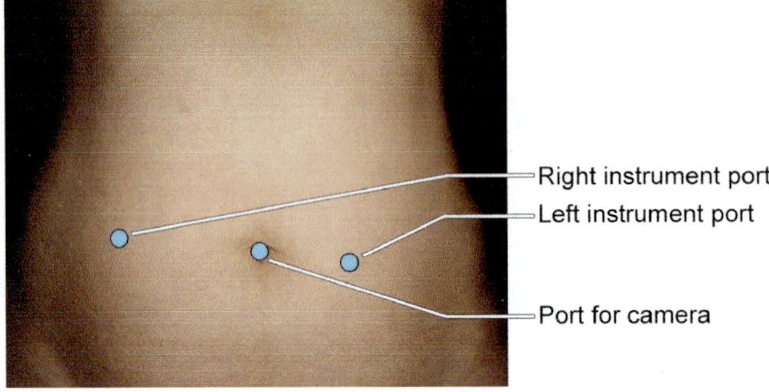

Fig. 15: Port position for bilateral hernia, laparoscopically assisted vaginal hysterectomy (LAVH), and most of the gynecological procedures.

- Rotation of an angled telescope allowing alteration in the position of the end of the telescope
- Withdrawal of the telescope
- Transposition of the operator's instruments
- Additional port placement
- Changing the instruments to a different port

■ CONCLUSION

The proper placement of ports in laparoscopic suturing and knotting is crucial for the success of minimally invasive surgeries. The position of instrument ports significantly affects the ergonomics, efficiency, and precision of surgical procedures. Instruments must mimic the natural hand-eye coordination observed in conventional surgeries, making correct port positioning essential for reducing surgeon fatigue and preventing musculoskeletal strain.

Laparoscopic instruments should act like first-class levers, with the correct proportion of the instrument inside and outside the abdominal cavity. This balance ensures optimal force transmission and movement control, thereby enhancing the surgeon's ability to perform complex tasks with precision. Incorrect port positioning can lead to various issues, such as reduced instrument control, increased physical strain on the surgeon, and the phenomenon known as "swording," where instruments obstruct each other.

A manipulation angle of 60° between instruments is ideal, promoting better visualization, reduced instrument conflict, and improved dexterity. This angle allows for a natural hand position, minimizing physical strain and enhancing the surgeon's comfort during lengthy procedures.

Overall, adhering to ergonomic principles and optimal port positioning is vital for the safety and success of laparoscopic surgeries, ensuring effective suturing and knotting while maintaining the surgeon's well-being.

■ BIBLIOGRAPHY

1. Bell ST, Roberts HP. Optimal Port Placement in Laparoscopic Surgery. London: Academic Press; 2022.
2. Davies JF, Kumar A. Ergonomic principles of port positioning in laparoscopic surgery. Surg Endosc. 2020;34(3): 1243-51.
3. Hernandez R, Lopez G. Laparoscopic Suturing Techniques: From Basics to Advanced Strategies. New York: Springer; 2019.
4. Morgan HL, Patel SB. Impact of port position on laparoscopic knot tying: A comparative study. J Laparoendosc Adv Surg Tech. 2021;31(5):568-74.
5. National Institute for Health and Care Excellence (NICE). (2021). Guidelines for Safe Port Placement in Laparoscopic Surgeries. [online] Available from https://www.nice.org.uk.
6. Singh V, Reddy MS. Advanced Laparoscopic Surgery: Techniques and Tips. Philadelphia: Elsevier; 2023.
7. Thompson CD, Anderson RE. Simulation Training for Effective Port Placement in Laparoscopic Suturing. Medical Education in Surgery. 2024;46(2):210-8.
8. Wu XJ, Zhang Y. Principles of Port Placement in Relation to Anatomical Landmarks and Internal Structures. Asian J Endosc Surg. 2018;11(4):308-16.
9. Yates DR, Moore FT. Technological Advancements in Laparoscopic Port Instruments: Enhancing Suturing and Knotting Techniques. J Minim Invasive Surg. 2022;29(1):47-54.
10. Zimmerman KA. Port Placement and Patient Positioning in Laparoscopic Surgery. Cham: Springer; 2020.

Comparison of Laparoscopic Knots

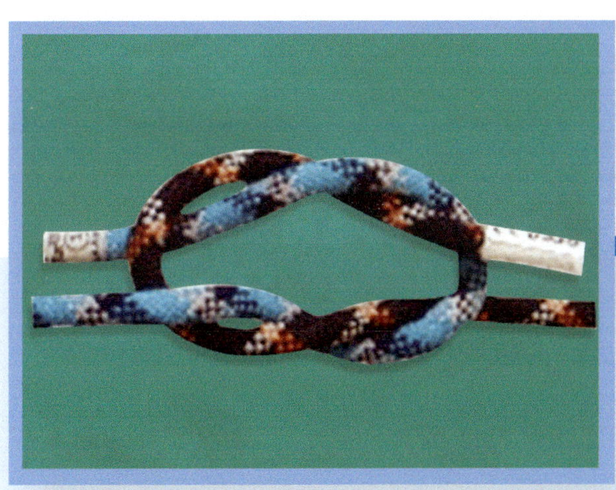

■ INTRODUCTION

The holding and tensile characteristics of five extracorporeal slip knots in relation to absorbable and nonabsorbable ligature materials have been evaluated in a standardized in vitro test rig. The knots studied—Tayside, Roeder, Melzer (modified Roeder), cross square, and blood knots—were tied with the following materials: silk, polyamide, Dacron, polydioxanone (PDS), and lactomer (Polysorb). Following construction and slippage (rundown) to a fixed-diameter loop around a cylinder, the knots were locked (tightened) using a standardized force after which they were removed from the test rig and subjected to holding strength (force required to induce reverse slippage) and other tensile characteristics (stress, strain, and elasticity) by a tensiometer. Analysis of the data has demonstrated the following:

- The safest slip knots (resist slippage) are the Tayside, Melzer, and Roeder knots tied with lactomer and Dacron.
- The holding strengths of the cross square and blood knots are weak with all ligature materials tested.
- PDS is a safe ligature material for the Melzer and Tayside but not for the Roeder knot.
- Extracorporeal slip knots tied with silk and polyamide are less secure than the equivalent knots tied with Dacron, lactomer, and PDS.

Although the majority of surgeons employ clips to occlude vessels and ducts during endoscopic surgery, this practice is unsafe when applied to tubular structures, especially vessels, that are larger than 3.0 mm and those surrounded by adipose tissue. The poor holding strength of metallic clips has been documented. Safe and reliable knotting is essential for the ligation of sizable ducts and vessels and for tissue approximation.

In endoscopic surgery, special techniques are required for this purpose. Intracorporeal knotting using the standard microsurgical (surgeon's) knot requires additional skills and is time-consuming. By contrast, extracorporeal knots are easier to master and are less time-consuming. The most commonly employed slip knot is the Roeder ligature, first described for use in tonsillectomy and introduced in endoscopic surgery by Semm. Studies with this knot have shown that it is very secure when tied in catgut. Furthermore, its holding strength increases as it swells by hydration due to absorption of tissue fluid, and for this reason, it is been recommended for ligature of the cystic duct in continuity during laparoscopic cholecystectomy.

A variety of slip knots are used by various professions and in certain leisure activities. Some of these have been adapted for use in endoscopic surgery. The holding strength of individual types of slip knots is influenced by a number of factors including the ligature material used and its caliber. Thus, a slip knot may be secure when tied in catgut but unsafe with other materials. In addition, some slip knots are difficult to tie or jam lock too easily for reliable placement by push rod before locking. The aim of the present study was to compare the performance of five slip knots in relation to type and size of commonly used.

■ TAYSIDE KNOT

This knot is used by fishermen along the east coast of Scotland. It consists of a single cross hitch (first loop) followed by three turns around the standing part (straight limb) forming the second loop. The bight is then reversed (third loop) and passed through the second and third loops in an up-and-under fashion. The steps involved in tying the Tayside slip knot are shown in **Figure 1**. The characteristics of this knot include ease of tying and smooth forward slipping during knot placement (rundown). It requires simultaneous pushing with the rod against traction on the standing part and lateral traction on the tail for locking.

■ ROEDER KNOT

This knot is well known and is used in the construction of preformed catgut endoloops. When used to ligate structures in continuity, the procedure that should be followed is outlined in **Figure 2**. The knot is easy to tie and locks simply by pushing with the push rod against traction on the standing part.

■ MELTZER KNOT

This is a modification of the Roeder slip knot and was described by Meltzer in 1991 for use with PDS. The most important configurational change in this knot is the

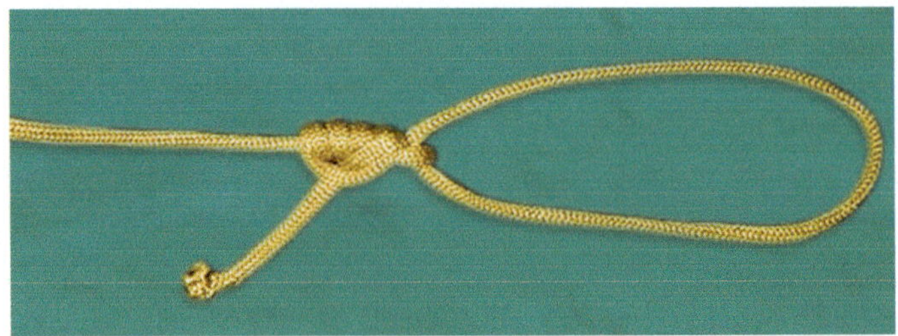

Fig. 1: Tayside knot.

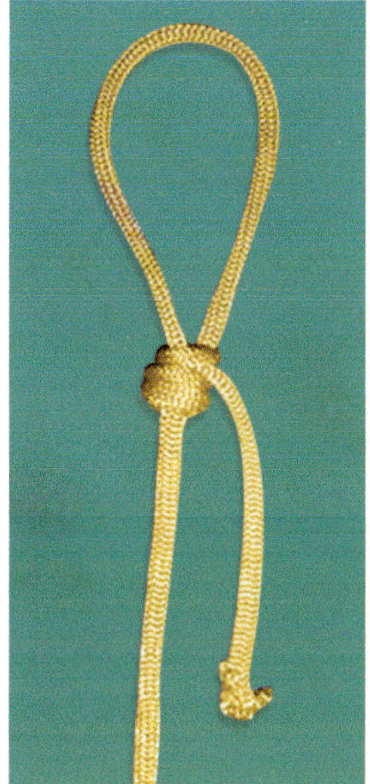

Fig. 2: Roeder knot.

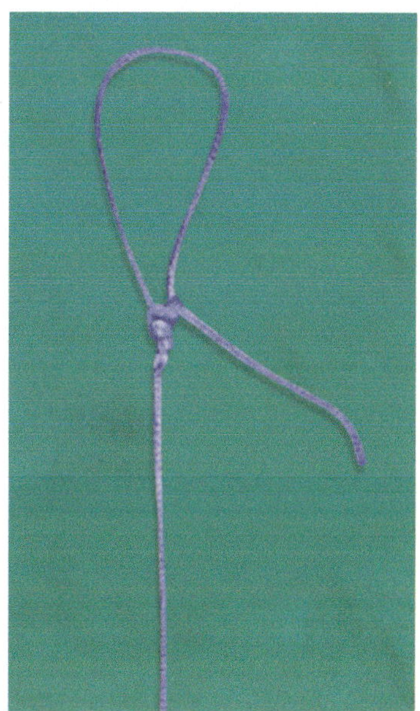

Fig. 3: Melzer knot.

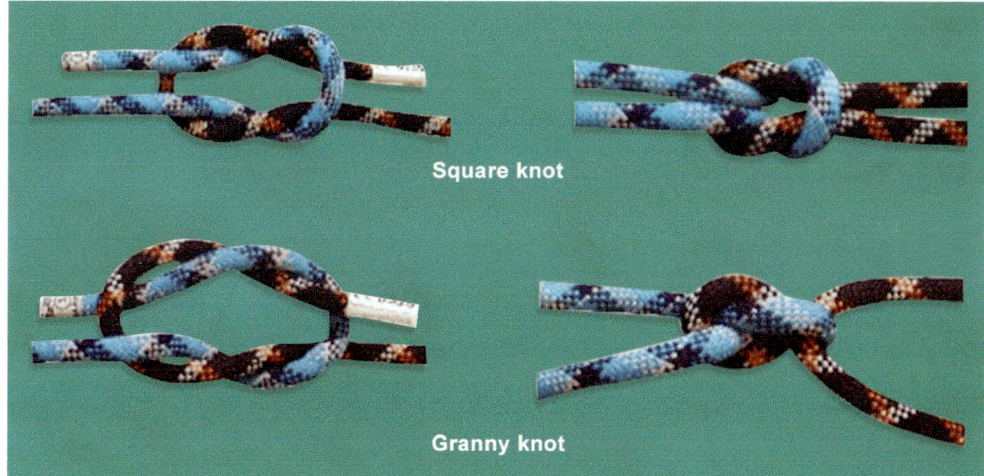

Fig. 4: Cross square slip knot.

double hitch used to construct the loop at the beginning of the knot **(Fig. 3)**.

■ CROSS SQUARE KNOT

In essence, this is a modified square knot. The second loop is twisted to form a crossed figure of eight, after which the bite (tail) is reversed and passed through the crossed loop in an up-and-under fashion. The steps involved in the fashioning of the cross square knot are shown in **Figure 4**. This knot is difficult to tie and can lock prematurely during knot rundown. Granny knot is just a variation of square knot.

■ BLOOD KNOT

This is a popular knot used by fishermen and is outlined in **Figures 5 and 6**. It is easy to tie and slides well during knot placement.

The "blood knot"— or more accurately, the term might be intended to mean a "slip knot" used in surgical contexts, including laparoscopic procedures—is a type of knot that is secure and can be tightened or loosened as needed. In the context of surgery, particularly in laparoscopic and robotic surgery, slip knots are essential for securing sutures without the need for excessive force or manipulation,

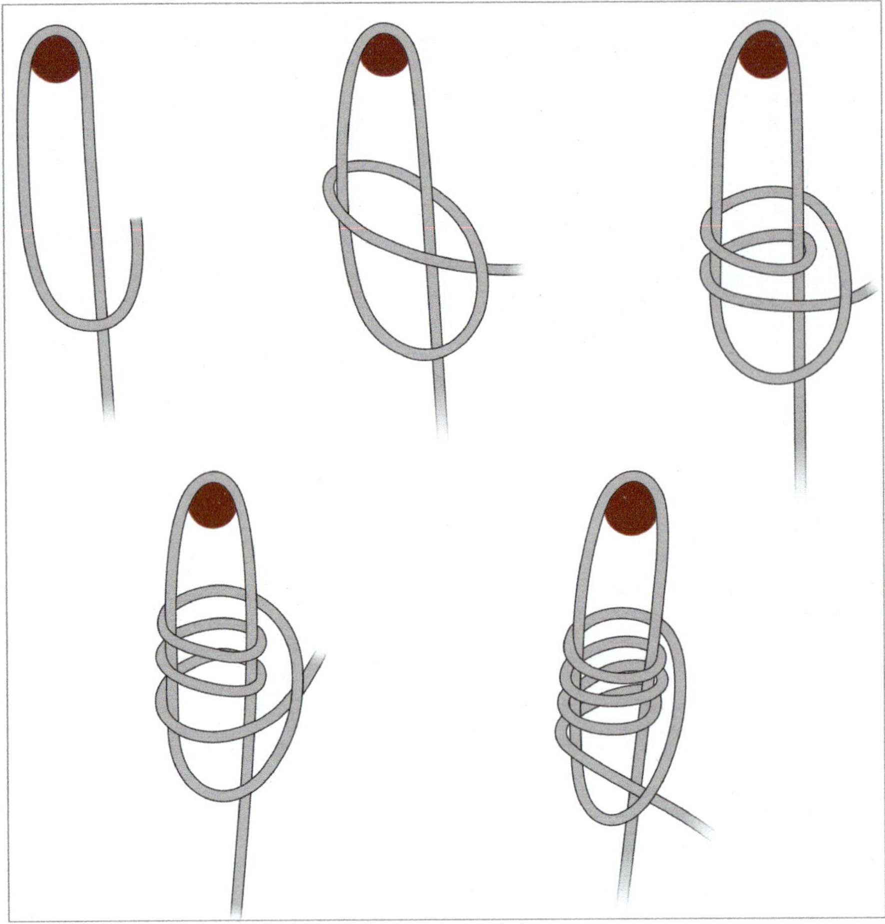

Fig. 5: Blood slip knot.

which is critical in the delicate environment of minimally invasive procedures.

In surgical practice, a slip knot (sometimes referred to informally as a "blood knot" in various clinical settings, though "blood knot" is more commonly associated with fishing) is designed to provide secure ligation of vessels or tissue with the ability to adjust the tightness of the knot after it has been placed. This is particularly useful in situations where precise control over the tension of a suture is necessary to ensure adequate hemostasis (control of bleeding) without compromising tissue integrity by overtightening.

Key characteristics of surgical slip knots include:

- *Adjustability:* The knot can be tightened or loosened as necessary after being initially placed, allowing for precise control over suture tension.
- *Security:* Once the desired tension is achieved, the knot can be locked in place to prevent slippage, which is crucial for maintaining hemostasis and tissue approximation without the risk of the knot coming undone.
- *Minimally invasive compatibility:* In laparoscopic surgery, where access to the surgical site is limited and maneuverability is restricted by the use of long instruments through small incisions, the ability to tie and adjust a slip knot remotely is invaluable. It reduces the need for additional instrument exchanges and manipulations, potentially decreasing operative time and risk of tissue trauma.

Slip knots in surgery are typically tied using specialized techniques and instruments, with surgeons often using tools like knot pushers in laparoscopic procedures to place and adjust these knots inside the patient's body. Mastery of these techniques is crucial for surgeons, particularly those specializing in minimally invasive procedures, as it directly impacts the efficacy and safety of the surgeries they perform.

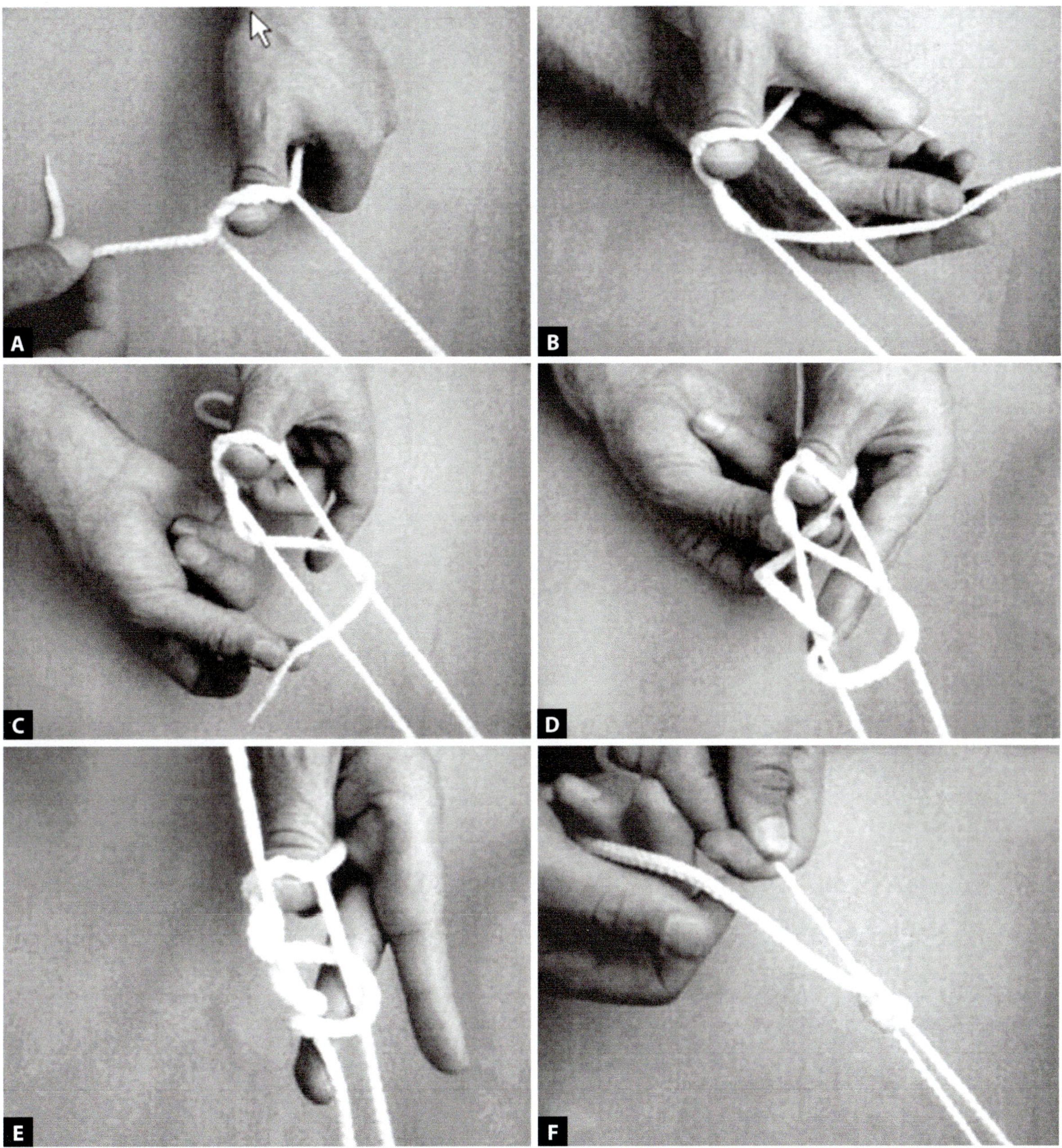

Fig. 6A to F: All the steps of the Blood slip knot.

■ TEST RIG

The slip knots were tied around a plastic cylinder 38 mm in diameter clamped at one end. The opposite end of the cylinder tapered gradually to a diameter of 35 mm. After the knot was tied, the standing part (long segment) of the ligature was threaded up the inside of a plastic carrier (10.3 cm long push rod) and then down the outside of the push rod, the assembly being held loosely in position by an outer 10 cm long cylinder with an internal diameter of 16 mm diameter. The outer holding tube was clamped in a perpendicular position to the tying cylinder.

The Gea extracorporeal knot, named after Dr Manuel Gea González, is a surgical technique designed to offer ease, speed, simplicity, and security in knot tying, particularly in laparoscopic procedures **(Fig. 7)**. This technique's key advantage lies in its controlled adjusting force, which minimizes the risk of tissue damage—a crucial consideration in delicate surgical environments.

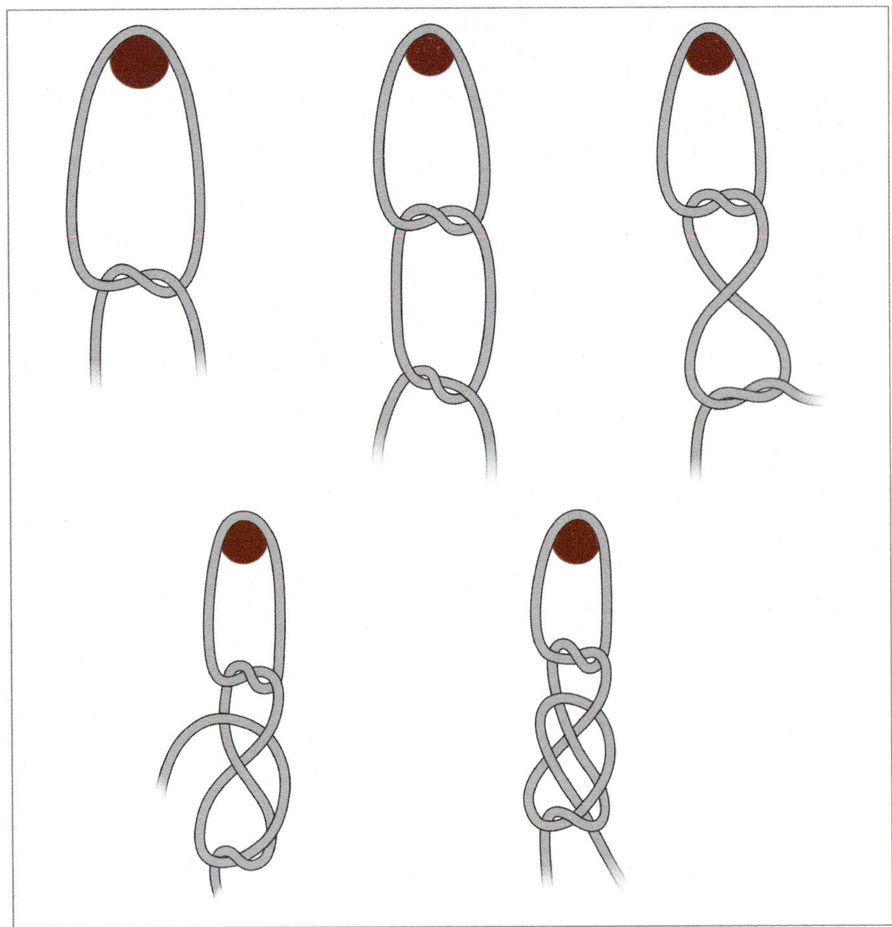

Fig. 7: Gea knot.

Extracorporeal knot-tying techniques, like the Gea knot, are especially valuable in minimally invasive surgeries where space is limited and direct hand access to the surgical site is not possible. In these scenarios, the ability to securely tie a knot outside the body and then introduce and tighten it inside the surgical site allows for precise control over suture tension. This is essential for ensuring the integrity of tissue approximation and hemostasis while avoiding excessive constriction that could lead to tissue ischemia or necrosis.

The Gea knot is adaptable and can be employed in various surgical contexts beyond laparoscopy, including endoluminal procedures where sutures must be placed within tubular structures of the body and open surgical procedures where its ease and security can also offer advantages. Its design allows for consistent and reliable suture tension, which is critical for surgical success and patient recovery.

Such extracorporeal knotting techniques underscore the evolution of surgical practices toward methods that prioritize patient safety, procedural efficiency, and the minimization of postoperative complications. The development and dissemination of techniques like the Gea knot represent the ongoing refinement of surgical skills and methodologies to enhance outcomes in the wide array of procedures performed in modern medicine.

Two weights, each 250 g, were then attached to the free ends of the assembled ligature for 3 minutes to achieve standardized tightening **(Fig. 8)**. The weights and nylon carrier were subsequently removed and the loop around the plastic cylinder was gently eased to the narrower end and removed. The free ligature ends were shortened to 10 mm each.

The 38 mm-diameter ligature loop was then divided at the opposite pole to the knot and the two ends were inserted between the jaws of the pneumatic clamps

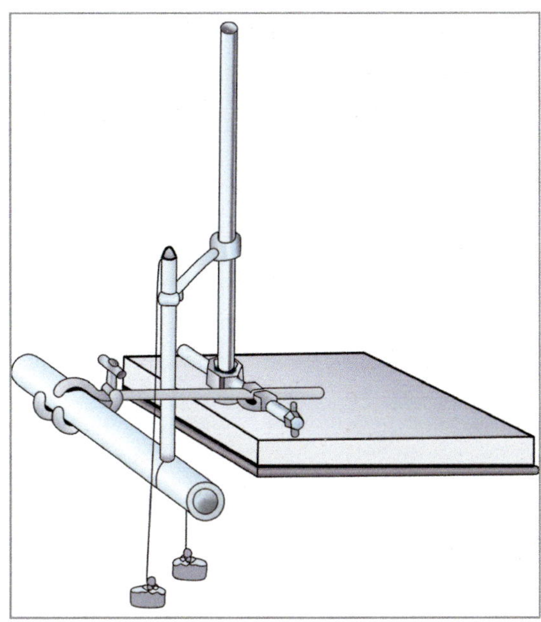

Fig. 8: Test rig used to test the different types of knots.

of an Instron tensiometer (model 1026, lnstron Ltd. Switzerland), the distance between the clamps being 13 mm. The tension load cell was 5 or 50 kg depending on the forces required: 50 kg for Tayside and Melzer slip knots using PDS, lactomer, and Dacron; 5 kg for other slip knots. The chart speed was set at 50 mm/min. For each experiment, the following were calculated:

- *Force required for reverse slipping* of the knot (F)
- *Stress* = *F/A,* where A is the cross-sectional area of the suture material used
- *Strain* = stretch/original length
- *Elasticity* = stress/strain

    Data on the cross-sectional area of the ligature materials was obtained from the manufacturer's specifications.

■ STATISTICAL ANALYSIS

The median and interquartile ranges of 10 measurements for each knot were obtained. Comparisons between the tensile characteristics of the various knots were performed using the Mann–Whitney U test.

■ RESULTS

Force required to induce reverse slippage: The data for the median force in Newton required to initiate reverse slipping of the slip-knots from the ligature materials used are tested in a laboratory setting. This data show that the force required to cause reverse slipping of the slip knots

is directly related to the diameter of the suture material used.

    Thus, reverse slippage of slip knots formed with ligature materials of sizes 1/0 or 0/0 is induced by forces that are generally twice as strong as those required to achieve the same endpoint for knots fashioned with the stress necessary to effect a standard elongation of the distance between the clamps prior to reverse slippage of the knot. Silk, polyamide, and Dacron manifested similar elasticity in all the knots examined. This was lower than the elasticity of lactomer and PDS. Melzer and Roeder knots had similar elasticity for the ligature materials tested but this was lower than the elasticity of Tayside, cross square, and blood knots (p <0.05). Slip knots tied with materials of small diameter (2/0) tended to be more elastic than those tied with thicker materials (1/0 and 0/0) although the differences between ligature sizes for this variable were not significant.

■ DISCUSSION

This in vitro study has identified key issues relating to extracorporeal slip knotting in endoscopic surgery. In the first instance, the holding strength of a slip knot is directly related to the material used and its cross-sectional area. There are no available data on the minimal holding strength required for a knot around a vessel except for the report by Nathanson et al. on the tension exerted by arteries and veins of different diameters perfused at a constant pressure of 147 mm Hg in an in vitro test rig. In this study, a 9.0 ram porcine artery under these test conditions was observed to exert a wall tension of 0.55 N. According to this, the minimal effective holding strength of a knot for securing a pressurized vessel of this caliber should be 1.2 N. If allowance is made for the systolic changes (maximum of 180–200 mm Hg), the calculated minimal holding strength in vivo is 1.6 N. A three-fold safety margin which would cover all arteries that could possibly be tied in surgical practice (open and endoscopic) yields a figure of 5.0 N. If one accepts this level of holding strength, then silk and polyamide provide less security when used for extracorporeal slip knots in endoscopic surgery than the other ligature materials examined in this study, although they exceed the safety margin of 5.0 N when used to tie Tayside and Melzer knots. This is in sharp contrast to their established safety when used in tying surgeon's knots during conventional open surgery. By the same criterion, the cross square and the blood knots are less secure than the other knots tested in this study and are therefore not recommended.

The effect of size of ligature material is demonstrated by the observation that a slip knot, irrespective of its configuration, fashioned with 1/0 has a holding strength double than that of the same slip knot tied with the same but smaller-caliber material (2/0). Factors other than surface area are involved since the average volumetric difference between the two gauges is 33–50%. These include surface frictional properties (roughness) and the weave, coating, and torsional stiffness. Overall the best absorbable material for extracorporeal slip knots is lactomer and this can be safely tied using the Tayside, Melzer, and Roeder techniques. PDS is safe with the Melzer knot, acceptable with the Tayside knot, and unreliable with the Roeder knot. Of the nonabsorbable materials tested, only Dacron provided a knot of sufficient security when tied by the Tayside, Melzer, or Roeder knot. The difference in strain between different suture materials for each slip knot relates to the surface friction properties, the torsional stiffness, and the flexibility of the suture material, all of which affect the stacking or tightening of the knot in addition to the elasticity of the suture material, which influences its ability to stretch. While some of these properties will be influenced by the diameter of the suture material, we found no difference in strain between different diameters of each suture material. PDS, Dacron, and lactomer are less flexible materials with relatively high torsional stiffness. The variability between the knots for each ligature material is an indication of the amount of additional tightening that a knot requires for its loops to be well stacked. The variability between the suture materials for each knot represents differences in elasticity, flexibility, and surface frictional properties of the different suture materials. It follows that for knots with high-stress measurements (Tayside, Melzer, and Roeder), a low strain indicates a well-stacked slip knot and vice versa. The Tayside slip knot had a relatively high stress and comparatively low strain. In the present study, the ligature materials that provided slip knots with a high-stress low-strain ratio (indicative of optimal stacking) were lactomer and Dacron. The "elasticity" of a knot is inversely related to its ability to stack. Thus, Tayside, cross square, and blood knots, which become maximally stacked when tightened, require higher stress to affect a standard elongation. Melzer and Roeder knots have a similar configuration, and for this reason, a similar "knot elasticity". For these two knots, less stress is required to affect a standard elongation since some of the

energy is expanded in incremental stacking of the knots. For a given slip knot tied with different ligature materials, the differences observed are a function of the elasticity of the various materials. Silk, polyamide, and Dacron are relatively inelastic materials and were found to have a lower elasticity than PDS or lactomer in all the knots examined. PDS exhibited the highest elasticity in all the knots. As expected, the smaller-diameter suture materials resulted in slightly more elastic knots. There are two limitations to the present study. The first relates to the experiments being performed on dry ligature materials. In vivo hydration by absorption of tissue fluid will vary with different materials. Hydration causes swelling of the ligature and may alter the surface frictional properties, torsional stiffness, and elasticity to varying extents depending on the nature and composition of the ligature material. The more a ligature swells by hydration the greater the subsequent increase in its holding strength. Although this effect can be reproduced in the in vitro situation by immersion in physiological solutions at 37°C, the influence of hydration on knot performance was not examined in the present study. The second limitation relates to the size of the loop demarcated by the slip knot. In the present study, the size of the loop was standardized to 38 mm to enable sufficiently long ends on either side of the knot for secure jamming within the pneumatic clamps of the tensiometer. The countertension that this wide loop exerted on the cylinder when the knots were tightened is less than the tension that would be applied if the knots were run down and tightened around vascular pedicles and ductular structures where the resulting diameter of the encircling loop would be much smaller. Thus, the tensiometric values recorded for the knots are representative of but different from those which apply when the same knots are employed to ligate vessels in vivo. However, this consideration does not invalidate the comparative performance of the various slip knots or the effect of the material used or its size.

■ CONCLUSION

In this chapter we have demonstrated that the holding strength of slip knots used in laparoscopic surgery is highly dependent on the type and size of the ligature material. The Tayside, Melzer, and Roeder knots tied with lactomer and Dacron showed superior resistance to slippage. In contrast, the cross square and blood knots exhibited weaker holding strengths across all tested materials, making them less reliable for clinical use. The findings underscore the importance of selecting the appropriate knot and material combination to ensure secure ligation during laparoscopic procedures. The results also highlight the significance of mastering knot-tying techniques to enhance the efficacy and safety of minimally invasive surgeries. Future studies should consider the effects of in vivo conditions, such as tissue hydration, on knot performance to provide a more comprehensive understanding of their clinical reliability.

■ BIBLIOGRAPHY

1. American College of Surgeons. Guidelines for Laparoscopic Suturing and Knot Tying. Chicago: ACS Publications; 2023.
2. Garcia E, Lopez RM. Impact of Knot Technique on Laparoscopic Procedure Outcomes: A Statistical Analysis. Journal of Clinical Laparoscopic Surgery. 2019;15(3):234-9.
3. Greenberg AS, Clark JM. Essentials of Laparoscopic Suturing and Knotting. New York: McGraw-Hill Education; 2024.
4. Liu Y, Wang G. Technical evolution of laparoscopic knot tying: A historical perspective. MITAT. 2018;27(2): 67-74.
5. Martinez JL, Smith RD. Innovations in Laparoscopic Suturing Technology. Cham: Springer; 2022.
6. Nathanson LK, Easter DW, Cuschieri A. Ligation of the structures of the cystic pedicle during laparoscopic cholecystectomy. Am J Surg. 1991;161(3):350-4.
7. Nathanson LK, Nathanson PD, Cuschieri A. Safety of vessel ligation in laparoscopic surgery. Endoscopy. 1991;23:206-10.
8. Nelson MT, NakashimaM, Mulvihill SJ. How secure are laparoscopically placed clips? An in vitro and in vivo study. Arch Surg. 1992;127(6):718-20.
9. Patel VR, Moran ME. A comparative analysis of laparoscopic knots and their clinical significance. J Endourol. 2019;33(10):794-802.
10. Raeder H. Die tecknik der mandelgesundungbestrebungen. Aertzl Rundschau: Munchen. 1918;57:16-171.
11. Robbins T, Kumar A. A comparative study of slip knots and square knots in laparoscopic surgery. Surg Laparosc Endosc Percutan Tech. 2020;30(2):150-5.
12. Semm K. Tissue-puncher and loop-ligation. New aids for surgical-therapeutic pelviscopy (laparoscopy)—endoscopic intraabdominal surgery. Endoscopy. 1978;10:11-124.
13. Singh K, Balakrishnan S. Laparoscopic Knot Tying: The Art and Science. London: Elsevier Health Sciences; 2021.
14. Thompson C, Gupta A. Efficacy and safety of intracorporeal and extracorporeal knots in laparoscopic surgery: A review of literature. Surg Innov. 2020;27(4):408-16.
15. Zhou J, Tan J. Simulation training for laparoscopic knot tying: effectiveness and skill transfer. Med Educ. 2022;56(1):95-103.

Prevention of Postoperative Adhesion Formation

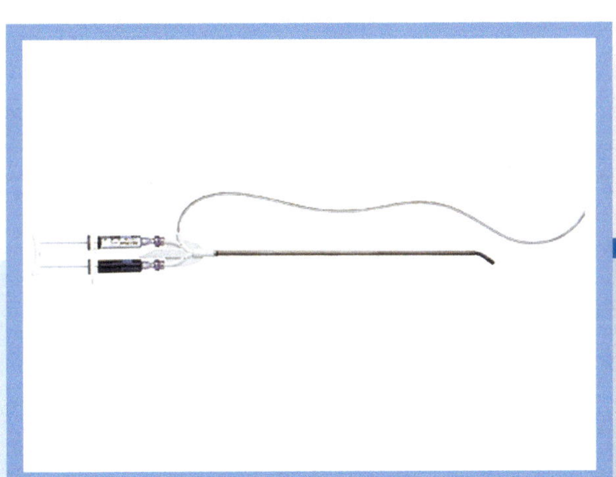

■ INTRODUCTION

Postoperative adhesions have long been recognized as a complication of general and gynecological surgery. As the frequency of abdominal and pelvic surgery has increased, the incidence of pelvic adhesions has risen in direct proportion. Postsurgical adhesions occur in 60–90% of women who had undergone major gynecological surgery. The morbidity of adhesion formation and its economic costs are substantial **(Table 1)**.

In an analysis of the burden of postoperative adhesions, studies showed that 35% of women having had open gynecological surgery were readmitted on average 1.9 times in the following 10 years for reoperation due to adhesions. Adhesions are the single largest cause of intestinal obstruction, accounting for 30–41% of all cases requiring further surgery. Further, it is estimated that 15–20% of cases of infertility in women are secondary to adhesions. Despite long-standing controversy regarding the association between adhesions and pelvic pain, there is increasing evidence to support such a relationship.

Surgical research in the prevention of postsurgical adhesions and its preventive strategies goes beyond a century. Historically, there has been difficulty in analyzing the literature on adhesion formation, since there is no single consistent model of adhesion formation and no standard and reliable means of measuring its formation. Further, there has been marked variability in the results from animal models and between the various means of inducing peritoneal injury. A lack of standardization has made the comparison of studies difficult.

■ PERITONEAL HEALING AND ADHESION FORMATION

Healing of the peritoneum following surgery is different from healing of the skin following injury. In the peritoneum, islands of regenerated peritoneum occur over the entire surface at once. This means that large peritoneal wounds heal as quickly as small ones. During surgery,

TABLE 1: Incidence of postsurgical adhesions.

Postsurgical adhesions	Incidence
Adhesiolysis	76%
Surgical treatment of endometriosis	82%
Ovarian surgery	75%
Myomectomy	68%
Tubal surgery	76%

the mesothelial injury exposes a denuded and acellular surface that serves as the nidus for wound healing and/or tissue–tissue adhesion. This submesothelial damage and exposure of the submesothelial matrix occurs with simultaneous activation of the coagulation cascade and deposition of fibrin at the site of injury. Under normal conditions, this fibrinous exudate serves as a platform for the progress of proper healing, but under certain circumstances, the deposited fibrin can instead serve as a bridge between unrelated, neighboring tissues. Within a short period of time, the wound and its surrounding area are invaded by inflammatory cells that migrate from the peritoneal vasculature or from the peritoneal fluid. The inflammatory exudate is initially composed of neutrophils; by 24 hours, the predominant cell is the macrophage. Next, the injured wound surface is evenly reperitonealized by the combined effort of multiple foci of proliferating mesothelial cells. Reperitonealization continues for 7–10 days during which time the entire surface becomes covered by a contiguous sheet of mesothelium. This process differs from the annular ingrowth of peripheral epithelial cells that occurs cutaneous wound healing. In the abdomen, the speed of reperitonealization remains the same (7–10 days), regardless of the initial wound size, since it is not limited by the rate of migration of cells from the periphery. The presence of mesothelial cells at the wound site corresponds to progressive wound healing and/or fibrosis and the deposition of an extracellular matrix (ECM) composed of fibronectin, hyaluronic acid, various glycosaminoglycans, and proteoglycans. The process of ECM deposition is directed by and maintained through the action of various growth factors and cytokines. Finally, the deposited matrix is strengthened and remodeled over time (1 week to 1 month). As the cells realign, the temporary ECM molecules are replaced by more permanent proteins such as collagens while revascularization continues.

The balance between fibrin deposition and degradation is critical in determining normal peritoneal healing or adhesion formation. If fibrin is completely degraded, normal peritoneal healing will occur. In contrast, if fibrin is not completely degraded, it will serve as a scaffold for fibroblasts and capillary ingrowth. Fibroblasts will invade the fibrin matrix and ECM will be produced and deposited. This ECM is normally completely degraded by matrix metalloprotease, leading to normal healing. If this process is inhibited by tissue inhibitors of matrix metalloprotease, peritoneal adhesions will form. In addition to fibroblast invasion and ECM deposition, the formation of new blood vessels has been universally claimed to be important in adhesion formation.

COFACTORS THAT CONTRIBUTE TO ADHESION FORMATION

The effects of carbon dioxide (CO_2) pneumoperitoneum have come under increased scrutiny. CO_2 pneumoperitoneum induces adverse effects such as hypercarbia, acidosis, hypothermia, and desiccation. It alters peritoneal fluid and the morphology of the mesothelial cells. Pneumoperitoneum is a cofactor in adhesion formation since adhesions increase with the duration of the pneumoperitoneum and with the insufflation pressure in animal models. It is recognized that pelvic inflammatory disease and endometriosis are additional potential causes of adhesions. The amount of raw peritoneal surfaces left following excision surgery may help us anticipate the likelihood of adhesion formation. It has been demonstrated that the pneumoperitoneum used during laparoscopy is a cofactor in adhesion formation. Reactive oxygen species (ROS) are produced in a hyperoxic environment and during the ischemia/reperfusion process. ROS activity is injurious to cells, which protect themselves by an antioxidant system known as ROS scavengers. Recent data also point to a role for ROS in adhesion formation since the administration of ROS scavengers decreases adhesion formation in several animal models. ROS activity increases during both laparotomy and laparoscopy.

Drying of tissues during surgery increases adhesion formation, a situation remedied by paying attention to the arid conditions and correcting them during the procedures. Intentional drying of the tissues, by applying gauze, is an otherwise desirable procedure to aid the surgeon's view of the area, but because of increased adhesions, it must be minimized. Laparotomy is more likely to produce adhesions than surgery performed via laparoscopy.

ADHESION PREVENTION STRATEGIES

Surgical Technique

There is no substitute for meticulous surgical technique. This includes minimizing injury to tissues through the careful use of atraumatic instruments that do not crush tissue or leave denuded surfaces. Preventing blood loss is important, as intra-abdominal blood can increase the chances of adhesion formation. Copious irrigation helps to remove any remaining intra-abdominal blood. In addition, the judicious selection of sutures may help in preventing foreign body reactions. Nonreactive suture material such as polyglycolic acid (Dexon), polyglactin (Vicryl), or polydioxanone (PDS) should be used, whereas using reactive material, such as catgut, should be discouraged. The surgical principles of adhesion prevention must be adhered to, i.e., the gentle handling of tissues, meticulous control of bleeding, avoidance of foreign materials, excision of necrotic tissue; minimization of ischemia and desiccation; and prevention of infection.

Peritoneal Closure

Several randomized trials have demonstrated that closure of the parietal or visceral peritoneum is not necessary. Peritoneal closure is associated with slightly longer operating times and greater postoperative pain and cause more adhesions. In a study by Tulandi et al., the rate of adhesion formation after laparotomy with peritoneal closure was 22.2%, compared with 16% without closure.

Access

The issue of whether laparoscopic surgery resulted in fewer adhesions as compared to open laparotomy has been assessed. Diamond et al. found that the incidence of de novo adhesion formation was lower when surgery was performed laparoscopically as compared to laparotomy. Similar finding were reported by Lundorff et al. While the concept of reduction in adhesion formation holds true in theory, there are few trials to support this in practice.

ADHESION PROTECTORS

An ideal adhesion barrier should be nonreactive but should protect tissue at risk during the critical wound healing period before being resorbed and cleared; it should remain adherent to the target tissue and be easily applicable during laparoscopic procedures performed on adhesiogenic organs such as ovaries and adnexa. Other properties of an ideal barrier are shown in **Box 1**.

> **BOX 1:** Properties of an ideal adhesion protector.
>
> - Noncytotoxic
> - Nonhemolytic
> - Nontoxic
> - Nonsensitizing
> - Nonirritating
> - Nongenotoxic
> - Nonpyrogenic
> - Should not potentiate infections
> - Should be easy to use at laparoscopy

Liquids

Crystalloids

Historically, crystalloids such as normal saline and Ringer's lactate were used to produce a "hydroflotation" effect by instilling 500 mL to 3 liters of fluid into the peritoneal cavity at the end of surgery in an attempt to prevent adhesion formation. Irrespective of the volume instilled, the absorption rate by the peritoneum ensures that all the fluid is reabsorbed into the vascular circulation in 24–48 hours, too short an interval to prevent adhesion formation.

Besides pure crystalloids, others have tried adding pharmacologic agents such as antihistamines, promethazine, heparin, and steroids to the solutions, either singly or in combination based on animal studies. However, none of these were shown to reduce the incidence of adhesion formation in randomized controlled human trials. Most studies that looked at using corticosteroid drugs to help prevent adhesions reported little success. The pharmacologic properties of corticosteroids suggest that they would be helpful in adhesion prevention. However, this is not the case; one possibility is that peritoneal surgery overwhelms the therapeutic benefits of the dose. If a higher dose is used, the effect on other organs, such as immunosuppression and delayed wound healing, would outweigh any positive benefit.

Nonsteroidal anti-inflammatory drugs (NSAIDs) are a class of drugs that ease the postsurgical inflammatory response. Some studies have shown a marked reduction in adhesion formation in animal models when the drug was given perioperatively. Others have not found them to be beneficial for that indication. Areas devascularized by surgery are hypoxic, thus permitting fibrin persistence and adhesion formation as devascularized sites are prime adhesion candidates. However, these sites are not readily available to drugs given systemically.

Recently, several liquid products have been developed in an attempt to combine hydroflotation, barrier and pharmacologic agents in a single product.

Dextran

Dextran is a water-soluble glucose polymer originally used as a plasma expander. The weight most often considered in adhesion studies is a 32% solution of dextran 70 suspended in glucose. Hyskon® is the best known brand name. Hyskon® is slowly absorbed in 5–7 days. It was proposed that by producing a "siliconizing" effect, hydroflotation, and effects on the clotting cascade, it would reduce adhesion formation. In studies, use of Hyskon® produced mixed results. Some workers found that patients treated with Hyskon® had fewer and less severe adhesions than patients treated with saline (Ringer's lactate). Other studies found no differences between treatments. Hyskon® carries with it side effects that include temporary weight gain, vulvar edema, leg edema, pleural effusion, and coagulopathy. Rarely, a patient may be allergic to it. Its use in gynecologic reconstructive surgery has been virtually eliminated.

Icodextrin Solution

One of the most recently developed peritoneal instillates is 4% icodextrin solution (Adept®, Baxter BioSurgery). Adept® is hypothesized to provide in preventing formation of adhesions by providing a physical separation of the peritoneal surfaces during the early phases of natural healing. Adept® is a single use, sterile, clear, colorless-to-pale yellow fluid for intraperitoneal administration containing icodextrin. Icodextrin is an α-1,4-linked glucose polymer, provided at a concentration of 4% w/v in an electrolyte solution. Icodextrin (glucose polymer) used in this device is generated via hydrolysis of corn starch. Adept®'s ability to draw and maintain a reservoir of fluid in the peritoneal cavity is by the process of colloidal osmosis, which is achieved through the presence of molecular weight species of icodextrin that are not rapidly absorbed across the peritoneal membrane.

It is Food and Drug Administration (FDA) approved for the reduction of adhesion reformation after laparoscopic adhesiolysis. In a randomized study during laparoscopic gynecologic surgery, it was found that instillation of 4% icodextrin solution decreased adhesion formation and reformation.

Hyaluronic Acid

Intergel® (Lifecore, Johnson & Johnson, Gynecare) is a cross-linked compound of hyaluronic acid with ferric ion. Intergel® provides a transient, viscous, lubricant coating on peritoneal surfaces following surgical procedures. It reduced the extent of adhesion formation following abdominal surgery. However, the product was withdrawn from the market after reports of late-onset postoperative pain requiring surgery.

Seprafilm® and Sepracoat®

Seprafilm® (Genzyme BV, Naarden, Netherlands) is a sterile translucent membrane comprising sodium hyaluronate and carboxymethylcellulose which temporarily separates potentially adherent surfaces, turning to a gel within 24 hours and cleared from the abdominal cavity in 7 days. While it degrades very rapidly in a few days, it is difficult to manipulate. It is fragile, brittle and impossible to use through a trocar in association with laparoscopy. Finally, it progressively loses its initial adherence and can migrate some distance, thereby leaving the wound unprotected. Sepracoat® (HAL-C Bioresorbable Membrane, Genzyme Corp) is a solution of hyaluronidase in phosphate-buffered saline, reabsorbed from the body cavity and excreted in 5 days. Its mechanism of action includes the reduction of tissue desiccation. In animal models and patients, these agents reduced adhesion formation by about 44% without any apparent increase in adverse events. However, it did not receive FDA approval for clinical use and was withdrawn from the market in 1997.

Hydrogel

A novel technique of substance delivery into the abdominal cavity is by combining two streams of liquid polymers, delivered via a catheter to the target tissue. When combined, the two streams produce a bright-blue solid polymer within minutes. Sprayable hydrogel (SprayGel®, Confluent Surgical) can be easily applied at laparoscopy; the solid polymer acts as an adhesion barrier. SprayGel® is a synthetic hydrogel which forms an absorbable, flexible, adherent gel barrier when two polyethylene glycol-based liquids are sprayed onto target tissue (**Fig. 1**).

In a European multicenter, randomized study, Mettler et al. evaluated 66 women who underwent myomectomy with or without SprayGel® application. When compared with initial surgery, the mean adhesion tenacity score of adhesions seen at second-look laparoscopy was 64.7% lower in patients receiving adhesion barrier than in control patients (0.60 vs. 1.7). Compared with initial surgery, mean adhesion extent score at second-look laparoscopy was 4.5 versus 7.2 cm^2 and mean adhesion incidence score was 0.64 versus 1.22. There were no adverse effects attributed to the adhesion barrier.

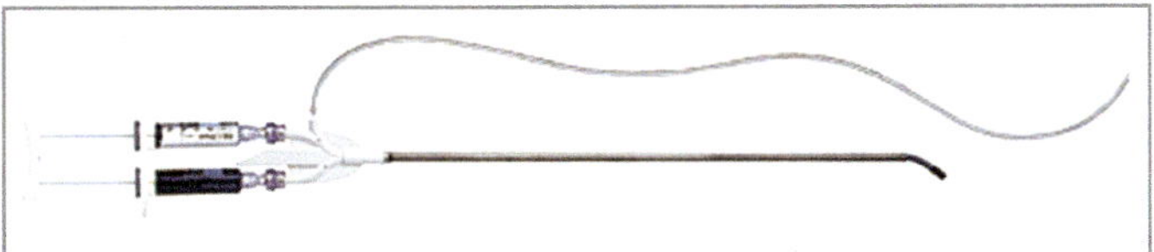

Fig. 1: Laparoscopic sprayer: SprayGel is applied to the surgical site through the SprayGel laparoscopic sprayer, designed for site-specific delivery. The SprayGel laparoscopic sprayer connects to the SprayGel air pump, which is a reusable, self-contained air pump. It remains intact where applied for approximately 5–7 days, protecting the target tissue during wound healing and then is hydrolyzed gradually into polyethylene glycol constituent molecules that are resorbed and rapidly cleared by the kidneys.

A similar product is a sprayable self-polymerizing gel called Adhibit® (Angiotech). Adhibit® is a spray gel applied at the time of surgery that binds directly to the tissue and creates a temporary barrier, preventing contact and adhesions from forming between tissue surfaces. Adhibit is a synthetic, self-polymerizing liquid hydrogel that is metabolized by the body in less than 30 days. A randomized, controlled, single-blind study of 71 women who had surgery to remove uterine fibroids (myomectomy) reported that 48 women who received Adhibit (0.8 ± 2.0) had a reduction in adhesions compared with 23 women in a control group who did not receive the gel (2.6 ± 2.2, $p = 0.01$). Adhesions were measured 8–10 weeks after the surgery, using the modified American Fertility Society score.

AdSurf® (Britannia Pharmaceuticals) is a new clinical approach to the prevention of surgical adhesions. It is administered as a sterile dry powder via aerosol prior to surgical closure, giving it a distinct ease of application. The powder melts at just below normal body temperature and coats the internal surface tissues, preventing the formation of adhesions. Furthermore, when applied to the tissues, AdSurf® disperses throughout the peritoneal cavity, creating a better chance for the prevention of adhesions. AdSurf® is a unique formulation of the naturally occurring phospholipids dipalmitoylphosphatidylcholine (DPPC) and phosphatidyl glycerol (PG).

■ ADHESION BARRIERS

Barrier Agents

Barrier agents include mechanical barriers and viscous solutions. Many different mechanical barriers have been tried, but they are generally inadequate because they interfere with the blood supply or produce foreign body reaction. The original "barriers" consisted of peritoneal and omental grafts placed over traumatized surfaces and sewn in place. This practice placed a layer of dead necrotic tissue on top of traumatized peritoneal surfaces, providing an abundant supply of substrate for adhesion formation. Subsequent animal studies have shown that placing devascularized tissue over damaged peritoneal surfaces increases rather than decreases adhesion formation. Although no human randomized trials have been performed, this practice has been abandoned.

Oxidized Regenerated Cellulose

One of the first barriers to be evaluated was Interceed® (Gynecare, Johnson & Johnson), a mesh-like product designed to be placed over or between injured surfaces.

A review published by Larsson in 1996 concluded that Interceed is "safe and effective in all controlled human clinical trials." Unfortunately, it did not eliminate adhesions in all patients and in all clinical situations. Some of the reviewed studies showed no benefit. It has been shown that the product was efficacious in limited situations, where injured areas or structures can be completely covered with the material. In addition, the entire area must be completely blood-free. The presence of blood in the matrix of the material completely negated any benefit. Postoperative adhesions may be induced by its application if adjacent tissues (e.g., ovary and tube) and structures are coapted or conjoined by the device or if it is folded, wadded, or layered. Care must be taken to apply Interceed® in single layers, interposed between adjacent anatomic structures at risk for adhesion formation. It is the easiest adhesion barrier to use at laparoscopy.

Expanded Polytetrafluoroethylene

Gore-Tex surgical membrane, constructed of expanded polytetrafluoroethylene (ePTFE) (Preclude®, WL Gore), is a nonabsorbable barrier and produced in thin sheets (0.1 mm), with an average pore size of <1 µm. It is sutured to the tissue so that it overlaps the incision by at least 1 cm. It prevents adhesion formation and reformation, independent of the type of injury. It is also effective in the presence of blood. In a randomized trial, ePTFE decreased postmyomectomy and pelvic sidewall adhesions.

It is not widely used, however, because it is nonabsorbable and has to be fixed to the tissue. This product must be sewn in place and is usually removed during a second surgical procedure. Its usefulness is limited by the nature of the product, in that, it must be sutured in place and removed at a subsequent surgery. It is very difficult to apply at laparoscopy.

Newer agents in development include carboxymethyl cellulose (CMC) and polyethylene oxide (PEO) composite gel (Oxiplex/AP, FrizoMed) and polylactide (PLa): copolymer of 70:30 Poly (L-lactide-co-D, L-lactide) film (SurgiWrap, Mast Biosurgery). More recently, recombinant human tissue plasminogen activator has been evaluated for its effectiveness in the prevention of postoperative adhesions. This group of agents holds significant promise. The development of new aids to prevent postsurgical adhesion formation is encumbered by the way the peritoneum heals, access to the peritoneal cavity, limitations of extrapolating results in humans as compared to animal models and the complexities of interperitoneal circulation and transperitoneal transport.

When barrier methods are used in conjunction with excellent surgical technique, meticulous hemostasis and careful tissue handling, the risk of adhesion formation is reduced, but not completely eliminated. There are three devices approved by the FDA for adhesion prevention: The site-specific Interceed® and Seprafilm® and the broad-covering Intergel®. These devices are FDA approved for laparotomy use. There are no approved devices in the United States for adhesion prevention by laparoscopic instillation.

■ THE FUTURE

Improved surgical training and tools are important considerations. Research designed to define the peritoneal wound environment would identify target molecules. This information could be used to design devices carrying wound-modifying factors to alter the wound healing process. There is growing literature on the visualization and quantification of adhesions that would greatly facilitate our ability to compare various interventional modalities. A study correlating functional cine magnetic resonance imaging (MRI) studies with later operative observations demonstrated the ability of this noninvasive imaging technique to visualize adhesions. Another active and potentially useful field of inquiry is into the origin and behavior of the premesothelial or stem cells responsible for reperitonealization. The discovery of tissue-derived stem cells in the adult has focused on the possibility of stem cell reactivation as a driving force for patterned tissue regeneration and healing. There may be cell-driven approaches to adhesion prevention involving stem cell therapies which theoretically would prevent denuded surfaces from adhering to one another. The possibility of a serum marker for adhesion formation could facilitate investigations of adhesion formation. The correlation of the presence of a marker protein in the serum for the formation of peritoneal adhesions would facilitate a way of predicting who would form adhesions, and thereby a means of noninvasively measuring the efficacy of any given intervention. As yet, there is no consistent correlation between protein levels and the presence or severity of adhesions.

■ CONCLUSION

The current evidence for the use of fluid and pharmacological agents for the prevention of adhesions is limited. There is insufficient evidence for the use of steroids, icodextrin 4%, SprayGel, and dextran in improving adhesions following surgery. There is some evidence that hyaluronic acid agents may decrease the proportion of adhesions and prevent the deterioration of preexisting adhesions. However, due to the limited number of studies available, this evidence should be interpreted with caution and further studies are needed.

There has been a wide range of adhesion-reducing substances evaluated in animal models. However, in clinical situations, no adhesion-preventing substance, material, or barrier is unequivocally effective. One key challenge is that these physical agents may reduce adhesions where they are placed but do not prevent adhesions developing elsewhere in the abdomen. The ideal adhesion-reduction agent should be easy to use in all types of surgical procedures and be capable of reducing adhesion formation at the operation site and throughout the peritoneum. A direct cause-and-effect relationship between adhesion prevention and outcome measures is difficult to establish. Screening of potential tools is time consuming and expensive. Besides, a disparity between preclinical animal results and clinical trials in humans is disappointing and costly. We are just beginning to understand the intricate role of the mesothelium in the early formation of adhesions and how mesothelial cells regulate the peritoneal fibrinolytic environment. More basic research into the mechanisms of adhesiogenesis is needed so that we can identify new opportunities for therapeutic intervention.

■ BIBLIOGRAPHY

1. Angiotech presents positive Adhibit™ data at the 19th Annual European Congress of Obstetrics and Gynecology: Surgical adhesion scores were threefold less in patients treated with Adhibit™. Vancouver: Angiotech Pharmaceuticals; 2006.
2. Becker JM, Dayton MT, Fazio MT, Beck DE, Stryker SJ, Wexner SD, et al. Prevention of postoperative abdominal adhesions by a sodium hyaluronate-based bioresorbable membrane: a prospective, randomized, double-blind multicenter study. J Am Coll Surg. 1996;183:297-306.
3. Becker JM, Dayton MT, Fazio VW. Prevention of Postoperative Adhesions by a Sodium Hyaluronate-Based Bioresorbable Membrane: A Prospective, Randomized, Double-Blind Multicenter Study. J Am Coll Surg. 2021;232(4):527-38.
4. Becker JM, Stucchi AF. Intra-abdominal Adhesion Prevention: Are We Getting Any Closer? Ann Surg. 2004;240(2):202-4.
5. Binda MM, Molinas CR, Koninckx PR. Reactive oxygen species and adhesion formation. Clinical implications in adhesion prevention. Hum Reprod. 2003;18(12):2503-7.
6. Burns JW, Colt MJ, Burgees LS, Skinner KC. Pre-clinical evaluation of Seprafilm bioresorbable membrane. Eur J Surg. 1997;577:40-8.
7. Cheong YC, Laird SM, Li TC, Shelton JB, Ledger WL, Cooke ID. Peritoneal Healing and Adhesion Formation/Reformation. Hum Reprod Update. 2022;28(2):234-49.
8. Diamond MP, Freeman ML. Clinical Implications of Postsurgical Adhesions. Hum Reprod Update. 2020;26(1):96-107.
9. diZerega GS. Contemporary adhesion prevention. Fertil Steril. 1994;61(2):219-35.
10. Diamond MP, Daniell JF, Feste J, Surrey MW, McLaughlin DS, Friedman S, et al. Adhesion reformation and de novo adhesion formation *after* reproductive pelvic surgery. Fertil Steril. 1987;47:864-6.
11. Diamond MP. Reduction of postsurgical adhesions by intraoperative pre coating with Sepracoat™ (HAL-C) solution: a prospective randomised, blinded, placebo controlled multicentre study. Fertil Steril. 1998;69:1067-74.
12. DiZerega GS, Verco SJ, Young P, Kettel M, Kobak W, Martin D, et al. A randomized, controlled pilot study of the safety and efficacy of 4% icodextri*n* solution in the reduction of adhesions following laparoscopic gynaecological surgery. Hum Reprod. 2002;17:1031-8.
13. diZerega GS. Biochemical events in peritoneal tissue repair. Eur J Surg. 1997;163(Suppl 577):10-6.
14. Ellis H. The cause and prevention of postoperative intraperitoneal adhesions. Surg Gynecol Obstet. 1971;133:497-511.
15. Ellis H. Intraabdominal and postoperative peritoneal adhesions. J Am Coll Surg. 2005;200:641.
16. Ellis H. The magnitude of adhesion-related problems. In: diZerega GS (Ed). Peritoneal Surgery. New York: Springer; 2000. pp. 297-306.
17. Fazio VW, Cohen Z, Fleshman JW, Van Goor H (Eds). Adhesion Prevention in Surgery: Guidelines and Clinical Practice. New York: Springer; 2018.
18. Franklin R, Haney A, Kettel L, Lo*t*ze AA, Murphy JA, Rock G, et al. An expanded polytetrafluoroethylene barrier (Gore-Tex surgical membrane) reduces post-myomectomy adhesion formation. Fertil Steril. 1995;63:491-3.
19. Franklin R; the Ovarian Adhesion Study Group. Reduction of ovarian adhesions by the use of Interceed. Obstet Gynecol. 1995;86(3):335-40.
20. Gehlbach DL, Sousa RC, Carpenter SE, Rock JA. Abdominal myomectomy in the treatment of infertility. Int J Gynaecol Obstet. 1993;40(1):45-50.
21. Gutt CN, Oniu T, Schemmer P, Mehrabi A, Büchler MW. Fewer Adhesions Induced by Laparoscopic Surgery? Surg Endosc. 2023;37(3):1123-9.
22. Genevieve M, Boland BA, Weigel RJ. Formation and prevention of postoperative abdominal adhesions. J Surg Res. 2006;132(1):3-12.
23. Gray RI, Ott DE, Henderson AC, Cochran SA, Roth EA. Severe local hypothermia from laparoscopic gas evaporative jet cooling: a mechanism to explain clinical observations. JSLS. 1999;3:171-7.
24. Holmdahl L, Risberg B, Beck DE, Burns JW, Chegini N, DiZerega GS, et al. Adhesions: Pathogenesis and Pre*v*ention—Panel Discussion and Summary. Eur J Surg. 2019;584:56-62.

25. Haney A, Hesla J, Hurst B, Kettel LM, Murphy AA, Rock JA, et al. Expanded polytetrafluoroethylene (Gore-Tex surgical membrane) is superior to oxidized regenerated cellulose (Interceed TC7) in preventing adhesions. Fertil Steril. 1995;63:1021-6.

26. Hazebroek EJ, Schreve MA, Visser P, De Bruin RW, Marquet RL, Bonjer HJ. Impact of temperature and humidity of carbon dioxide pneumoperitoneum on body temperature and peritoneal morphology. J Laparoendosc Ad Surg Tech A. 2002;12:355-64.

27. Hill-West JL, Dunn RC, Hubbell JA. Local release of fibrinolytic agents for adhesion prevention. J Surg Res. 1995;59:759-63.

28. Johns A. Evidence-based prevention of post-operative adhesions. Hum Reprod Update. 2001;7(6):577-9.

29. Johns DA, Ferland RR, Dunn R. Initial Feasibility Study of a Sprayable Hydrogel Adhesio$_n$ Barrier System in Patients Undergoing Laparoscopic Ovarian Surgery. J Am Assoc Gynecol Laparosc. 2003;10(3):334-8.

30. Kumar S, Wong PF, Leaper DJ. Intra-Abdominal Adhesions: Cause, Consequence, and Management. Am J Surg. 2024;227(5):889-98.

31. Kavic SM. Adhesions and adhesiolysis: the role of laparoscopy. J Soc Laparoendosc Surg. 2002;6(2):99-109.

32. Khaitan E, Scholz S, Richards WO. Laparoscopic adhesiolysis and placement of Seprafilm: a new technique and novel approach to patients with intractable abdominal pain. J Laparoendosc Adv Surg Techniques. 2002;12(4):241-7.

33. Liakakos T, Thomakos N, Fine PM, Dervenis C, Young RL (Eds). Prevention and Management of Postoperative Adhesions. Amsterdam: Elsevier; 2019.

34. Larsson B. Efficacy of Interceed in adhesion prevention in gynecologic surgery: A review of 13 clinical studies. J Reprod Med. 1996;41:27-34.

35 Lienemann A, Sprenger D, Steitz HO, Korell M, Reiser M. Detection and mapping of intraabdominal adhesions by using functional cine MR imaging preliminary results. Radiology. 2000;217:421-5.

36. Lower AM, Hawthorn RJS, Ellis H, O'Brien F, Buchan S, Crowe AM. The impact of adhesions on hospital readmissions over ten years after 8849 open gynaecological operations: an assessment from the Surgical and Clinical Adhesions Research Study BJOG. Int J Obstet Gynaecol. 2000;107(7):855-62.

37. Lundorff P, Hablin M, Källfelt B, Thorburn J, Lindblom B. Adhesion formation after laparoscopic surgery in tubal pregnancy: a randomized trial versus laparotomy. Fertil Steril. 1991;55:911-5.

38. LeGrand EK, Rodgers KE, Girgis W, Campeau JD, diZerega GS. Comparative efficacy of nonsteroidal anti-inflammatory drugs and anti-thromboxane agents in a rabbit adhesion-prevention model. J Invest Surg. 1995;8(3):187-94.

39. Menzies D, Ellis H. Intestinal Obstruction from Adhesions—How Big is the Problem? Ann Royal Coll Surg Eng. 2022;104(2):123-7.

40. Menzies D. Peritoneal adhesions. Incidence, cause, and prevention. Surg Ann. 1992;24:27-45.

41. Menzies D. Postoperative adhesions: their treatment and relevance in clinical practice. Ann R Coll Surg Engl. 1993;75:147-53.

42. Mettler L, Audebert A, Lehmann-Willenbrock E, Schive-Peterhansl K, Jacobs VR. A randomized, prospective, controlled, multicenter clinical trial of a sprayable, site-specific adhesion barrier system in patients undergoing myomectomy. Fertil Steril. 2004;82:398-404.

43. Metwally M, Watson A, Lilford R, Vandekerckhove P. Fluid and pharmacological agents for adhesion prevention after gynaecological surgery. Cochrane Database Syst Rev. 2006;2:CD001298.

44. Molinas CR, Koninckx PR. Hypoxaemia induced by CO2 or helium pneumoperitoneum is a co-factor in adhesion formation in rabbits. Hum Reprod. 2000;15:1758-63.

45. Molinas CR, Mynbaev O, Pauwels A, Novak P, Koninckx PR. Peritoneal mesothelial hypoxia during pneumoperitoneum is a cofactor in adhesion formation in a laparoscopic mouse model. Fertil Steril. 2001;76:560-67.

46. Monk BJ, Berman ML, Montz FJ. Adhesions after extensive gynecologic surgery: clinical significance, etiology and prevention. Am J Obstet Gynecol. 1994;170:1396-403.

47. National Institute for Health and Care Excellence (NICE). (2021). Surgical Management of Intra-abdominal Adhesions. Available from https://www.nice.org.uk [Last accessed May, 2024].

48. Nordic Adhesion Prevention Study Group. The efficacy of Interceed (TC7) for prevention of reformation of postoperative adhesions on ovaries, fallopian tubes, and fimbriae in microsurgical operations for fertility: a multicenter study. Fertil Steril. 1995;63(4):709-14.

49. Ott DE. Laparoscopy and tribology: the effect of laparoscopic gas on peritoneal fluid. J Am Assoc Gynecol Laparosc. 2001;8:117-23.

50. Reich H. (2011). Laparoscopic surgery for adhesiolysis. [online] Available from https://www.contemporaryobgyn.net/view/laparoscopic-surgery-adhesiolysis [Last accessed May, 2024].

51. Sinervo K. Adhesions: An Update. [online] Available from https://centerforendo.com/adhesions-update [Last accessed May, 2024].

52. Soules MR, Dennis L, Bosarge A, Moore DE. The prevention of postoperative pelvic adhesions: an animal study comparing barrier methods with dextran 70. Am J Obstet Gynecol. 1982;143:829-34.

53. Tulandi T, Al-Jaroudi D. Non-closure of peritoneum: a reappraisal. Am J Obstet Gynecol. 2003;189:609-12.

54. Tulandi T, Al-Shahrani A. Adhesion prevention in gynecologic surgery. Minimally invasive gynecologic procedures. Curr Opin Obstet Gynecol. 2005;17(4):395-8.

55. Tulandi T, Hum HS, Gelfand MM. Closure of laparotomy incisions with or without peritoneal suturing and second-look laparoscopy. Am J Obstet Gynecol. 1988;158:536-7.

56. West MA, Hackam DJ, Baker J, Rodriguez JL, Bellingham J, Rotstein OD. Mechanism of decreased in vitro murine macrophage cytokine release after exposure to carbon dioxide: relevance to laparoscopic surgery. Ann Surg. 1997;226:179-90.

Glues and Adhesive in Laparoscopic Tissue Approximation

■ INTRODUCTION

More than four million surgical procedures are done annually worldwide with traditional sutures and staplers. To seal a wound, biological and synthetic glues, in surgery as a tissue adhesive to replace traditional suturing techniques, are promising. Potential benefits of glues include better cosmetics, a significant reduction in percutaneous injuries from suture needles, which would in turn reduce the risk of transmission of infectious diseases. The field of surgical tissue adhesive is rapidly developing with multiple products now available with respect to bleeding. However, it must be said that the use of fibrin sealant is not a substitution for excellent surgical technique.

■ HISTORY AND DEVELOPMENT

Tissue adhesives can be categorized into three types: fibrin-based, collagen-based, and gelatin-based. Additionally, they can be classified as natural or synthetic.

Natural adhesives: Include fibrin and collagen-based products. They are effective in adhesion but have limited availability due to autologous tissue isolation and poor tensile strength.

Synthetic adhesives: Include cyanoacrylates and resorcinol/formaldehyde. They offer strong mechanical properties, low degradation rates, and better adhesion than natural adhesives but have disadvantages such as low bio-absorption, low adherence to wet surfaces, cytotoxic degradation products, and potential heat generation during curing.

Protein-based adhesives: Include fibrins and gelatins. They are biocompatible but have low wet adhesive strength.

Surgical adhesives: Used to hold tissues together and support wound healing. They are less painful than stitches or staples and take less time to apply. The adhesive eventually breaks down and is absorbed internally or peels off externally.

Examples of surgical adhesives:
Biologically derived adhesives: Fibrin glue, matrix protein adhesives

Synthetic adhesives: Cyanoacrylate, various polymer hydrogels

Vascular sealing adhesives: BioGlue, ArterX. These glues are used largely as hemostatic agents for bleeding surface and vascular anastomosis. There is a wide range of fibrin product varieties, but in essence, they fall into 2 types: two-component fibrin and cryoprecipitate-based glues. The composition of the two component types is basically the same, despite several different product proprietary names; the many different preparations vary in the source of the fibrinogen (usually human) and the thrombin (usually bovine).

Gelatin-based Glues

These are alternative resorbable biological glues that have greater bonding strength than fibrin-based glue. Gelatin–resorcinol–formaldehyde–glutaraldehyde (GRFG) was the first generation. The second generation of gelatin hydrogel glues is much less toxic as the formaldehyde has been substituted with other cross-linking agents.

Fibrin adhesives can be created from autologous sources or pooled blood. They are typically used for hemostasis and can seal tissues while they do not have adequate tensile strength to close skin. Commercial preparations such as Tisseel and Hemaseel are Food and Drug Administration (FDA) approved. Gelatin-based glues are photochemically activated surgical tissue. "Bonding or soldering" technology involves using photoreactive gelatins and a water-soluble dysfunctional macromer [polyethylene glycol diacrylate (PEGDA)]. Photoreactive groups, for example, ultraviolet light-reactive benzophenone or visible light-reactive xanthene dyes (e.g., fluorescein sodium salt, eosin Y, and rose Bengal) are incorporated in the gelatins, which are then suspended in a saline solution containing PEGDA forming a viscous. This forms an adhesive hydrogel within 1 minute when irradiated with the appropriate light. The resulting gel is tightly adherent to soft tissues such as the liver. Experimentally, this photocurative gelatin glue has been used to seal effectively arteriotomies in canine abdominal or thoracic aortas. This glue has great potential application in laparoscopic surgery, as the percutaneous delivery of the glue followed by in situ photogelatin will result in prompt, safe, and effective hemostasis (Nakaymama et al, 1999).

Synthetic Glues (Cyanoacrylates)

Cyanoacrylates (CAs) have been available since 1960 but their clinical use has been limited because of the thermal damage and scarring to the tissues (hence, strictures in anastomoses work) they produce and also because of unsubstantiated concerns regarding mutagenicity and carcinogenicity. There is no doubt that CAs are cytotoxic, but this varies with the chemistry and the formulation. Experiments have consistently shown that polymerized CAs are cytotoxic to human fibroblasts and inhibit cell proliferation, but this cytotoxicity varies considerably between the various cyanoacrylates.

Histoacryl blue was the first cyanoacrylate glue to be used clinically for the closure of skin incisions in Europe in the early 1980s. It is *n*-butyl-2 cyanoacrylate monomer colored by a blue dye. It is now the favored adhesive embolic agent used by interventional radiologists and for endoscopic control of bleeding varices and gastroduodenal lesions. Histoacryl and two-component fibrin glue have been used successfully and without complications in the endoscopic sealing of bronchopulmonary fistulae after pulmonary surgery.

Dermabond was the first synthetic cyanoacrylate used in the United States of America (USA) and is now approved by the FDA for closure of trauma-induced skin lacerations and small surgical incisions. The chemical formulation of Dermabond is 2-octyl cyanoacrylate monomer. When applied to skin, Dermabond polymerizes within 45–60 seconds to form a more pliable bond than Histoacryl, which sloughs off after 7–10 days. Under current regulations, the glue is for surface application to the wounds, i.e., not in the base of the wound or between the wound edges. Clinical trials have demonstrated equivalent cosmetic results following healing to that achieved following wound closure by sutures.

The main advantage of all fibrin-based glues is their lack of toxicity and complete compatibility such that healing is not disturbed. Fibrin glues have been used effectively in the laparoscopic management of patients with blunt hepatic trauma. In one report of 61 patients, 55 patients were successfully treated without recourse to laparotomy (Chan et al 1998). Thus, the selective use of laparoscopy and fibrin glue can reduce the nontherapeutic laparotomy rate among blunt hepatic trauma patient; also fibrin can be used to fix the prosthesis during percutaneous endoscopic external ring inguinal hernia repair (Waldron et al, 1998). Fibrin glue is very effective in preventing bleeding from surface liver cracks that form during hepatic laparoscopic cryotherapy for in situ ablation of liver tumors (Cuschieri et al, 1995).

In a comparative experimental study of cryoprecipitate glues, fibrin sealant, and gelatin glue, the cryoprecipitate glue and fibrin glue were equally effective in controlling bleeding from the aortic and atrial suture lines whereas gelatin did not provide total control at either site. The cryoprecipitate glue and fibrin caused minimal adhesion in contrast to extensive fibroblastic proliferation induced by gelatin-based glues.

The limitation of all fibrin-based and gelatin glues is that they are only effective in the absence of active bleeding, this problem has been overcome by the development of hybrid biological sealants.

Adhesive Based on Protein Engineering

These polymers are still at the experimental stage but show great promise as biocompatible and biodegradable internal sealants; they are based on proprietary protein engineering based on DNA gene technology. Epithelization and healing with absorption of the material were observed at 28 days, the wound strength was equivalent to sutured controls.

Drying the area with a sponge and using the gas-driven spray applicator are effective methods to create a dry field. The use of gas from the applicator to remove blood prior to adding the component of fibrin sealant is an excellent technique for rapidly achieving a dry field. The spray technique is particularly valuable for the diffuse area of capillary bleeding often encountered at the time of reoperative surgical dissection or when diffuse capillary or venous bleeding is encountered from inflamed tissue.

The spray technique is particularly useful to cover large surface area of bleeding. It also results in the most efficient use of the fibrin sealant, thus reducing the cost associated with the use of the agent.

If a localized area of bleeding is encountered, it may be best to use the needle or tip applicators provided by the manufacturer for specific application of the fibrin sealant at a small site.

■ SURGICAL APPLICATIONS

Benefits of fibrin sealants include tissue compatibility, lack of toxicity, natural bioabsorption, and superior adhesiveness. These advantages contribute to the versatility of fibrin sealants as an alternative to suturing in some surgical procedures given as follows.

- Cardiovascular surgery for various vascular abnormalities
- *Spleen repair:* Reducing the number of splenectomies
- *Colostomy closure:* Reducing complications in temporary colostomies when used directly over the suture lines

- Control of hemorrhage
- Closure of intestinal fistula
- Control of variceal bleeding and obliteration of esophageal varices
- *Thoracic surgery:* Closure of pulmonary leaks and laparoscopic vascular surgery
- *Pediatrics endoscopic surgery:* Inwound closure and tissue approximation
- Urological application of fibrin sealant in hemostasis (laparoscopic nephrectomy)
- Urinary tract sealant (open and laparoscopic pyeloplasty)
- Tissue adhesive (fistula closure and skin grafting).

Although the three FDA approved indications for fibrin sealant are reoperative cardiac surgery, colon anastomosis, and treatment of splenic injury, fibrin sealants have been successfully employed in countless surgical procedures including hepatic resection, bowel and vascular anastomosis, enterocutaneous and anorectal fistula closure, and neurosurgery. Fibrin sealant can be used to assist with a variety of tissue apposition and adherence indications. The classical example is the use of fibrin sealant to eliminate potential space at the time of lymphatic dissection in the axilla or groin associated with tumor resection; the goal is to achieve adherence of the skin to underlying tissue after removal of lymphatics and soft tissue so that a potential space for seroma formation or bleeding is eliminated.

USE OF FIBRIN SEALANT IN SURGERY

Safety Consideration

Little has been published concerning the toxicity of cyanoacrylate adhesive; in other research, direct toxicity of cyanoacrylate was thought to be an important contributor to postoperative arterial occlusion lesion in seven patients who had undergone surgery for nonruptured cerebral aneurysms using cyanoacrylate. Currently, however, there are no published reports with clinical data on the long-term toxicity and carcinogenicity effect of synthetic glues. Another problem with fibrin glues isa wrong believe that such blood products have the potential to transmit disease, although numerous studies have shown otherwise. The effectiveness of these products has not been compelling enough to override lingering concerns.

CONCLUSION

Fibrin sealant has been used with increasing frequency in a variety of surgical fields for its unique hemostatic and adhesive abilities as this sealant mimics the last step of coagulation cascade. With rapid advances in minimal access surgery, the potential use of this type of biological and synthetic material is expanding from reinforcing gastrointestinal anastomosis to repair perforated duodenal ulcer to mesh fixation in laparoscopic hernia repair. Although fibrin sealant is gaining increasing acceptance among surgeons in various surgical procedures, suturing still taking place by most surgeons worldwide.

BIBLIOGRAPHY

1. Banett P, Jarman FC, Goodge J, Silk G, Aickin R. Randomized trial of histoacryl blue tissue adhesive glue versus suturing in the repair of pediatric laceration. J Pediatr Child Health. 1998;34(6):548-50.
2. Bayfield MS, Spotnitz WD. Fibrin sealant in thoracic surgery. Chest Surg Clin N Am. 1996;6(3):567-83.
3. Canby-Hagino ED. Fibrin sealant treatment of splenic injury during open and laparoscopic left radical nephrectomy. J Urol. 2000;164(6):2004-5.
4. Chen Y, Wong T. Glues and Adhesives in Clinical Surgery. Singapore: World Scientific Publishing; 2021.
5. Cuschieri A, Crosthwaite G, Shimi S, Pietrabissa A, Joypaul V, Tair I, et al. Hepatic cryotherapy for liver tumors. Surg Endosc. 1995;9:483-9.
6. Donkerwolker M, Burny F, Muster D. Tissue and bone adhesive-historical aspect. Biomaterial. 1998;19:1461-6.
7. Garcia AL, Sutherland I. Cyanoacrylate adhesives in laparoscopic surgery: A review of applications and outcomes. Surg Endosc. 2022;36(1):45-54.
8. Goldberg JM, Vargas HD. Surgical Adhesives and Sealants: Current Technology and Applications. Cham: Springer; 2023.
9. Hvass U, Chatel D, Frikha I. Long-term result with pericardial patch and fibrin glue repair. Eur J Cardiothoracic Surg. 1995;9:75.
10. Kumar A, Gupta V. Efficacy of fibrin sealants in laparoscopic partial nephrectomy: A systematic review and meta-analysis. Am J Surg. 2019;217(4):682-90.
11. Matthew TL. Closure of small bronchopleural fistula using fibrin sealant. Chest. 1988;94.
12. Mckay TC. Laparoscopic ureteral anastomosis using fibrin glue. J Urol. 1994;152.
13. Morris JD, Joehl RJ. Application of polyethylene glycol (PEG) based adhesives in laparoscopic surgery:

Techniques and outcomes. J Laparoendosc Adv Surg Tech. 2024;34(2):213-21.

14. Mortia T. Successful endoscopic closure of radiation induced vesicovaginal fistula with fibrin glue. J Uro. 1999;162.

15. Patel PK, Smith LB. Bioadhesives for tissue approximation: Innovations in laparoscopy. J Biomed Mater Res B Appl Biomater. 2020;108(2):327-36.

16. Richardson JD, Franklin GA. A Comparative Study of Tissue Adhesives in Laparoscopic Procedures. J Am Coll Surg. 2018;226(5):891-7.

17. Santini M, Fiore T. Innovations in Surgical Sealants: Focus on Laparoscopic Applications. New York: Nova Science Publishers; 2020.

18. Spotnitz WD, Welker RL. Clinical use of fibrin sealantin. In: Mintz PD (Ed). Transfusion Therapy: Clinical Principles and Practice. AABB, Bethesda; 1999. pp. 199-220.

19. Spotnitz WD. History of tissue adhesives. In: Sierra D, Saltz R (Eds). Surgical Adhesives and Sealants: Current Technology and Applications. Lancaster (PA): Technomic; 1996. pp. 3-11.

20. Thompson JN, Patel J. Biological adhesives for wound closure: The future of tissue adhesion in laparoscopic surgery. Wound Repair Regen. 2019;27(6):662-70.

21. Zhang X, Lee NP. The Role of Adhesives in Minimizing Postoperative Complications in Laparoscopic Surgery. Surg Innov. 2022;29(3):304-12.

Impact of Training on Laparoscopic Suturing and Knotting

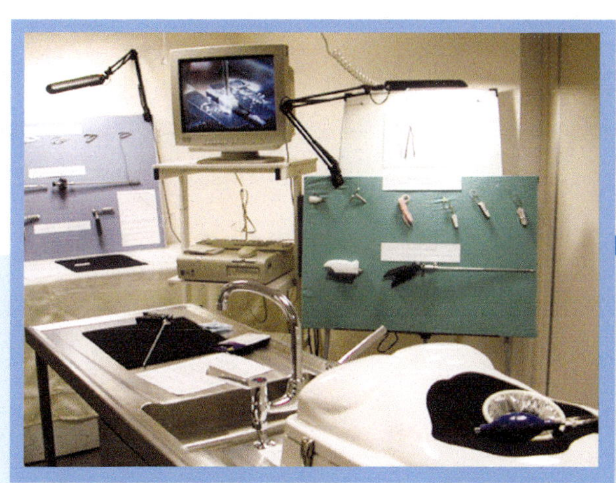

■ INTRODUCTION

Minimal access surgery represents a rapidly increasing component of gynecological and general surgery. Surgical competence entails a combination of knowledge, technical skills, decision-making, communication skills, and leadership skills. Of these, dexterity or technical proficiency is considered to be of paramount importance among surgical trainees. Surgical proficiency must, therefore, be acquired in less time, with the risk that some surgeons may not be sufficiently skilled at the completion of training. The benefits of laparoscopic surgery in terms of lower morbidity, shorter hospital stays, and quicker recovery times are well established. On the other hand, a common criticism of laparoscopic surgery is that it is time-consuming and complex. This has been associated with significant under-reporting of complications and deaths following laparoscopic surgery.

Laparoscopic surgery requires specific skills in hand–eye coordination and due to the lack of manual contact with the tissue and the restricted instrument mobility, the need for specific training was obvious. It has been shown that the complication rate decreases sharply as more laparoscopic procedures are performed. Similarly, the operation time is longer during the learning phase and decreases with experience. Formal training courses using graded exercises on pelvic simulators and exercises on animal models have been offered. This allows the basic skills required for laparoscopic surgery to be acquired before using them in a clinical setup, and provides an avenue whereby the learning curve may be partially circumvented. This kind of training is accepted as useful and even necessary. Therefore, the current training programs need to be assessed to ascertain their efficacy and establish their optimal content.

The skill development of trainees also needs to be monitored. This particular experiment prospectively investigated the effect of training on the speed and quality of endoscopic knot tying in trainees in obstetrics and gynecology and studied inter and intraoperator differences according to previous laparoscopic experience and according to several personal characteristics.

■ ENDOSCOPIC TRAINING

The effect of training on endoscopic knot tying was investigated in obstetrics, gynecology, and surgery trainees. All trainees participated on a voluntary basis. During the observation period, they performed 100 identical knots in

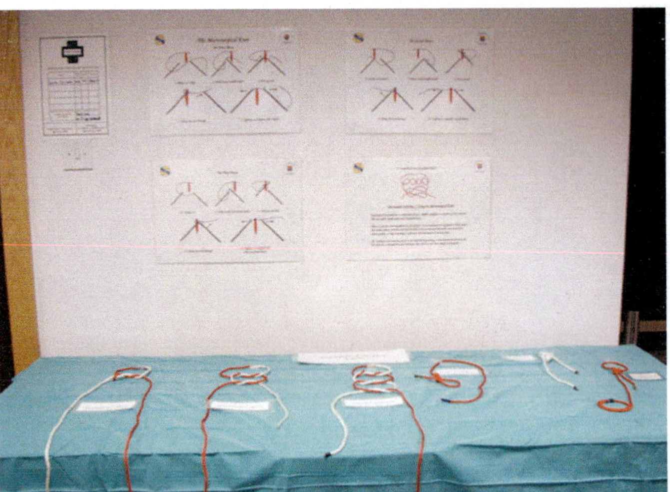

Fig. 1: Demonstration of different types of knots to keep them in memory.

3–4 training sessions of 2 hours over a period of 4 weeks **(Fig. 1)**. During this period, they were not exposed to any other additional training in endoscopic surgery, except clinical activities. Using an endotrainer (Ethicon, Cincinnati, USA) with a fixed camera, a 5 mm needle holder, and 5 mm forceps (Ethicon) a series of 10 knots were performed with Dexon® threads, 13 cm in length that had been fixed to a flat 10,310 red rubber surface. Prior to the study, a video was shown demonstrating the technique of tying two-turn, flat, square knot. During the study, trainees were allowed to rewatch the video demonstration, and an instructor was present during all training sessions in order to give advice, if required.

Proficiency-based training in laparoscopic suturing and knot tying translates to the operating room. Medical students with no previous laparoscopic or simulator experience were enrolled in an Institutional Review Board (IRB)-approved randomized controlled trial. All subjects were trained to proficiency on a previously validated suturing model (Fundamentals of Laparoscopic Surgery video trainer). Subjects were then randomized to a control group, which received no additional training, and an ongoing training group, which trained again to proficiency at 1 and 3 months (immediately after testing). Simulator testing was repeated at 2 weeks, 1 month, 3 months, and 6 months after initial training.

Simulator-based Training

A simulator defines a task environment with sufficient realism to serve a desired purpose.

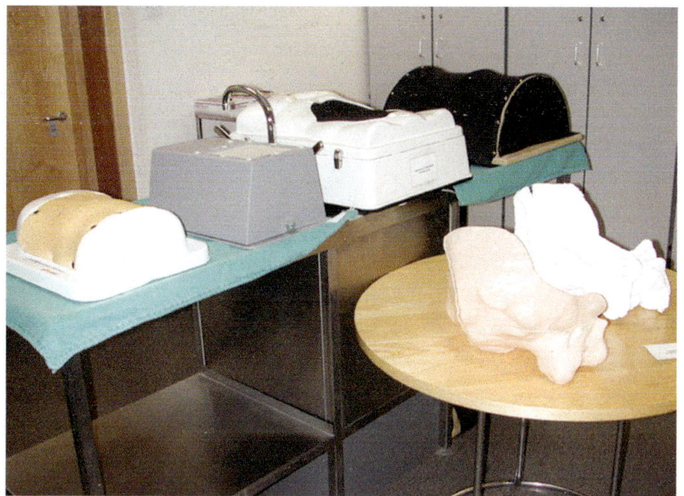

Fig. 2: Different types of simple pelvitrainers.

Novices underwent structured training in basic skills on the minimally invasive surgical trainer simulator (Mentice AB, Gothenburg, Sweden) followed by knot-tying training on the LapSim simulator (Surgical Science, Gothenburg, Sweden) **(Fig. 2)**. They were assessed pre- and post-training on a video trainer, which consists of an electromagnetic field generator and two sensors that are attached to the dorsum of the surgeon's hands at standardized positions. The advanced Dundee endoscopic psychomotor trainer (ADEPT) was originally designed as a tool for the selection of trainees for endoscopic surgery, based on the ability of psychomotor tests to predict the innate ability to perform relevant tasks. Studies have shown the validity and reliability of the trainer.

Optical motion tracking systems consist of infrared cameras surrounded by infrared light-emitting diodes.

■ VIRTUAL REALITY

Virtual reality (VR) is defined as a collection of technologies that allow people to interact efficiently with three-dimensional computerized databases in real time by using their natural senses and skills. Surgical VR systems allow interaction to occur through an interface, such as a laparoscopic frame with modified laparoscopic instruments. The minimally invasive surgical trainer-VR (MIST-VR) system was one of the first VR laparoscopic simulators developed as a task trainer. One of the main advantages of VR systems, in comparison to dexterity analysis systems, is that they provide real-time feedback about skill-based errors.

The popularity of laparoscopic techniques has led to a new domain in surgical training, with a move away from the apprenticeship model, toward structured programs of teaching new skills outside the operating room. Hands-on courses enabling young surgeons to practice techniques on synthetic, porcine, or more recently VR models are now commonplace. The aim has been to ensure trainees are armed with basic laparoscopic skills, such as hand–eye coordination and depth perception prior to entering the operating room. The success of these initial courses led to the development of similar courses for the advanced laparoscopic skills required for gastric and colonic surgery.

Compared to aviation, where VR training has been standardized and simulators have proven their definite benefit in increasing skills, the objectives, needs, and means of VR training in minimal access surgery (MAS) is established.

Rasmussen distinguishes three levels of human behavior:
1. Skill-based level
2. Rule-based level
3. Knowledge-based behavior

Skill-based Behavior

This represents surgeon's behavior that takes place without conscious control. Task execution is highly automated at this level of behavior and is based on the fast selection of motor programs, which control the appropriate muscles. The motor programs are based on an accurate internal representation of the task, the system dynamics, and the environment at hand (e.g., learned by training and experience). An example of an everyday skill is walking. Many tasks in surgery can be considered as a sequence of skilled acts. For example, an experienced surgeon performs a suturing task smoothly, without conscious control over his or her movements.

In minimal access surgery, suturing can also be considered a skill-based behavior. However, because of the indirect access to the tissue, it is a much more complicated skill because of reduced depth perception and difficult hand–eye coordination.

Rule-based Behavior

At the next level of human behavior, rule-based behavior is applied. During rule-based behavior, task execution is controlled by stored rules or procedures. These may have been derived empirically from previous occasions or communicated from other persons' expertise as instructions or as a cookbook recipe. Appropriate rules are selected according to their "success" in previous experiences. For example, procedural steps and the recognition of anatomy and pathology in minimal access surgery require rule-based behavior. At the rule-based level, the information is typically perceived as discrete signs. A sign serves to activate or trigger a stored rule. Stopping your car in front of a red light is a good example of a sign (red light) that triggers a stored rule (stop car). In laparoscopic cholecystectomy, having fully established the critical view of safety is the sign that triggers the rule that the appropriate structures may be clipped next.

Knowledge-based Behavior

In unfamiliar situations, faced with a task for which no rules are available from previous encounters, human behavior is knowledge-based. During knowledge-based behavior, the goal is explicitly formulated, based on an analysis of the overall aim. Different plans are developed, and their effects are mentally tested against the goal. Finally, a plan is selected. Serious complications that occasionally occur during surgery demand a great deal of knowledge-based behavior from the surgeon. He or she has to analyze the complication and the aim the surgical procedure in order to develop strategies to counter the complication. Then, he or she has to select the best strategy and consequently take the appropriate actions.

At the knowledge-based level, information is perceived as symbols. Symbols refer to chunks of conceptual information, which are the basis for reasoning and planning. Pathological symptoms are a good example of symbols in medical practice.

Training in laparoscopic surgery is beginning to evolve into a stepwise, curricular approach that is not organ or procedure-specific. Instead, it is necessary to learn manipulative skills, which are then combined to achieve proficiency in tasks such as laparoscopic suturing or division of a vessel **(Fig. 3)**. The constituent parts can then be combined with anatomical knowledge to enable the completion of a specific procedure. Basic psychomotor skills can be learned with a simple, cheap version of a video-box trainer. Higher level skills such as dissection and use of high-energy instruments will necessitate the use of more realistic tissues, which can be achieved on porcine or human cadaveric models.

Recent advances in VR simulation are also beginning to produce realistic simulations of complete procedures, for example, laparoscopic cholecystectomy.

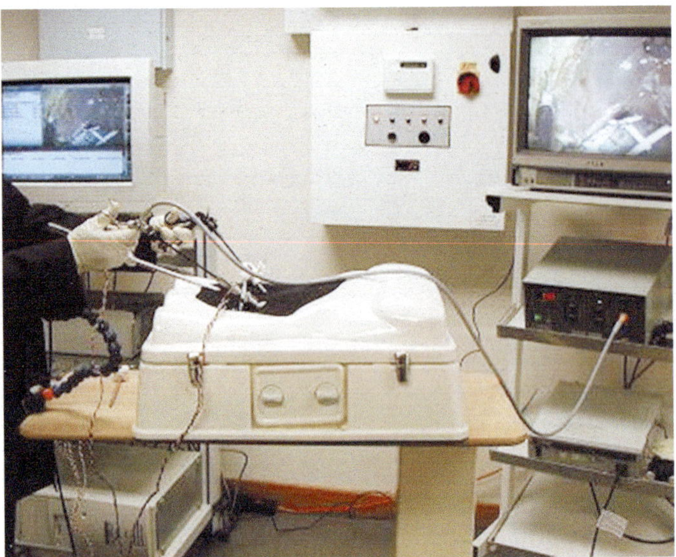

Fig. 3: Pelvitrainer exercises to improve skill.

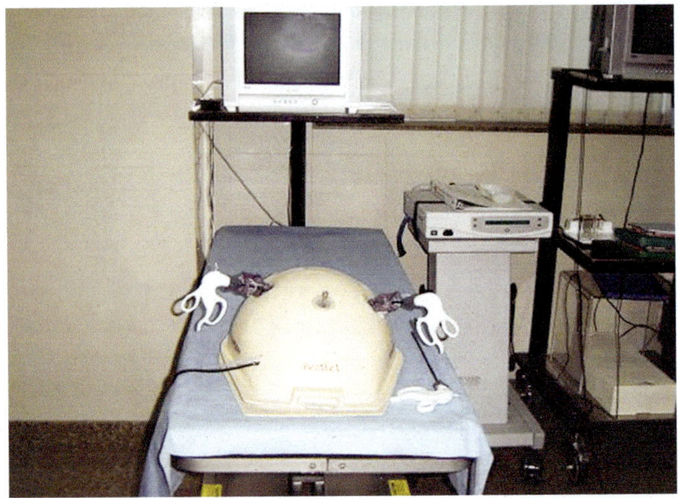

Fig. 4: The simple pelvitrainer can be used for improving suturing skill.

It would be rational to assume that a high-fidelity simulation model, such as anesthetized animal tissue, would be superior in terms of training outcome to a synthetic plastic model **(Fig. 4)**.

In fact, a study comparing two groups learning to perform microanastomotic repair of a transected spermatic cord on either the animal or synthetic model found no difference in the eventual outcome of the two groups. The synthetic model is obviously cheaper and does not require specialized storage facilities. It can be assumed that as the subjects were using real sutures and instruments, the nature of the task was learned regardless of the fidelity of the simulated tissue.

TRAINING OBJECTIVES, NEEDS, AND MEANS

To enable the design and evaluation of an effective and efficient training method, it is of utmost importance to determine the training objectives, needs, and means, since they provide an answer to the questions:

- What is the end goal of the training?
- What should be trained?
- How can we train it?

The objectives represent the level of competence that is expected of the trainee after he or she has completed the training. Training needs are the difference between the initial level of competence of the trainees and the required level of competence after successful completion of the training defined in the objectives. Ultimately, demands for effectivity and efficiency, on the one hand, and the state-of-the-art in technology, on the other hand, determine the tools and methods for training, i.e., the training means. Effective training ensures that all training objectives are met. Efficient training ensures that the training means are cost effective and that the required training time is minimized. Since safety and patient outcome are the most important criteria in surgery, training effectivity should be of primary importance.

The complexity and the costs of the training means are largely determined by the training objectives that have been set. Fulfilling all training needs of laparoscopic residents with only one training method will require a highly complex and probably very expensive trainer in which all three levels of behavior can be trained. Such a trainer is not yet available. The complexity and the cost of a training means are relatively low if the training objectives comprise skill-based behavior only, since this can be trained with simple models such as Pelvitrainers **(Figs. 3 and 4)**. Evidently, the cost and complexity of a training means increase when the training objectives advance from the training of skill-based behavior to the training of knowledge-based behavior. Fortunately, the overall effectiveness of training increases as well when higher levels of behavior, such as knowledge-based behavior, are incorporated into the training objectives.

PRESENT TRAINING IN LAPAROSCOPY

A closer look at the training program of laparoscopic residents provides an indication of the training needs that are addressed and the training means that are available today. Much as in conventional surgery, the laparoscopic surgeon must effectively combine the three levels of behavior. Instrument handling and dissection techniques require skill-based behavior, whereas the recognition of surgical anatomy requires a great deal of rule-based behavior. Complications such as uncontrollable bleeding or unsuspected situations such as the encountering of aberrant anatomy require problem-solving on a knowledge-based level.

Obviously, training in skill-based behavior in laparoscopic surgery is highly desired as laparoscopy combines unusual hand–eye coordination with the use of complex instruments. Surgical residents are usually trained in laparoscopic surgery during a 2-day introduction course. Basic skill-based behavior such as instrument–tissue handling and minimally invasive suturing are trained. Additionally, rule-based behavior is trained through lectures, textbooks, and video instructions. After the resident has successfully completed this course, he or she will receive training in the operating room. It is only in the operating room that most knowledge-based behavior necessary to deal with complications and emergencies is acquired. Currently, a living animal model provides the only way to effectively train rule- and knowledge-based behavior outside the operating room. Training on living animal models is very useful in the training curriculum of resident surgeons. However, at the same time, the use of laboratory animals for training is discouraged by many government policies. Technological innovations, such as VR simulation, will change the way laparoscopic surgery is trained **(Figs. 5 and 6)**. Current accomplishments in surgical simulation envision the dawning of the next-generation surgical education. In this respect, the aviation industry provides excellent examples of the effectiveness and efficiency of VR simulators as a means of training.

Simulator training in aviation in contrast to surgery: The training needs in aviation has explicitly been defined by regulatory authorities like the Federal Aviation Administration (FAA), and the training means are certified accordingly. The training objectives, needs, and means in pilot training have been investigated in depth, and models of pilot behavior have been developed as a tool to design, evaluate, and optimize training methods. Half a century of extensive research has resulted in many training tools, from basic flight training devices to the high-tech full flight simulator (FFS).

After the introduction of VR training methods in the 1990s, the training of surgeons has often been compared to

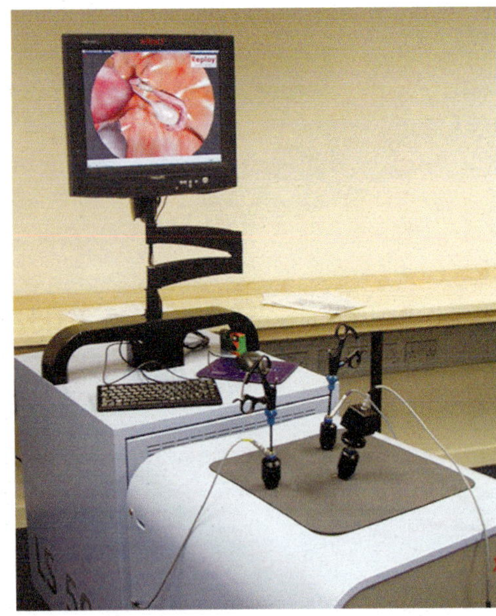

Fig. 5: The programming of virtual reality (VR) simulator will increase the rule-base level.

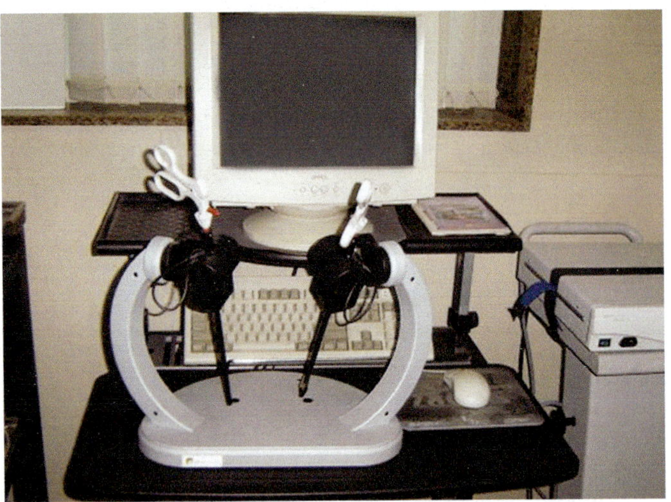

Fig. 6: Prototype virtual reality (VR) pelvitrainers.

the training of pilots. The training of laparoscopic residents can best be compared to the type-conversion training of pilots.

During type-conversion training, young pilots who have finished flight training at the academies and have recently joined an airline are trained to fly a particular type of aircraft.

The general objective of type conversion training is to teach the trainee how to safely control, navigate, and manage a particular operational aircraft. Since the trainees have already acquired much of the skill-based

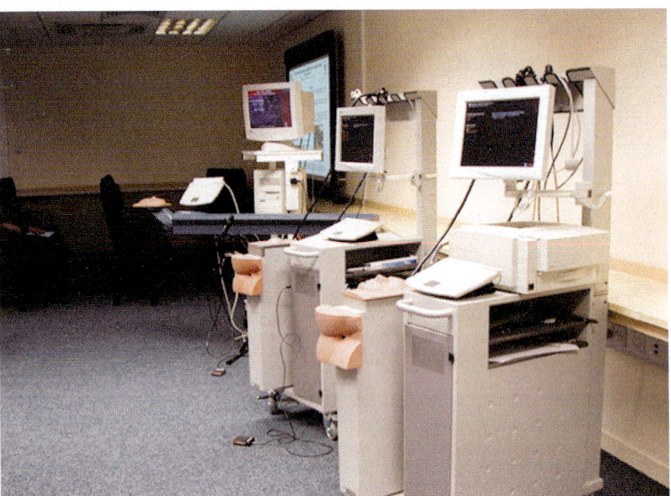

Fig. 7: Different types of virtual reality systems for endoscopy.

behavior required to fly a multiengine aircraft, the training needs mainly consist of acquiring additional rule- and knowledge-based behavior. The trainees have to learn the new checklists and the specific procedures during takeoff and landing, and they have to become familiar with all the aircraft systems like electronics and hydraulics. Furthermore, they have to train for all sorts of emergency scenarios that may occur during an actual flight. Training for this knowledge-based behavior is very important since it significantly improves flight safety. This training provides an excellent training tool to accomplish all the specified training needs. The high level of realism during the training of a pilot has even made zero flight time training possible, during which type conversion training takes place completely outside a real aircraft.

Defining the training objectives, needs, and means, for the sake of proper training and safety of our patients, the objectives, needs, and means in laparoscopy training should be defined. Along with this guideline, VR simulators should be developed. An explicit formulation of the training objectives facilitates the development and certification of a simulator since it determines what the simulator should be capable of. For example, pilots spend many hours training on low-cost simulators.

The laparoscopy simulators that have been developed during the past decade can all be considered as laparoscopy training devices **(Fig. 7)**. Most of these simulators specifically aim at training skill-based behavior, such as endoscopic manipulation and endoscopic camera navigation **(Fig. 8)**. However, performing safe laparoscopy also requires a professional level of rule and

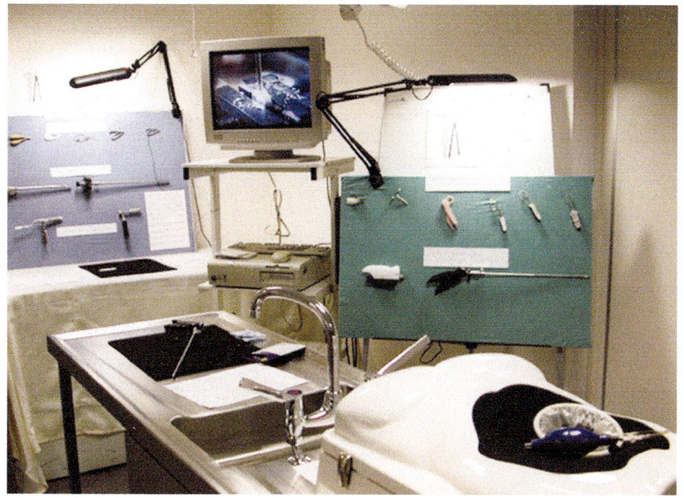

Fig. 8: Hand-assisted laparoscopic surgery (HALS) training box.

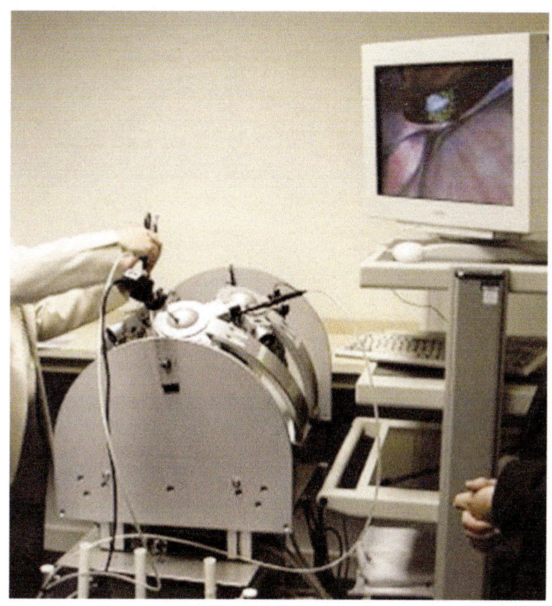

Fig. 9: Virtual reality trainer with programmable circuit.

knowledge-based behavior from the surgeon. Ideally, these should also be trained outside the operation theatre. Currently, the training of rule- and knowledge-based behavior outside the operation theater is only possible on living animal models.

However, technological innovations like increasing computing power, detailed anatomical models, soft-tissue modeling, and force feedback will enable the integration of all levels of behavior in a VR training simulator for laparoscopy. In the future, this might result in a full-scale laparoscopy simulator (FLS), comparable to the FFS in pilot training. Perhaps an FLS even introduces zero operating time training as the ultimate objective.

The medical society should establish detailed objectives for training. Recently, experts have begun to investigate what level of professional behavior is required to perform a safe laparoscopy. In addition, they are establishing the training needs of laparoscopic residents by determining what should be trained to accomplish the training objective. The question of which aspects of skill, rule, and knowledge-based behavior should be trained is addressed. Currently, there is no such standard available. Once the training objectives have been standardized and the training needs at the different levels of behavior have been identified, the simulator society will have clear guidelines as to what their training devices should be capable of.

One of the most obvious training needs of laparoscopic residents is the training of manual skills. The manual skills required during laparoscopy are rather different from those in conventional surgery. Training for skill-based behavior

is feasible with basic trainers such as a Pelvitrainer. The VR basic skill trainers that are commercially available usually simulate a generic abdomen and endoscopic instruments on a computer monitor. Basic tasks, such as pick and place tasks, are implemented to train endoscopic manipulation. The training of skill-based behavior does not require a highly realistic anatomical environment; for example, the organs do not necessarily have to be simulated realistically. For example, the VR trainer simulates basic manipulation tasks in a highly simplified environment similar to the pelvitrainer box. Several studies have reported that training on the VR facilitated the learning of skill-based behavior.

An advantage of VR simulators over simple pelvitrainers is the capability to easily extend the training to the rule-based level of behavior, since textbook theory, instructions, and training videos can easily be integrated into the simulator software **(Fig. 9)**. Much textbook material and many training videos that provide rule-based behavior training have been made available on the internet.

Laparoscopy simulators are capable of training skill- and rule-based behavior **(Fig. 10)**. To train knowledge-based behavior, a laparoscopy simulator should be capable of accurately imitating the surgical environment encountered during laparoscopic surgery.

The perceived information from the environment should be simulated accurately to ensure effective training **(Fig. 11)**. The training of knowledge-based behavior on a

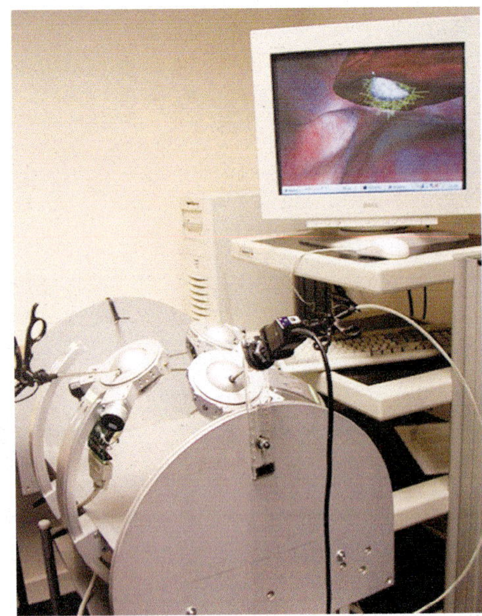

Fig. 10: Virtual reality trainer with software control.

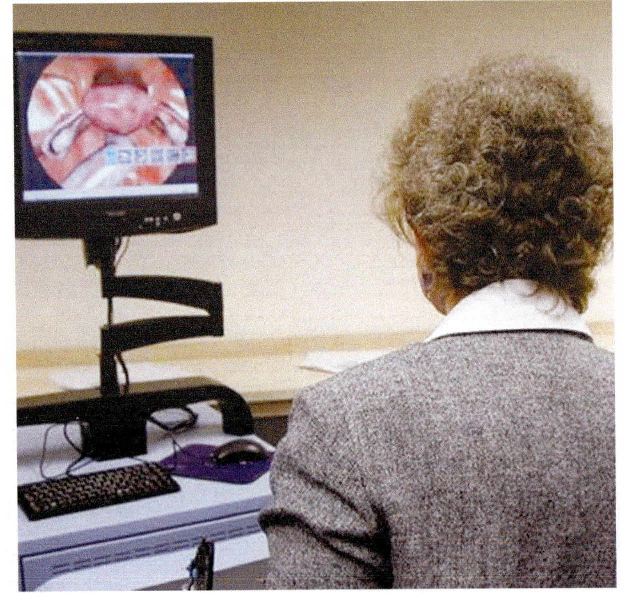

Fig. 11: Virtual reality trainer for laparoscopically assisted vaginal hysterectomy (LAVH).

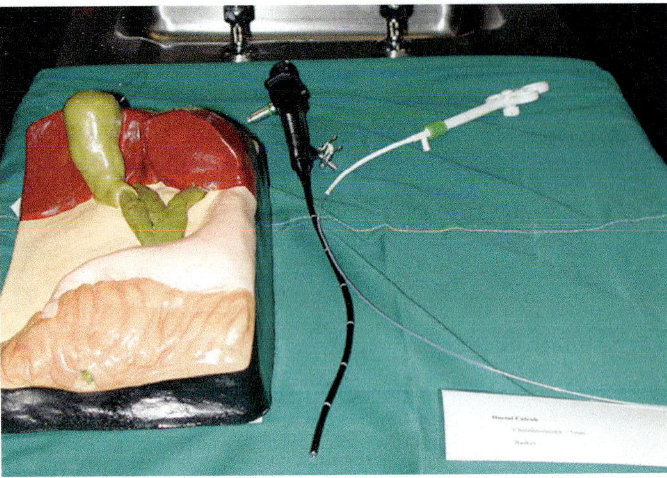

Fig. 12: Simulated models of gallbladder (GB) and common bile duct (CBD) to improve choledocoscopic skill.

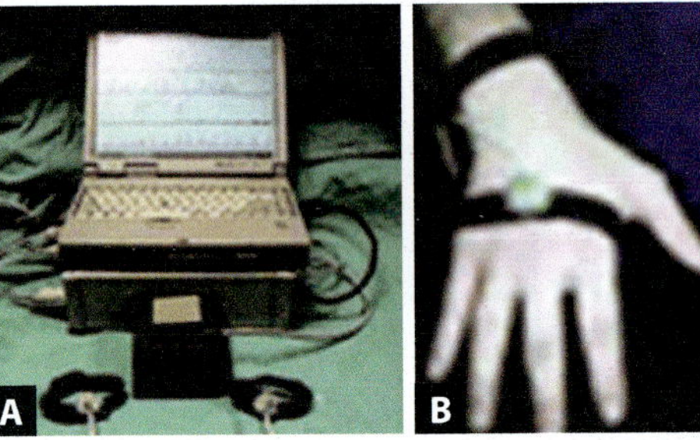

Figs. 13A and B: Imperial College surgical assessment device (ICSAD); (A) Signal generator; (B) Sensors.

simulator still poses a huge challenge. Two fundamental problems occur. Whereas the physics that determines the behavior of an aircraft is fairly well known and described mathematically, the physics that describes the behavior of soft-tissue organs is highly complicated and many parameters are simply still missing. Additionally, each aircraft roughly has the same flight characteristics and cockpit layout, but each new patient has a different anatomical layout than the previous one. Laparoscopy simulators have to be able to generate "random" patients **(Fig. 12)**.

The integration of knowledge-based behavior training in a future simulator would enhance safety levels in laparoscopy, and then every possible surgical complication could be trained beforehand. As in aviation, intensive training can reduce a situation that at first required improvising at a knowledge-based behavior level from the trainee, to a situation that can be solved by applying trained rules **(Figs. 13A and B)**.

Basic Surgical Skills

Surgical residents attended the Brightlands Smart Services Campus (BSSC) Leiden and Eindhoven, the Netherlands; before and after the course participants performed on the Xitract LS500, featuring standardized laparoscopic cholecystectomy clip and cut task **(Fig. 14)**.

Box Trainers

Training involves the use of box trainers with either innate models or animal tissues; it lacks objective assessment of

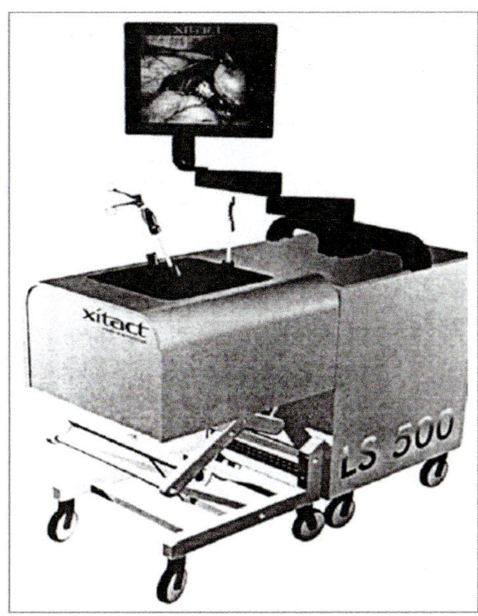

Fig. 14: Xitact LS500 simulator.

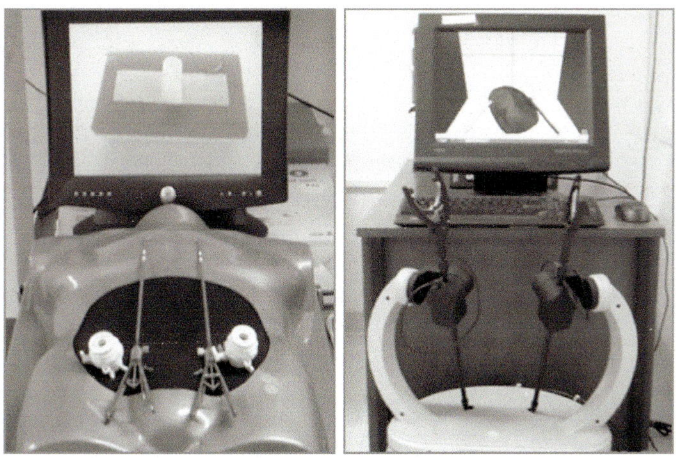

Fig. 15: Minimally invasive surgical trainer-virtual reality (MIST-VR).

skill acquisition **(Fig. 15)**. VR simulators have the ability to teach laparoscopic psychomotor skills, and objective assessment is now possible using dexterity-based and video analysis systems.

Bench Model Fidelity

Impact of bench model fidelity on the acquisition of technical skill using clinically relevant outcome measures: All participants were assessed on the high- and low-fidelity bench models. Immediate outcome measures included procedure times, blinded, expert assessment of videotaped performance using checklists and global rating scales, anastomotic patency, suture placement precision, and final product ratings.

■ RESULTS

Regarding the duration of knot tying, an obvious learning curve was observed. The mean time required to tie a knot decreased from the first 10 to the last 10 knots. The initial time was slightly higher, while the calculated time for the last knots was slightly lower, and the time to tie a knot continued to decrease slowly. For the quality of endoscopic intracorporeal knots, a learning curve was also noted: as the tying times decreased, the quality of the knots increased **(Fig. 16)**, from 2.0 ± 0.4 SD for the first 10 knots to 2.2 ± 0.97 SD for the last 10 knots.

Final knot scores were higher for more experienced (p = 0.01) and more practically oriented trainees, particularly those practicing handicrafts (p = 0.05).

All participants completed a correct knot as compared to only 25% completing the knot before training. Time to completion was 66% faster and knot quality was 45% better after training. Significant reduction was noticed in the number of movements (p = .006) and distance traveled (p < .000) by both hands after training.

Trained group performed significantly better than the control group at post-testing confirming curriculum effectiveness.

Training on the bench model simulators were higher among subjects who received hands-on training, irrespective of model fidelity.

No significant difference for the parameters time and score outcome pre- and post-BSSC was observed.

■ DISCUSSION

This study was undertaken to demonstrate the effect of training on the speed and quality of knot tying. Training for knot tying was efficient and the learning curves of all trainees were remarkably similar, which is considerably faster than generally accepted. These data are indicative of the minimum necessary time trainees should be provided with to achieve this particular skill. As expected, more experienced trainees were clearly characterized by lower initial tie times, as well as slightly lower final tie times. The effect of previous experience was, however, limited compared to the overall effect of the actual training. The observation shows that more experienced trainees were characterized by lower initial and persistently lower final tie times, whereas their speed of learning was slightly

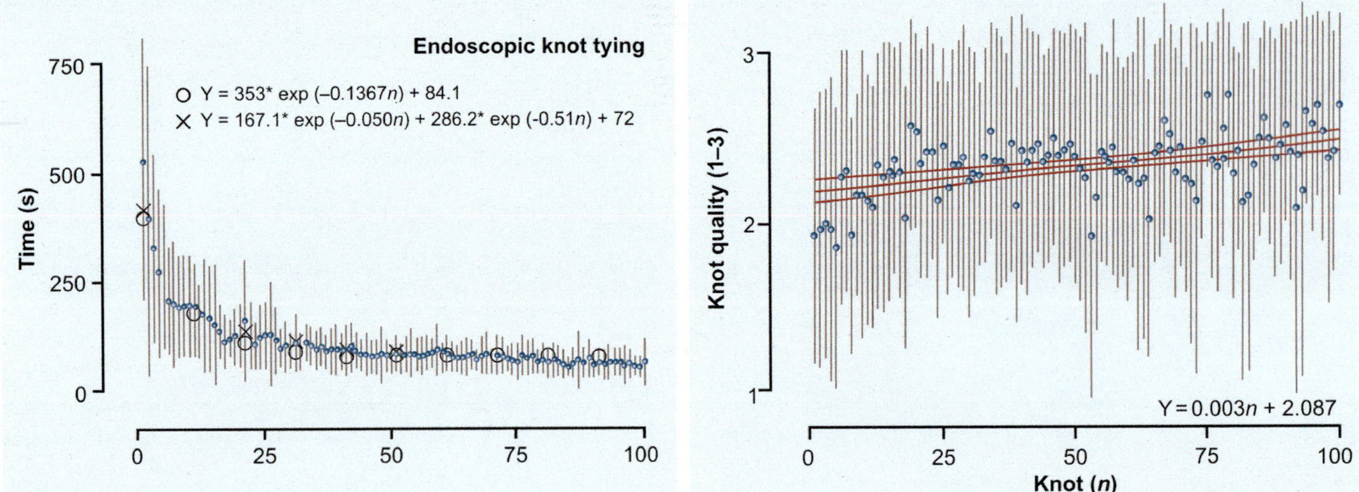

Fig. 16: Learning curve of the duration of endoscopic knot tying and the quality of the knots. The means and standard deviation (SD) are indicated. For the duration of knot tying, the calculated duration using a monoexponential (O) or bi-exponential decay model (X) is indicated. For the knot quality, the regression line and 95% confidence limits are indicated.

lower suggests other differences between these two groups, such as long-term and cumulative effects of training. To explain this, our knowledge of the neurophysiology of learning and memory is not yet sufficient; hence, learning takes months, rather than hours, as seen in sports, for example, tennis, where beginners make dramatic improvements in a few days but take much more time and practice to become skilled. The fundamental issues of training in endoscopy, however, are not speed but quality of surgery and prevention of accidents.

The assumption was that the sequential training up to a plateau of all different tasks of endoscopic surgery could be advantageous in comparison to the current apprenticeship model, where trainees start by watching and assisting surgery, then perform minor surgical interventions and gradually proceed to more extensive laparoscopic procedures. If, however, the training effect of watching and assisting surgery is limited, this observation should impact upon training program of residents. It might be that video endoscopy of pure diagnostic procedures only trains depth of vision cues, not eye–hand coordination. The former emphasizes hours of training with simple procedures up to a certain speed and quality, whereas the latter emphasizes difficulty by performing multiple tasks from the beginning. It is assumed that adequate training can minimize the complication rate because complications were particularly seen during the early part of the learning curve.

It has been claimed that laparoscopic procedures could be safely introduced to young inexperienced residents provided that they were having properly supervised training.

CONCLUSION

These data demonstrated similar and important learning effects in all trainees in endoscopic knot tying over a period of a few hours and showed that more experienced trainees at the beginning of the training were able to tie better quality knots faster than the inexperienced trainees. Following this learning period, the differences between inexperienced and experienced trainees, although small, persist. Surprisingly, assisting and watching surgery did not contribute to the training effect. Specific consecutive training in each aspect of endoscopic surgery may be more appropriate.

BIBLIOGRAPHY

1. Aggarwal R, Moorthy K, Darzi A. Laproscopic skill training and assessment. Br J Surg. 2004;91:1549-58.
2. Aharoni A, Guyot B, Salat-Baroux J. Operative laparoscopy for ectopic pregnancy: How experienced should the surgeon be? Hum Reprod. 1993;8(12):2227-30.
3. Airan MC. Letter to the editor. Am J Surg. 1990;159:619.
4. Alaker M, Wynn GR, Arulampalam T. Virtual reality training in laparoscopic surgery: a systematic review and meta-analysis. Int J Surg. 2022;29:85-94.
5. Altman LK. When patient's life is the price of learning new kind of surgery. New York Times. 1992a;Section C:3.
6. Champion JK, Hunter J, Trus T, Laycock TW. Teaching basic video skills as an aid in laparoscopic suturing. Surg Endosc. 1996;10:23-5.

7. Cuschieri A, Francis N, Crosby J, Hanna GB. What do master surgeons think of surgical competence and revalidation? Am J Surg. 2001;182:110-6.

8. Cushieri A, Berci G, McSherry CK. Laparoscopic cholecystectomy. Am J Surg 1990;159(3):273.

9. Derossis AM, Fried GM, Abrahamowicz M, Sigman HH, Barkun JS, Meakins JL. Development of a model for training and evaluation of laparoscopic skill. Am J Surg. 1998;175(6):482-7.

10. Diaz R, Quintero L. Innovations in Surgical Education: Laparoscopic Suturing and Knotting. Cham: Springer; 2021.

11. Friedman Z, You-Ten KE, Bould MD, Naik V. Deliberate practice for surgical skill acquisition: a look at laparoscopic suturing and knot tying. Am J Surg. 2020;219(4): 643-50.

12. Gallagher AG, O'Sullivan GC. Metrics for performance measurement in advanced laparoscopic surgery. Surg Innov. 2024;31(1):15-25.

13. Grober ED, Hamstra SJ, Wanzel KR, Reznick RK, Matsumoto ED, Sidhu RS. The education: impact of bench model *fi*delity on the acquisition of technical skill: the use of clinically relevant outcome measures. Ann Surg. 2004;374-81.

14. Jha AK, Duncan BW, Bates DW. Simulator-based training and patient safety. Making health care safer: A critical analysis of patient safety practices. Agency for Health care. Research and Quality: United States Department of Health and Human Services; 2001. pp. 511-7.

15. Kavic MS, Segan RD. Laparoscopic Suturing. Philadelphia: Lippincott Williams & Wilkins; 2020.

16. Korndorffer JR. Proficiency maintenance-impact training on laparoscopic. Am J Surg. 2006;599-603.

17. Korndorffer JR Jr, Dunne JB, Sierra R, Stefanidis D, Touchard CL, Scott DJ. Simulator training for laparoscopic suturing using performance goals translates to the operating room. J Am Coll Surg. 2005;201(1):23-9.

18. Martin JA, Regehr G, Reznick R, MacRae H, Murnaghan J, Hutchison C, et al. Objective structured assessment of technical skill (OSATS) for surgical residents. Br J Surg. 2018;105(2):121-7.

19. Moorthy K, Munz Y, Sarker SK, Darzi A. Objective assessment of technical skills in surgery. BMJ. 2003; 1032-37.

20. Munz Y, Almoudaris AM, Moorthy K, Dosis A, Liddle AD, Darzi AW. Curriculum-based solo virtual reality training for laproscopic knot tying: objective assessment of the transfer of skill from virtual reality to reality. Am J Surg. 2007;193(6):774-83.

21. Muresan C 3rd, Lee TH, Seagull J, Park AE. (2010). "Transfer of training in the development of intracorporeal suturing skill in medical student novices: a prospective randomized trial." Am J Surg. 200:537-4*1*.

22. Nduka CC, Darzi A, Teaching laparoscopic surgery. Training courses are popular and valuable. BMJ. 1994;308:1435.

23. Palter VN, Grantcharov TP. Laparoscopic Skills Training and Assessment. New York: Springer; 2023.

24. Shijven M, Klaassen R, Jakimowicz J, Terpstra OT. The intercollegiate basic surgical skills course. Surg Endosc. 2003;17(12):1979-84.

25. Smith ST, Jacobs LM. The effectiveness of simulation-based training on laparoscopic suturing: a meta-analysis. Surg Endosc. 2019;33(6):1872-80.

26. Spruit EN, Band GP, Hamming JF. "Increasing efficiency of surgical training: effects of spacing practice on skill acquisition and retention in laparoscopy training." Surg Endosc. 2014;29(8):2235-43.

27. Turner CE, Williams RG. Competency-based training in laparoscopic surgery: shaping the future of surgical education. Surgery. 2019;166(5):907-11.

28. Vossen C, Van Ballaer P, Shaw RW, Koninckx PR. Effect of training on endoscopic intracorporal knot tying. Human reproductive. 1997;12(12):2658-63.

Robotic Suturing and Knotting

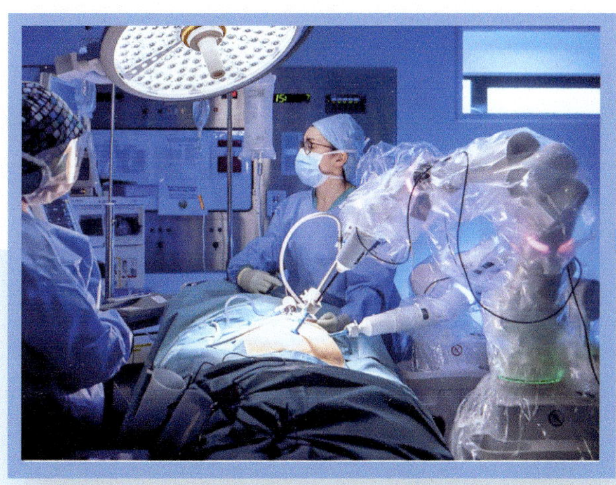

■ INTRODUCTION

In the realm of traditional open surgery, suturing techniques have long relied on the use of a needle holder and forceps, aiming for the precise joining of wound edges and ensuring a secure knot is tied. However, with the advent of laparoscopic surgery, these conventional methods underwent significant adaptation to accommodate the limitations posed by the rigid, less flexible laparoscopic tools, which offer restricted movement. This evolution took a notable leap forward with the advent of three-dimensional (3D) robotic suturing, which has simplified the learning curve for intracorporeal suturing. This advancement is largely attributed to the intuitive nature of robotic systems and the enhanced mobility provided by the robotic wrists. As the medical field has seen a rise in the use of therapeutic endoscopic procedures, especially for the early stages of gastrointestinal cancers, there has been a drive to develop devices capable of suturing endoscopically. However, the application of these devices presents its own set of challenges, including the need for dual-channel endoscopes and the absence of the additional movement flexibility found in robotic wrists. Unfortunately, robots can only tie intracorporeal knots **(Fig. 1)**. The integration of robotics into endoscopic suturing marks a significant progression, offering promising solutions to these challenges. This chapter delves into the evolution and adaptation of suturing techniques across different surgical platforms, encompassing laparoscopic, robotic, and endoscopic methods.

■ SURGICAL ROBOTS CURRENTLY AVAILABLE

The advent of surgical robots has revolutionized the way surgeries are performed, offering enhanced precision, reduced recovery times, and minimized surgical trauma. As this technology continues to evolve, a variety of robotic systems have emerged, each with its unique features and capabilities. This chapter provides an extensive overview and comparison of the surgical robots currently available, focusing on their design, functionalities, clinical applications, and the comparative advantages they offer in the operating room (OR).

da Vinci Surgical System (Fig. 2)

Manufacturer: Intuitive Surgical

Launch year: 2000

Key features:
- Multiarm robotic platform offering a high degree of dexterity and control
- 3D high-definition vision system
- Instruments with EndoWrist capabilities allowing seven degrees of motion
- Various models are available, including the da Vinci Xi—the most advanced with overhead instrument

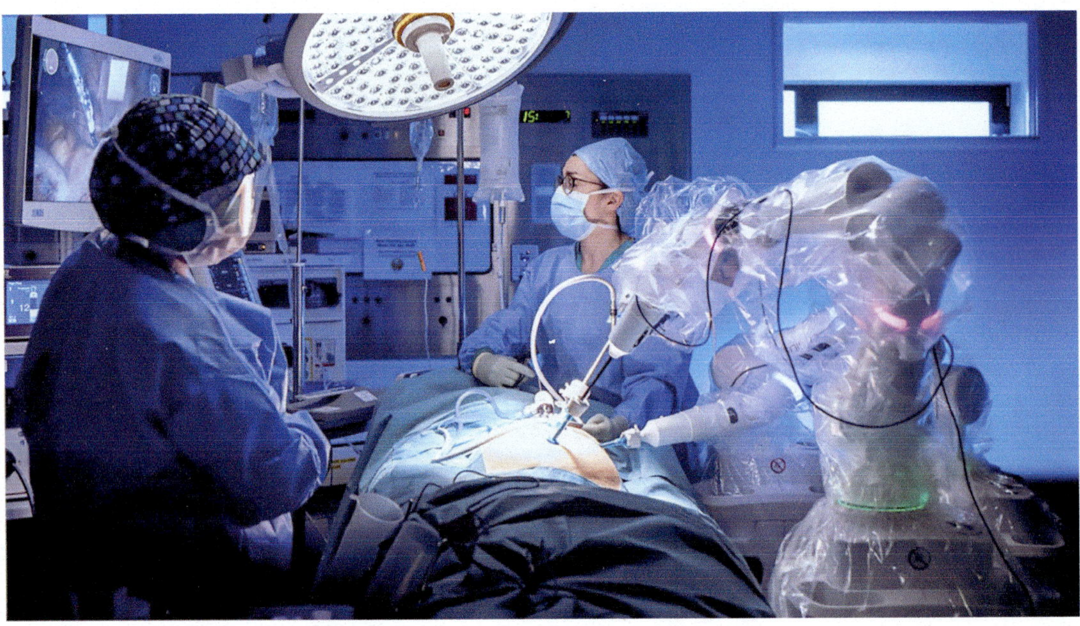

Fig. 1: Robot can only do intracorporeal knots.

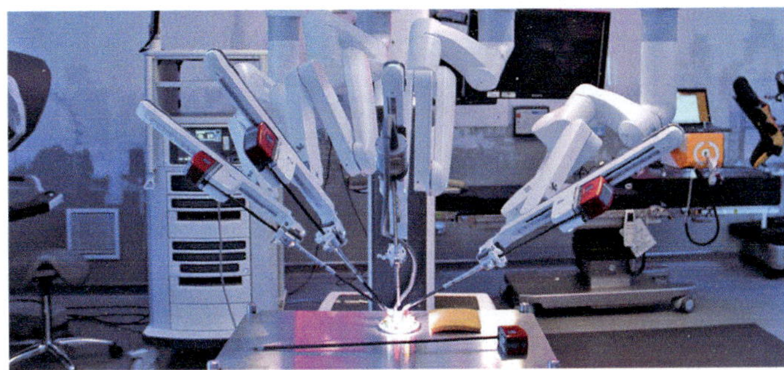

Fig. 2: da Vinci Robot.

arms that facilitate anatomical access from virtually any position.

Clinical applications: It is used across a broad spectrum of minimally invasive procedures including urology, gynecology, general surgery, cardiothoracic, and head and neck surgery.

Comparative advantage: The da Vinci system is the most widely adopted surgical robot, with a vast array of specialized instruments and a large body of clinical outcome data supporting its use.

Senhance Surgical System (Fig. 3)

Manufacturer: Asensus Surgical

Launch year: 2017 [Food and Drug Administration (FDA) approval]

Key features:
- Offers haptic feedback, allowing surgeons to feel the force applied during surgery
- Eye-tracking camera control for hands-free operation
- Utilizes standard laparoscopic instruments, potentially reducing the cost per procedure
- Smaller arms designed for easy setup and integration into the OR

Clinical applications: Primarily focused on general abdominal surgeries such as colorectal and gynecological procedures.

Comparative advantage: Senhance's haptic feedback is a significant differentiator, offering surgeons a more intuitive control and potentially reducing fatigue.

Versius Surgical Robotic System

Manufacturer: CMR (Cambridge Medical Robotics) Surgical

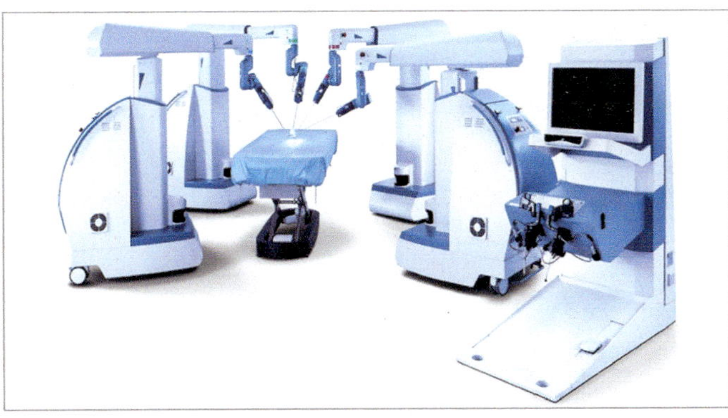

Fig. 3: Senhance Surgical System.

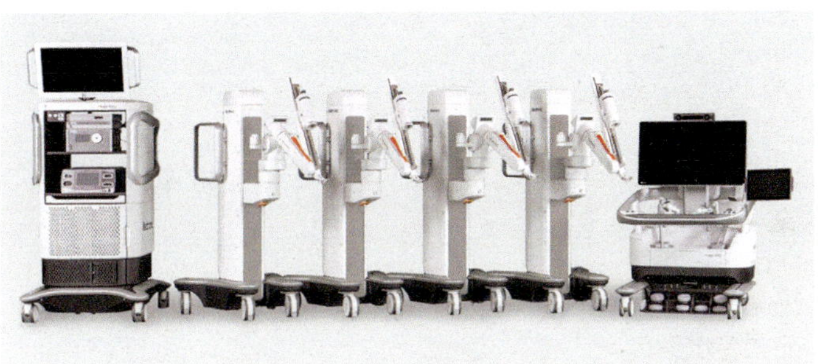

Fig. 4: Hugo Robotic-Assisted Surgery (RAS) System.

Launch year: 2019

Key features:
- Modular design with individually cart-mounted, small, and versatile robotic arms
- Designed to mimic the human arm, offering flexibility in port placement and ease of use across various surgical procedures
- Portable and easy to integrate into existing OR workflows

Clinical applications: Versatile for use in a wide range of abdominal surgeries, including colorectal, gynecological, and urological procedures.

Comparative advantage: Versius stands out for its modular, portable design, making it adaptable to a variety of surgical settings and potentially lowering barriers to robotic surgery adoption.

Hugo Robotic-Assisted Surgery System (Fig. 4)

Manufacturer: Medtronic

Launch year: 2021

Key features:
- Modular, multiquadrant platform designed for a wide array of soft-tissue surgeries
- Incorporates the Touch Surgery Enterprise system, offering preoperative planning and virtual training tools
- Uses individual arm carts, similar to Versius, for flexibility in the OR setup

Clinical applications: Aimed at a broad range of procedures, including bariatric, gynecological, thoracic, and urologic surgeries

Comparative advantage: Hugo's integration with digital tools for training and planning, along with Medtronic's established presence in the healthcare field, positions it as a strong contender in the robotic surgery market.

Cambridge Medical Robotics Surgical's Robotic System (Fig. 5)

In the rapidly evolving landscape of medical technology, CMR Surgical's Versius robotic system stands out as a beacon of innovation in minimally invasive surgery. Designed with the intention to make robotic surgery universally accessible and cost-effective, Versius has carved a niche for itself in the competitive arena of surgical robotics. This chapter delves into the features, clinical applications, and the transformative potential of the Versius system, highlighting its role in the future of surgical procedures.

Genesis of Versius: Cambridge Medical Robotics, known as CMR Surgical, introduced the Versius Surgical Robotic System as a response to the growing need for more adaptable and scalable solutions in laparoscopic surgery.

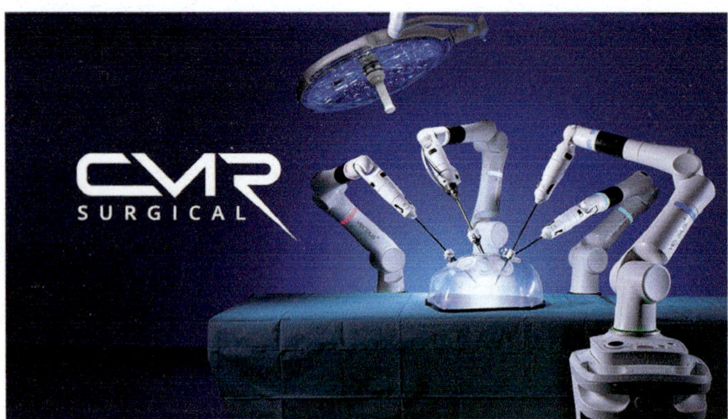

Fig. 5: Cambridge Medical Robotics (CMR) Surgical's Robotic System.

The system's development was driven by the goal of providing a versatile, easy-to-use platform that could bring the benefits of robotic surgery to hospitals and patients globally. With its launch, Versius has set a new standard in surgical precision, safety, and flexibility.

Key features of Versius:
- *Modular design:* One of the most striking features of Versius is its modular design, comprising small, individually cart-mounted robotic arms. This design offers unparalleled flexibility in the OR, allowing for easy setup and reconfiguration based on the specific requirements of each surgery.
- *Human-like dexterity:* The robotic arms of Versius mimic the range of motion of a human arm, providing surgeons with intuitive control and the ability to perform complex maneuvers with ease. This is complemented by the system's 3D high-definition visualization, ensuring precision in tissue manipulation.
- *Portable and scalable:* Versius' compact size and portability make it an ideal solution for hospitals of varying sizes and capacities. Its scalability allows for the system to be tailored to the hospital's specific needs, whether it involves a single robotic arm for minor procedures or multiple arms for complex surgeries.
- *Enhanced ergonomics:* Recognizing the physical toll that laparoscopic surgery can take on surgeons, Versius is designed to offer improved ergonomics. The system's console and controls reduce surgeon fatigue, potentially leading to better outcomes and increased surgeon well-being.

Clinical applications: Versius has been engineered to support a wide range of surgical procedures, including but not limited to colorectal, gynecological, urological, and general surgeries. Its versatility and ease of use make it particularly suitable for hospitals looking to introduce or expand their robotic surgery programs without the extensive overhead and space requirements of larger systems.

Transformative potential: The introduction of Versius into the surgical robotics market represents a significant step forward in making minimally invasive robotic surgery more accessible and cost-effective. By addressing some of the limitations of previous systems, such as size, complexity, and cost, Versius opens the door to a broader adoption of robotic assistance in surgery. This not only has the potential to improve patient outcomes through more precise and less invasive procedures but also to democratize access to state-of-the-art surgical care across different regions and healthcare systems.

As CMR Surgical continues to innovate and expand the capabilities of the Versius system, the future looks promising for the field of robotic-assisted surgery. Ongoing research and development are focused on enhancing the system's capabilities, including the integration of artificial intelligence (AI) and machine learning (ML) for predictive analytics and surgical planning. With a commitment to improving surgical outcomes and patient care, Versius is poised to play a pivotal role in the future of minimally invasive surgery.

Mantra Robotic System (Fig. 6)

Vision for innovation: The "Mantra" robotic system could be envisioned as the next leap in surgical robotics, emphasizing ultra-precision, adaptability, and seamless integration with surgical workflows. Its design might incorporate AI-driven analytics, enhanced dexterity, and intuitive control mechanisms, setting new standards for patient outcomes and surgical efficiency.

Core features:
- *AI and ML:* Utilizing AI to provide real-time analytics, the "Mantra" system could offer predictive modeling for surgical planning and intraoperative decision-making, enhancing the surgeon's capabilities with data-driven insights.
- *Enhanced dexterity and control:* Building on the limitations of existing systems, "Mantra" could feature advanced robotic arms that offer a greater range of motion and finer control, mimicking the nuanced movements of the human hand with even greater accuracy.
- *Immersive 3D visualization:* High-definition, 3D visualization systems could provide surgeons with immersive views of the surgical field, potentially integrated with augmented reality (AR) to overlay critical information directly onto the surgical view.
- *Customizable modular design:* Recognizing the diverse needs across surgical specialties, "Mantra" could adopt a modular design, allowing for customization and scalability across a range of surgical procedures from general surgery to highly specialized microsurgery.
- *Ergonomic surgeon interface:* Prioritizing surgeon comfort and reducing fatigue, the interface could be ergonomically designed for optimal usability during long procedures, incorporating feedback mechanisms to simulate tactile sensations.

Clinical applications: The potential applications of a system like "Mantra" would be broad, spanning general surgery, urology, gynecology, cardiothoracic surgery, and beyond. Its advanced features could particularly benefit procedures requiring high precision and control, such as microsurgical techniques or surgeries in anatomically complex regions.

Impact on surgical care:
- *Reduced patient trauma:* By enhancing precision and control, "Mantra" could minimize surgical trauma, leading to quicker recovery times and reduced complications.
- *Democratization of robotic surgery:* If "Mantra" was designed to be cost-effective and easy to integrate into existing hospital infrastructure, it could help democratize access to advanced surgical care, making robotic-assisted procedures available to a wider patient population.
- *Education and training:* With integrated simulation capabilities, "Mantra" could also serve as a powerful tool for surgical education and training, preparing the next generation of surgeons with hands-on experience in robotic-assisted techniques. While the "Mantra" robotic system is a conceptual exploration based on current trends and future possibilities in surgical robotics, the ongoing innovation in this field is very real. New systems and technologies are continually being developed to overcome the limitations of existing platforms, enhance surgical precision, and improve patient outcomes. As the landscape of surgical robotics evolves, systems such as the imagined "Mantra" represent the ambitious goals and innovative spirit driving the future of minimally invasive surgery.

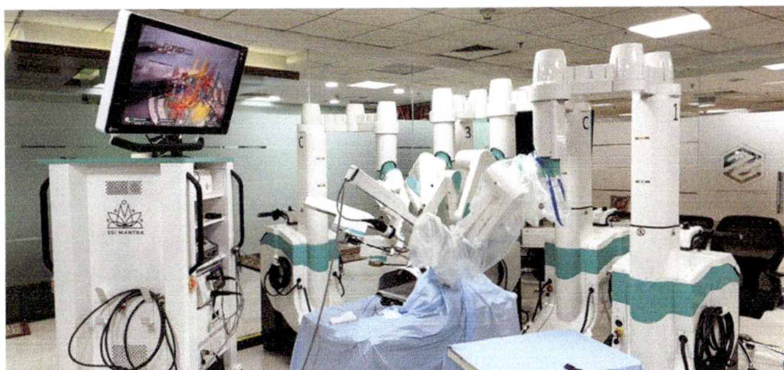

Fig. 6: Mantra robotic system.

Comparison and conclusion: The choice of a surgical robot is influenced by various factors, including the type of procedures performed, cost considerations, the learning curve for the surgical team, and the specific advantages each system offers. For instance, the da Vinci system's extensive track record and wide array of instruments make it a go-to choice for hospitals performing a diverse range of minimally invasive surgeries. Meanwhile, systems such as Senhance and Versius offer unique features such as haptic feedback and modular design, respectively, which may be particularly appealing for specific clinical applications or hospital settings.

The future of robotic surgery looks promising, with ongoing advancements aimed at increasing the capabilities of these systems, reducing costs, and expanding their use into more surgical specialties. As the technology progresses, surgical robots are expected to become even more integrated into the fabric of surgical care, offering enhanced outcomes for patients and new capabilities for surgeons. The key to successful integration lies in careful consideration of each system's strengths and limitations, ongoing surgeon training, and a clear understanding of the clinical benefits they offer.

IMPORTANCE OF SUTURING IN ROBOTIC SURGERY

In traditional open surgery, suturing involves using a needle holder in one hand to penetrate the tissue with a comprehensive stitch and employing forceps in the other hand to invert the wound's edge. The primary objectives are twofold: First, to achieve a precise alignment of the wound edges to facilitate healing through primary intention and second, to secure a knot that remains intact without causing undue tension on the tissues.

With the advent of laparoscopic surgery, suturing techniques have evolved to address the unique challenges presented by this approach, such as the restricted movement afforded by the rigid instruments used in laparoscopic procedures. The introduction of robotic technology has further enhanced suturing techniques, making intracorporeal suturing more accessible and easier to master. The advantages of using a 3D robotic system for suturing include its intuitive operation and the increased mobility provided by the robotic wrists.

Despite the less invasive nature of laparoscopic and robotic surgeries, these procedures still necessitate surgical incisions and can result in scarring. In the 1990s, Japanese physicians pioneered the use of endoscopic surgery for the gastrointestinal tract to remove early-stage cancers in a minimally invasive manner. The development of endoscopic submucosal dissection (ESD) techniques has enabled patients to avoid major surgeries, thereby shortening hospital stays and reducing medical resource usage.

However, one significant risk associated with ESD is the potential for iatrogenic perforation. Given this risk, it is crucial for endoscopists to have access to endoscopic suturing devices, enabling them to repair perforations endoscopically rather than resorting to surgical intervention. The field of endoscopic suturing, being relatively new, faces challenges with the current devices which are often difficult to use. These challenges include the necessity for a double-channel endoscope and the absence of the additional mobility that robotic wrists offer.

WHY ROBOT CANNOT TIE EXTRACORPOREAL KNOT?

Robotic systems, especially in the context of minimally invasive surgery such as robotic-assisted laparoscopy, are primarily designed for intracorporeal procedures due to their precise control, dexterity, and ability to manipulate instruments within a confined space. The task of tying extracorporeal knots, on the other hand, presents specific challenges for robotic systems for several reasons:

- *Design and functionality:* Robotic surgical systems such as the da Vinci Surgical System are engineered to mimic and extend the capabilities of the human hand inside the patient's body. They excel in tasks that require intricate movements and high precision, such as suturing or dissection within the body cavity. These systems are not designed to perform tasks outside the body, such as tying extracorporeal knots, which traditionally rely on the surgeon's tactile feedback and manual dexterity.
- *Lack of tactile feedback:* One of the limitations of current robotic systems is the reduced tactile feedback, which is crucial for tying knots extracorporeally. When surgeons tie knots manually, they rely on touch to gauge the tension of the suture and the integrity of the knot. Although some robotic systems offer haptic feedback, it may not be sufficient for the nuanced adjustments required for extracorporeal knot tying.
- *Complexity and efficiency:* Tying extracorporeal knots involves manipulating the suture outside the patient's

body and often requires the surgeon to adjust the tension and position of the knot manually. This task can be more efficiently and effectively performed by the surgeon's own hands or with the assistance of specialized tools designed for extracorporeal knot tying. In contrast, the robotic system's strengths lie in performing tasks within the surgical field where its precision and control offer the most benefit.

- *Operational constraints:* Robotic arms are constrained by their range of motion and the need to operate through trocars (small ports through which robotic instruments are inserted). These constraints make it impractical for the robot to perform tasks outside the body, such as tying knots, which can be more easily and quickly accomplished by the surgical team in the OR without the need for robotic assistance.

While robotic surgery continues to evolve, with advancements in technology expanding the capabilities of surgical robots, the current focus remains on enhancing their performance for intracorporeal procedures rather than tasks like extracorporeal knot tying.

UNRAVELING THE WORLD OF SURGICAL ROBOTICS: A GUIDE TO COMMON KNOTS

In the ever-evolving landscape of medical technology, surgical robots have carved a niche, revolutionizing the way surgeries are performed. Among the plethora of tasks these mechanical marvels are designed for, suturing remains a cornerstone of surgical procedures, demanding precision, steadiness, and efficiency. Central to this task is the art of knot tying, a skill that ensures the integrity and security of sutures. This chapter delves into the common knots tied by surgical robots, highlighting their importance and application in robotic surgery.

Intracorporeal Knot

As the name suggests, the intracorporeal knot is tied within the body, utilizing the dexterity and precision of robotic arms. This knot is particularly advantageous in minimally invasive procedures, where space is limited and direct manual manipulation is challenging. The robotic system, equipped with high-definition 3D vision and instruments that mimic the movements of the human wrist, allows for precise control and placement of sutures, followed by the secure tying of knots. The intracorporeal knot is often used in delicate procedures such as tissue approximation, vessel ligation, and organ repair.

Slip Knot

Adapted for use in robotic surgery, the intracorporeal slip knot such as Dundee jamming knot and Aberdeen Termination slip knot, is a versatile and secure option for surgeons. It can be tightened or loosened as needed before it is locked into place, providing flexibility during the suturing process. This knot is particularly useful in situations where the tension of the suture needs to be adjusted after placement. Robotic systems facilitate the tying of slip knots with precision, ensuring that the tension is just right for optimal wound healing.

Square Knot

The square knot, a staple in both manual and robotic surgery, is prized for its simplicity and effectiveness. In robotic surgery, the square knot is executed with a series of movements that replicate those of a surgeon's hands but with enhanced steadiness and precision. This knot is commonly used to secure tissue layers together and is known for its reliability in maintaining suture tension over time.

Surgeon's Knot

The surgeon's knot, a variation of the square knot, adds an extra twist, which increases the initial friction and holds the knot in place as additional throws are made. This knot is particularly useful in situations where there is a risk of the suture slipping before the knot is fully secured. Robotic surgery systems excel at tying surgeon's knots, offering consistency and reliability in each knot's formation, which is crucial for maintaining the integrity of the suture.

Tying the Surgeon's Knot in Robotic Surgery: A Step-by-Step Guide

Robotic surgery represents the pinnacle of technological advancement in the field of minimally invasive procedures, offering unparalleled precision, flexibility, and control. Among the myriad of skills essential for a robotic surgeon, mastering the art of knot tying, particularly the surgeon's knot, is crucial. The surgeon's knot is favored for its initial locking mechanism, providing extra security in holding tissue together compared to the traditional square knot. This chapter offers a comprehensive guide on how to proficiently tie a surgeon's knot during robotic surgery, ensuring both newcomers and seasoned professionals can enhance their suturing repertoire.

Understanding the Surgeon's Knot

The surgeon's knot, akin to a reinforced square knot, involves an additional twist on the first throw, creating a tighter initial hold and more friction. This is particularly useful in situations where tension might cause a simple square knot to loosen before the second throw can be completed. In robotic surgery, where the surgeon operates remotely, the enhanced control and dexterity provided by robotic arms make the tying of a surgeon's knot both feasible and highly effective.

Step-by-Step Guide for Tying a Surgeon's Knot in Robotic Surgery

Positioning and setup:
- Ensure the robotic arms are correctly positioned for optimal access to the suturing site. Utilize the 3D visualization capabilities of the robotic system to get a clear view.
- Prepare the suture material, making sure it is properly loaded onto the needle driver and suture cutters are within reach.

First throw (double wrap):
- Grasp the needle with the robotic arm equipped with the needle driver. Pass the needle through the tissue to be sutured, leaving enough suture length on the short end to tie the knot.
- Using the robotic controls, wrap the long end of the suture around the needle driver twice. This double wrap is what differentiates the surgeon's knot from a standard square knot and ensures the initial locking mechanism.

Tightening the first throw:
- Carefully transfer the suture's long end to the other robotic arm (not holding the needle) if necessary, ensuring the double wrap remains intact.
- Gently pull both ends of the suture to tighten the first throw against the tissue, ensuring the knot lies flat and the double wrap provides the intended locking effect.

Second throw (single wrap):
- Wrap the long end of the suture around the needle driver once, creating a single loop.
- Tighten this loop against the first throw, effectively completing the square knot. This second throw secures the locking mechanism created by the first double-wrapped throw.

Additional throws (if needed): Depending on the surgical requirements, additional single-wrap throws can be added for extra security. Typically, one or two additional throws are sufficient.

Cutting the suture: Once the knot is securely tied, use the robotic suture cutters to trim the excess suture material, leaving enough tail to ensure the knot does not unravel.

Tips for mastery:
- *Practice:* Utilize simulators to practice the surgeon's knot in a robotic surgery setting. Repetition will enhance muscle memory and familiarity with robotic controls.
- *Tension control:* Pay careful attention to the tension applied during each throw. Overtightening can damage tissue, while undertightening may lead to knot failure.
- *Coordination:* Develop a rhythm between your hands and the robotic controls. Effective coordination is key to smooth, efficient knot tying.
- *Visualization:* Always maximize the use of the robotic system's 3D visualization for precise placement and tightening of knots.

Tying a surgeon's knot in robotic surgery combines the traditional principles of secure suturing with the advanced capabilities of robotic technology. By following this step-by-step guide and incorporating the provided tips into your practice, you can refine your technique, ensuring that each knot tied contributes to the success of the surgical procedure. Mastery of such skills not only enhances surgical outcomes but also paves the way for the continued evolution of minimally invasive surgery.

Tumble Square Knot

In the intricate world of surgical knot tying, the ability to execute a secure and reliable knot can be as critical as the surgical procedure itself. Among the plethora of knots at a surgeon's disposal, the tumble square knot stands out for its efficacy and security, particularly in minimally invasive procedures such as laparoscopic and robotic surgery.

The tumble square knot is a variant of the traditional square knot, adapted for use in situations where direct manual access is limited. It is especially favored in robotic surgery due to its combination of simplicity, strength, and the minimal tension it places on the tissue. The "tumble" aspect refers to the method by which the knot is tightened, ensuring equal and distributed tension, which is crucial for wound healing and tissue integrity.

Application and Advantages of Tumble Square Knot

The primary application of the tumble square knot is in minimally invasive surgical procedures, where space constraints and the need for precision and control are paramount. Its advantages are manifold as follows:

- *Security:* The tumble square knot, when tied correctly, is less prone to slippage compared to other knots, providing a secure approximation of tissue.
- *Tension distribution:* It allows for uniform tension distribution across the knot, reducing the risk of tissue necrosis or tearing.
- *Adaptability:* This knot can be tied using a variety of materials, from absorbable sutures to nonabsorbable ones, making it versatile across different surgical disciplines.
- *Efficiency:* In the hands of a skilled surgeon, the tumble square knot can be tied quickly, improving operative efficiency without compromising on safety.

Technique Overview of Tumble Square Knot

Mastering the tumble square knot requires practice and understanding of its steps. Following is a simplified overview:

- *Preparation:* The suture is passed through the tissue as per the requirement of the surgical procedure.
- *Initial loop:* Create an initial loop by crossing the free end of the suture over and under the standing part.
- *Tumble motion:* The key to the tumble square knot is the specific "tumble" motion applied to the suture ends. This involves flipping one end of the suture (typically using a needle holder or similar instrument) to create a loop through which the other end will be passed.
- *Final tightening:* After the tumble motion, pull both ends of the suture to tighten the first throw. Repeat the process for the second throw, ensuring the suture ends are crossed in the opposite direction to the first throw to complete the square knot.
- *Confirmation:* Ensure the knot is squared by pulling on the suture ends and visually confirming the knot's symmetry and tension.

Tips for Mastery

- *Practice:* Regular practice on simulators or during supervised surgical procedures is essential.
- *Visualization:* Use high-definition monitors during laparoscopic procedures for clear visualization.

- *Instrument familiarity:* Become adept at handling laparoscopic instruments, as this will significantly impact your ability to tie knots accurately and efficiently.

The tumble square knot is a cornerstone in the repertoire of surgical knot-tying techniques, particularly valued in laparoscopic surgery for its reliability and security. Mastery of this knot enhances a surgeon's ability to perform safe and efficient suturing in minimally invasive procedures, ultimately contributing to better surgical outcomes and patient care. As with all surgical skills, proficiency in tying the tumble square knot comes with practice and a deep understanding of its mechanics and applications.

Future Knots and Technological Advancements

As surgical robotics continue to advance, so do the techniques and knots that can be employed. Researchers and engineers are constantly working on enhancing the capabilities of surgical robots, including the development of new suturing techniques and knots that can be tied with even greater precision and efficiency. The future may see the introduction of knots specifically designed to leverage the unique capabilities of robotic systems, further expanding the possibilities in the field of robotic surgery.

■ FUTURE OF ROBOTIC SUTURING

A groundbreaking development in surgical robotics emerged as a robot successfully performed suturing on the soft tissue of a pig without any human intervention, marking a significant leap toward the future of fully automated human surgeries **(Fig. 7)**. This achievement was realized by the Smart Tissue Autonomous Robot

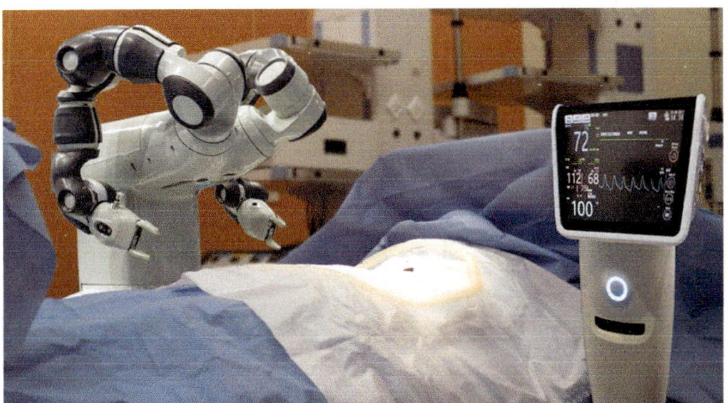

Fig. 7: Robot performs first robotic surgery without human help.

(STAR), developed by researchers from Johns Hopkins University and highlighted in the journal Science Robotics.

Led by Axel Krieger, an assistant professor of mechanical engineering at the Whiting School of Engineering, Johns Hopkins University, the team demonstrated that automation could adeptly handle one of surgery's most complex tasks—intestinal anastomosis. This procedure, crucial in reconnecting intestinal ends, demands exceptional precision and consistency, traits that STAR exhibited surpassingly well compared to human surgeons across four animal trials.

Intestinal anastomosis is renowned for its difficulty due to the necessity for meticulous suturing, where even minor errors can lead to severe patient complications. The robot's prowess in executing this delicate operation underscores the potential for surgical robots to enhance patient outcomes through precision and reliability.

The project, a collaboration that included experts from the Children's National Hospital in Washington, DC, and Jin Kang, a professor of electrical and computer engineering at Johns Hopkins, evolved from a 2016 prototype. The initial model demonstrated accuracy in intestinal repair but required significant human guidance and a large incision for access. The updated STAR version boasts advanced autonomy, surgical precision enhancements, specialized suturing tools, and sophisticated imaging systems for improved visualization during surgery.

The challenge of soft tissue surgery lies in its unpredictability, necessitating a system capable of real-time adjustments akin to human surgeons. STAR's novel control system meets this challenge, adapting the surgical plan on-the-fly with minimal human oversight. Hamed Saeidi, a visiting research scientist of mechanical engineering at Johns Hopkins and the study's first author, emphasized STAR's unique capability for planning, adapting, and executing surgical strategies in soft tissue autonomously.

The robot's enhanced capabilities are powered by a structural light-based 3D endoscope and a ML-based tracking algorithm developed by Kang and his team, emphasizing the crucial role of advanced machine vision in the evolution of intelligent surgical robots.

As laparoscopic surgical methods become increasingly prevalent, the necessity for automated systems such as STAR becomes evident. Such technologies promise to standardize high-precision surgical tasks, potentially making surgical outcomes less dependent on individual surgeon skills and more predictable across all patients.

The Johns Hopkins team, including Justin D Opfermann, Michael Kam, Shuwen Wei, Simon Leonard, and contributions from Michael H Hsieh, director of Transitional Urology at Children's National Hospital, anticipates that robotic anastomosis will democratize surgical practices, ensuring consistent, high-quality care for every patient. This vision represents a transformative step in surgical care, offering a glimpse into a future where robots play a crucial role in enhancing surgical precision and patient safety.

The dawn of autonomous robotic bowel suturing:
Shaping the future of surgery: In the ever-evolving landscape of medical technology, the realm of surgery stands on the brink of a monumental shift with the introduction of fully autonomous robots capable of performing complex surgical tasks, such as bowel suturing, without direct human intervention. This breakthrough heralds a new era in healthcare, where precision, efficiency, and patient outcomes are dramatically enhanced by advancements in robotic surgery. This chapter explores the implications, challenges, and future prospects of autonomous robotic bowel suturing.

The pioneering leap: Recent developments in AI and ML, combined with sophisticated robotic platforms, have made it possible for surgical robots to perform intricate procedures such as bowel suturing autonomously. These robots are equipped with advanced sensors, high-definition cameras, and AI algorithms that enable them to navigate the complex anatomy of the human body, identify suturing sites, and execute precise stitches with unparalleled accuracy.

The promise of autonomy: The primary allure of autonomous robotic surgery lies in its potential to minimize human error, thereby enhancing surgical outcomes. Traditional surgeries, even those assisted by robots, rely heavily on the surgeon's skill, experience, and stamina, all of which can vary significantly. In contrast, an autonomous robot can perform with consistent precision, unaffected by fatigue or subjective variations.

Furthermore, autonomous robots can potentially reduce the duration of surgeries and the risk of complications, leading to quicker recovery times for patients. They also hold promise for democratizing high-quality surgical care, making complex procedures accessible in remote or underserved regions by supplementing the shortage of highly skilled surgeons.

Challenges and considerations: Despite the optimism, the journey toward fully autonomous surgical robots is fraught with challenges. Ethical considerations, liability issues, and the need for robust regulatory frameworks are at the forefront of discussions among medical professionals, ethicists, and legal experts. Ensuring patient safety and building trust in robotic autonomy are paramount.

Technical hurdles also abound, including the need for advanced AI capable of real-time decision-making and adapting to the dynamic surgical environment. The development of fail-safe mechanisms and emergency protocols for human intervention is crucial to address unforeseen complications during surgery.

The road ahead: As research and development in this field accelerate, extensive clinical trials and validations are underway to establish the efficacy and safety of autonomous robotic systems. Collaborations between engineers, surgeons, and regulatory bodies are essential to navigate the complex pathway from laboratory innovations to clinical practice.

The future of autonomous robotic bowel suturing and other surgical procedures looks promising, with potential benefits that could revolutionize healthcare delivery. However, the successful integration of these technologies into routine surgical practice will require a careful balance between innovation and ethical responsibility, ensuring that patient welfare remains at the heart of technological advancement.

Conclusion: The advent of autonomous robotic surgery, particularly in complex tasks such as bowel suturing, marks a significant milestone in the field of medicine. While challenges remain, the potential for improved surgical outcomes, increased accessibility to quality care, and the advancement of surgical science is immense. As we stand on the cusp of this new era, the collective efforts of the medical community, technologists, and policymakers will be crucial in shaping a future where autonomous robots become trusted partners in surgery, enhancing the art and science of healing.

■ CONCLUSION

The transition from manual to robotic surgery has not only transformed the surgical landscape but also the intricacies of tasks such as knot tying. The common knots tied by surgical robots, including the intracorporeal, slip, square, and surgeon's knots, play a pivotal role in the success of minimally invasive surgeries. With ongoing advancements in robotic technology, the repertoire of knots and suturing techniques is set to expand, paving the way for even more precise and effective surgical interventions.

■ BIBLIOGRAPHY

1. Chen MH, Woo YL. Robotic suturing and knotting in gynecologic surgery: techniques and outcomes. Gynecol Oncol Rep. 2024;33:100645.
2. Fisher RA, Montero PN (Eds). Innovations in Robotic-Assisted Suturing. Ann Thorac Surg. 2018;106(2):560-6.
3. Gomez R, Fernandez R. Robotic suturing in pediatric surgery: techniques, challenges, and future directions. Pediatr Surg Int. 2022;38(3):345-51.
4. Gupta P, Smith RB. Efficacy of robotic suturing techniques: a comparative analysis. Surg Endosc. 2019;34(7):3072-9.
5. Hamilton EC, Scott DJ. Assessment tools for robotic suturing: validating skills in the era of minimally invasive surgery. Surgery. 2022;171(4):895-901.
6. Kim JY, Khanna A (Eds). Learning robotic suturing and knotting: a step-by-step guide for surgeons. Cham: Springer; 2022.
7. Lerner MA, Aydin H, Heller N. Comparative effectiveness of robotic versus laparoscopic suturing: a systematic review and meta-analysis. Surg Laparosc Endosc Percutan Tech. 2020;30(5):415-22.
8. Liang T, Tsai PH. Future perspectives on robotic suturing: challenges and opportunities. Int J Med Robot. 2021;17(1):e2187.
9. Lu B, Li B, Chen W, et al. "Toward image-guided automated suture grasping under complex environments: a learning-enabled and optimization-based holistic framework." IEEE Transactions on Automation Science and Engineering, 2022;19(4):3794-808.
10. Mayer HK, Bowers SP. Training programs and simulators for robotic suturing and knotting: a review. J Surg Educ. 2021;78(1):178-86.
11. O'Connor AM, Talamini MA. Innovative methods for teaching robotic suturing to surgical residents. Acad Med. 2019;94(9):1293-8.
12. Patel HRH, Joseph JV (Eds). Advances in Robotic-Assisted Urological Surgery. Cham: Springer; 2023.
13. Patel VR, Palmer KJ. The evolution of robotic suturing and knotting devices. J Robot Surg. 2019;13(4):549-57.
14. Quinn TM, Meara JG. Barriers to adoption of robotic suturing in low-resource settings: a global perspective. Global Surg. 2021;5(1):30-5.
15. Rajasekaran M, Jones DB. Robotic Surgery: Smart Materials, Robotic Structures, and Artificial Muscles. Singapore: World Scientific; 2020.

16. Ramos AS, Smith CD. The role of augmented reality in robotic suturing: enhancing precision and control. Ann Surg. 2022;275(4):e626.

17. Simmons MN, Gill IS. Decreasing suturing time: techniques and tips for robotic renal reconstruction. Urology. 2019;129:204-9.

18. Sutton C, Link RE (Eds). Robotic-Assisted Suturing in Surgery. New York: Springer; 2023.

19. Vickers AJ, Satava RM. High-fidelity virtual reality simulators for robotic suturing: bridging the gap between skill acquisition and operating room proficiency. J Robot Surg. 2023;17(2):255-61.

20. Wang Y, Mariani A. Robot-assisted microsurgical suturing: overcoming challenges in reconstructive urology. Eur Urol Focus. 2021;7(1):132-8.

21. Wright AS, Seagull FJ. The role of haptic feedback in robotic-assisted suturing. J Urol. 2019;202(2):239-44.

22. Zorn KC, Gofrit ON. The impact of suture material on knot integrity in robotic pyeloplasty. J Endourol. 2018;32(9):822-7.

Index

Page numbers followed by *f* refer to figure and *t* refer to table.